T0351133

Genetic Research on Addiction

Ethics, the Law, and Public Health

Genetic Research on Addiction

Ethics, the Law, and Public Health

Edited by

Audrey R. Chapman
Healey Professor of Medical Ethics and Humanities,
Department of Community Medicine and Health Care,
University of Connecticut School of Medicine,
Farmington, CT, USA

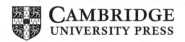

CAMBRIDGE
UNIVERSITY PRESS

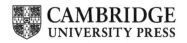

Shaftesbury Road, Cambridge CB2 8EA, United Kingdom

One Liberty Plaza, 20th Floor, New York, NY 10006, USA

477 Williamstown Road, Port Melbourne, VIC 3207, Australia

314–321, 3rd Floor, Plot 3, Splendor Forum, Jasola District Centre, New Delhi – 110025, India

103 Penang Road, #05–06/07, Visioncrest Commercial, Singapore 238467

Cambridge University Press is part of Cambridge University Press & Assessment, a department of the University of Cambridge.

We share the University's mission to contribute to society through the pursuit of education, learning and research at the highest international levels of excellence.

www.cambridge.org
Information on this title: www.cambridge.org/9781107653344

© Cambridge University Press 2012

First published 2012

A catalogue record for this publication is available from the British Library

Library of Congress Cataloging-in-Publication data
Genetic research on addiction : ethics, the law, and public health / edited by Audrey R. Chapman.
    p. ; cm.
Includes bibliographical references and index.
ISBN 978-1-107-65334-4 (hardback)
I. Chapman, Audrey R.
[DNLM: 1. Genetic Research–ethics.   2. Substance-Related Disorders–genetics.
3. Human Experimentation–ethics.   4. Informed Consent.   5. Public Policy. WM 270]
616.02′7–dc23
2012014544

ISBN   978-1-107-65334-4   Hardback

....

Every effort has been made in preparing this book to provide accurate and up-to-date information which is in accord with accepted standards and practice at the time of publication. Although case histories are drawn from actual cases, every effort has been made to disguise the identities of the individuals involved. Nevertheless, the authors, editors and publishers can make no warranties that the information contained herein is totally free from error, not least because clinical standards are constantly changing through research and regulation. The authors, editors and publishers therefore disclaim all liability for direct or consequential damages resulting from the use of material contained in this book. Readers are strongly advised to pay careful attention to information provided by the manufacturer of any drugs or equipment that they plan to use.

Contents

Section 4   Conclusions

Contributors

Peter J. Adams
Associate Professor of Social and Community Health, University of Auckland, Auckland, New Zealand

Paul Appelbaum
Elizabeth K. Dollard Professor of Psychiatry, Medicine & Law and Director, Division of Law, Ethics & Psychiatry, Department of Psychiatry, Columbia University, New York, NY, USA

Thomas F. Babor
Physicians Health Services Chair in Community Medicine and Public Health, Professor, and Chair, Department of Community Medicine and Healthcare, University of Connecticut Medical School, Farmington, CT, USA

Adrian Carter
National Health and Medical Research Council (NHMRC) Post-Doctoral Research Fellow, University of Melbourne and Honorary Research Fellow, University of Queensland Centre for Clinical Research in New Zealand, New Zealand

Audrey R. Chapman
Healey Memorial Chair of Medical Ethics and Humanities and Professor of Community Medicine and Healthcare, University of Connecticut School of Medicine, Farmington, CT, USA

Karen L. Dugosh
Quantitative Psychologist, Section on Law and Ethics Research, Treatment Research Institute on the Organization and Management of Addiction Treatment, University of Pennsylvania School of Medicine, Philadelphia, PA, USA

David S. Festinger
Director, Section on Law and Ethics Research, Treatment Research Institute on the Organization and Management of Addiction Treatment, and Adjunct Professor of Psychiatry, University of Pennsylvania School of Medicine, Philadelphia, PA, USA

Carl Erik Fisher
Resident in the Department of Psychiatry at Columbia University, New York, NY, USA

Amy Gaviglio
Research Project Coordinator, Department of Health Behavior and Health Education, University of Michigan, Ann Arbor, MI, USA

Alicia Giordimaina
Genetic Counselor in the Minnesota Department of Public Health, MN, USA

Wayne Hall
Professor and National Health and Medical Research Council Australia Fellow, University of Queensland Centre for Clinical Research; and Visiting Fellow at the Queensland Brain Institute, Queensland, Australia

Deborah Hasin
Professor of Clinical Epidemiology, Department of Psychiatry, College of Physicians and Surgeons and Mailman School of Public Health, Columbia University, New York, NY, USA

Toby Jayaratne
Assistant Research Scientist, Department of Health Behavior and Health Education, University of Michigan, Ann Arbor, MI, USA

Jonathan M. Kaplan
Associate Professor of Philosophy, Oregon
State University, Corvallis, OR, USA

Zita Lazzarini
Associate Professor of Health Law,
Department of Community Medicine and
Healthcare, University of Connecticut,
Farmington, CT, USA

Bruce G. Link
Professor of Epidemiology, Mailman
School of Public Health and Professor of
Sociomedical Sciences, Department of
Psychiatry, Columbia University, New York,
NY, USA

Rebecca Mathews
Senior Research Assistant, University of
Queensland Centre for Clinical Research,
Queensland, Australia

Thomas J. McMahon
Associate Professor, Department of
Psychiatry, Yale University School of
Medicine, New Haven, CT, USA

Jo C. Phelan
Associate Professor of Sociomedical
Science, Mailman School of Public
Health, Columbia University, New York,
NY, USA

David B. Resnik
Bioethicist and Institutional Review
Board Chair, National Institute of
Environmental Health, National
Institutes of Health, Bethesda, MD,
USA

Katherine Robaina
Research Assistant, Department of
Community Medicine, University
of Connecticut School of Medicine,
Farmington, CT, USA

Mark A. Rothstein
Herbert F. Boehl Chair of Law and
Medicine and Director, Institute of
Bioethics, Health Policy, and Law,
University of Louisville Medical
School, Louisville, KY, USA

Preface

This volume has a dual focus: identifying the ethical issues and requirements related to carrying out genetically based research on addiction and specifying the ethical, legal, and public policy implications of the interpretation, translation, and application of this research. It is hoped that the book will contribute to more ethically sensitive research and more socially responsible policies.

A motivating factor in the development of the volume was the desire to fill an important gap in the literature. It has been thought that a better understanding of the genetic contributions to addiction could lead to more effective drugs to assist in cessation of alcohol and drug use with fewer adverse side effects and that genotyping could better match patients to existing pharmacological treatments for addiction. These hopes have fueled medical investment in this field of research. Like other types of behavioral genetics research, the manner in which genetics research associated with addiction is conducted, interpreted to the public, and then translated into clinical practice and policy initiatives raises important ethical, social, and legal issues. Given the sensitivity of genetic research, its potential for stigmatization, its implications beyond the individual subject for the family and in some cases a broader community of membership, there is a need to guard against genetic research being misunderstood and misused. Yet there has been little literature exploring the ethical requirements of this research and its implications for public policy.

A grant from the National Institute on Alcohol Abuse and Alcoholism (NIAAA) of the US National Institutes of Health awarded to the Alcohol Research Center of University of Connecticut Health Center, for "Dissemination, and Educational Activities Related to Alcohol Research," afforded me the time to work on this volume. I have also had financial assistance from the Alcohol Research Center for the preparation of the volume. I would like to thank Professor Victor Hesselbrock, the Scientific Director of the Alcohol Research Center, for his support.

I would like to take this opportunity to thank other people who assisted with the development of this volume. I am grateful to Professor Thomas Babor, the Chairman of the Department of Community Medicine and Health Care at the University of Connecticut Health Center, who generously gave of his time and expertise. The role of the contributing authors of the chapters in the volume is obvious. Without their time and effort it would not have been possible to prepare and develop a multi-disciplinary volume incorporating a wide range of expertise. I would like especially to thank Jonathan M. Kaplan and Adrian Carter for their participation in the process of drafting the guidelines. I am also appreciative of the assistance of Joanna Chamberlin, my editor at Cambridge University Press, and Dr. Matthew Davies of Out of House Publishing Solutions who oversaw the copyediting, typesetting, and proofreading of the volume.

Introduction to the volume

Audrey R. Chapman

The misuse of alcohol and illicit drugs inflicts a major toll on individual users, their families, and the wider society. Addictive disorders contribute to excess morbidity and mortality and are economically costly. They also disproportionately affect people in the prime of life (Merikangas and Risch, 2003). The World Health Organization (WHO) divides the adverse effects of alcohol, opioids, and other psychoactive substances into four categories: chronic health effects (such as the toxic effect of alcohol in producing liver cirrhosis); the acute or short-term biological health effects of the substance (such as the effects of drug and alcohol overdose); the adverse social consequences of substance use (such as criminal activity to obtain access); and chronic social problems (such as the impact on family life) (WHO, 2004: 10–11). In addition, alcohol and drug consumption is associated with widespread psychosocial consequences, including violence, absenteeism in the workplace, and child neglect and abuse (WHO, 2011: 24). WHO estimates that alcohol ranks eighth among global risk factors for death and is the third leading global risk factor for disease and disability (WHO, 2011: 34). Of the ten leading risk factors of avoidable burden of ill-health, tobacco was fourth and alcohol fifth in 2000 (WHO, 2004: 16–17). Alcohol-related disability is a condition that affects more than 12% of the population in the United States at some point in their life. The majority of individuals with alcohol dependence (AD) – about three-quarters – never receive treatment (Heilig et al., 2011: 670–671).

Dependence on psychoactive substances has long been thought to have a biological basis, as suggested by observations of its prevalence in some families. The breaking of the genetic code in the 1960s and the inception of the Human Genome Project to sequence the human genome in 1990 have spurred efforts to identify the genetic basis of predispositions to drug and alcohol dependence. Given the high costs and difficulties in successfully treating addiction (Sellman, 2009), there has been interest in discovering more effective approaches to treatment. It has been thought that a better understanding of the genetic contribution of addiction could lead to more effective drugs to assist in cessation of drug use with fewer adverse side effects. Relatedly, it is assumed that genotyping could also better match patients to existing pharmacological treatments for addiction (Hall et al., 2002: 1482). This volume briefly describes such scientific research as well as current progress in identifying the genetic contributions to AD and other forms of addiction.

Like other behavioral genetics research, the manner in which genetics research associated with addiction is conducted, interpreted to the public, and then translated into clinical practice and policy initiatives raises important ethical, social, and legal issues. This volume

Genetic Research on Addiction, ed. Audrey R. Chapman. Published by Cambridge University Press.
© Cambridge University Press 2012.

has a dual focus: identifying the ethical issues and requirements related to carrying out genetically based research on addiction and specifying the ethical, legal, and public policy implications of the interpretation, translation, and application of this research. There are four sections in the volume. Section 1 consists of this introduction and two other chapters, one an overview of genetic research on AD and the other on the promises and risks for participants in studies. Section 2 addresses research issues, both human subject protection issues in genetically focused addiction research and issues related to seeking or accepting support for addiction research from industry. Section 3 explores ethical and policy issues in translating addiction research for public understanding and into public policy. The concluding chapter, which constitutes Section 4, uses the key issues raised in the volume and the recommendations made by the various chapter authors to develop guidelines for research and its policy applications.

Conceptualizing addiction

Criteria for addiction

To start at the beginning, what is addiction? According to one dictionary definition, addiction is the "compulsive need for the use of a habit-forming substance (like heroin, nicotine, or alcohol) characterized by tolerance and by well-defined physical symptoms upon withdrawal" (Merriam-Webster Dictionary). Addiction is often used interchangeably with the terms "substance dependence" or the "dependence syndrome." Although, as noted below, there is ongoing debate among philosophers, ethicists, public health specialists, scientists, and the general public about the conception of addiction, there is considerable consensus about the criteria for identifying someone who is addicted. As noted from the descriptions below, the two major medical classifications of dependence have considerable overlap. Both emphasize a strong desire or sense of compulsion to take the substance in question and difficulties in controlling the pattern of use and its termination, despite clear evidence of overtly harmful consequences.

The *International Classification of Mental and Behavioral Disorders*, 10th revision, usually referred to as the ICD-10, was endorsed by the 43rd World Health Assembly in 1990 and came into use in 1994. The ICD-10 lists six criteria for substance dependence, some of which are measurable in biological terms whereas others are not. To be diagnosable as "dependent," three or more of the following must have been experienced or exhibited together at some time during the previous year:

1. strong desire or sense of compulsion to take the substance
2. difficulties in controlling substance-taking behavior in terms of its onset, termination, or levels of use
3. physiological withdrawal state when substance use has ceased or been reduced, as evidenced by the characteristic withdrawal syndrome for the substance; or use of the same (or a closely related) substance with the intention of relieving or avoiding withdrawal symptoms
4. evidence of tolerance, such that increased doses of the psychoactive substance are required in order to achieve effects originally produced by lower doses
5. progressive neglect of alternative pleasures or interests because of psychoactive substance use, increased amount of time necessary to obtain or take the substance or to recover from its effects

6. persistance with substance use despite clear evidence of overtly harmful consequences, such as harm to the liver through excessive drinking, depressive mood states consequent to heavy substance use, or drug-related impairment of cognitive functioning (WHO, 2004: 13).

The second major source of criteria for identifying substance dependence is the fourth edition of the *Diagnostic and Statistical Manual* (DSM-IV) of the American Psychiatric Association. According to the DSM-IV, substance dependence is "a maladaptive pattern of substance use, leading to clinically significant impairment or distress, as manifested by three (or more) of the following, occurring at any time in the same 12-month period":

1. tolerance, as defined by either of the following:
   a. a need for markedly increased amounts of the substance to achieve intoxication or desired effect
   b. markedly diminished effect with continued use of the same amount of the substance

2. withdrawal, as manifested by either of the following:
   a. the characteristic withdrawal syndrome for the substance
   b. the same (or a closely related) substance is taken to relieve or avoid withdrawal symptoms

3. the substance is often taken in larger amounts or over a longer period than was intended
4. there is a persistent desire or unsuccessful efforts to cut down or control substance use
5. a great deal of time is spent in activities necessary to obtain the substance
6. important social, occupational, or recreational activities are given up or reduced because of substance use
7. the substance use is continued despite knowledge of having a persistent or recurrent physical or psychological problem that is likely to have been caused or exacerbated by the substance (American Psychiatric Association, 1994).

Conceptions of addiction

There are currently two major approaches to conceptualizing addiction, both of which were developed primarily in reference to patterns of opioid drug misuse and not AD. Presumably the conception would apply to AD, as well as nicotine addiction. The traditional and popular understanding of addiction, sometimes labeled as the moral model, presents addiction as an issue of moral impropriety based on a choice that individuals voluntarily make and for which they should be held responsible. By contrast, the more recently developed medical model holds that addiction is primarily a psychiatric or brain disorder that requires treatment. Some researchers propose a third psychological approach. Chapter 13 by Toby Jayaratne, Alicia Giordimaina, and Amy Gaviglio in this volume, for example, discusses the tendency for some individuals with a propensity for AD to attempt to decrease the threat this poses to their self-esteem by employing genetic explanations as a psychological coping tactic. There are more- and less-nuanced proponents of each of these models, as well as a small number of analysts who take the position that addiction is both a disease and a moral condition (Cochrane, 2007). Conceptions of addiction have implications for how society should treat addicts and whether addicts are considered to have the capability to exercise rational or responsible agency – for example, to make an autonomous decision to participate in a genetic research study of addiction.

The dominant moral model of addiction holds that addicts knowingly and willingly choose to use drugs or alcohol without regard for the adverse consequences for themselves and others. According to this view, the choice that individuals make to use psychoactive substances springs from a weak will. Some adherents of this position recognize that in a minority of cases the decision to use harmful substances develops into an addictive pattern. Others believe that addiction is just an excuse for continuing to use drugs while avoiding responsibility for the consequences of doing so (Carter et al., 2009: 25). This perspective is sometimes also referred to as the "skeptical" view, because it discounts the relevance of biogenetic mechanisms and recent neuroscience research as well as the need for medical treatment for addiction. According to one proponent, "addiction is no more a treatable medical problem than is unemployment, lack of coping skills, or degraded communities and despairing lives…More treatment will not win our badly misguided war on drugs. It will only distract our attention from the real issues in addiction" (Peele, 1990). Many of those who subscribe to this approach to addiction contend that most addicts have the capacity to stop drug use on their own (Peele, 2004, cited in Carter et al., 2009: 25). Some of those who argue that addiction is best conceptualized as a moral condition rather than a compulsion requiring medical treatment base their views on the fact that drug seeking and drug taking involve a series of actions that require rational planning; they therefore draw the conclusion that addicts rationally decide to continue to use drugs. Others worry that medicalization might encourage drug use or lead addicted persons to fatalism about their condition (Hyman, 2007: 8–9). The common belief that drug use is a voluntary choice that results in significant personal and social harm has led most societies to adopt punitive laws to discourage drug use and to impose significant penalties for purchase and use of illegal substances or if addicts engage in harmful or illegal acts while under the influence of an addictive substance.

There are conceptions of addiction that share many of the premises of the moral model while not explicitly presenting addiction as a moral issue. Bennet Foddy and Julian Savulescu (2007) offer a self-labeled reductive account that characterizes addiction as pleasure-seeking, individually based action that is rationally decided by its user. In their account, addictive desires differ from other desires for pleasure more in degree than in kind: they are especially strong; they occur in a particular context that triggers anticipation; and they are socially unacceptable because they threaten the welfare of the individual or challenge social norms. Foddy and Savulescu also compare addiction to substances with physical dependency syndromes and the addiction to other biological sources of pleasure such as sugar, sex, eating, or water. Like advocates of the moral model, they reject the view of addiction as a disease. For them pleasure is a healthy, necessary part of an individual's life. When it becomes excessive and out of control it may be considered to be a poor choice, but not a disease. They argue that very few addicts suffer brain damage that impairs their judgment, and for the most part, the changes in an addict's brain are comparable to those of a normal person when they engage in any normal rewarding activity (Foddy and Savulescu, 2010: 6). They relegate the concept of addiction to being nothing more than "an illiberal term invented to describe those who seek pleasure in a way that expresses our social disapproval" (Foddy and Savulescu, 2010: 20). Instead their "liberal account" of addiction advocates that the pleasure of addiction can be conceptualized as a legitimate human good and can be part of an autonomous, and even rational, life plan (Foddy and Savulescu, 2010: 19–20).

By contrast, the medical or disease model of addiction, informed by neuroscience research and brain-imaging studies, presents an addict's drug-seeking behavior as the direct result of changes in the structure and function of the brain caused by chronic substance use. Neurobiological research, particularly brain scans, suggests that chronic substance use can produce long-term disruptions of neurocognitive circuits involved in motivation and attention, decision making, and the ability to inhibit impulses. These alterations then increase cravings, impair appreciation of the consequences of substance use, and make it more difficult to resist urges to use the substance in question (Carter et al., 2009: 25–26). Some proponents of the medical model explicitly conceptualize addiction as a brain disease. The "chronic and relapsing brain disease" model of addiction put forward by Alan Leshner (1997) uses evidence that prolonged substance use causes pervasive and long-term changes in brain function to explain why an addicted person is vulnerable to relapse even after protracted periods of abstinence.

Acknowledging that the science is still in its early stages, Steven Hyman (2007) offers a nuanced and qualified interpretation of the neurobiology of addiction. He proposes that addictive drugs tap into and, in vulnerable individuals, usurp the potent neurotransmitter dopamine system in the brain that regulates rewards. The neural circuits "over learn" from excessive and distorted dopamine signals. This usurpation of the dopamine system makes drugs salient to the addict at the expense of other, more adaptive, goals. The result is a brain in which drug cues powerfully activate drug seeking and create craving if use is delayed, thus undermining the addict's ability to avoid seeking and using. Nevertheless Hyman cautions that this model does not reduce afflicted individuals to "zombies" who are permanently controlled by external cues or devoid of other goals. He also suggests that despite likely multiple relapses, addicts can regain a good measure of control over their drug taking.

Recognition of the important contribution of neuroscience does not necessarily lead to a reductive neuro-essentialist conception of addiction. Many proponents of this perspective acknowledge the importance of social, environmental, and cultural factors as well. For example, an approach that includes a neuroscientific component, but also goes beyond it, termed a "biopsychosocial systems model," proposes that psychological and sociological factors complement and are in dynamic interplay with neurobiological and genetic factors (Buchman et al., 2010: 37).

Like the moral model, the medical model has implications for how society approaches and deals with addicted individuals. Many proponents hope it will decrease the stigma associated with addiction and will incline society to treat addicts more humanely. Other advocates believe that treating addiction more as a disease than a moral failing could encourage greater societal investment into medical research into addiction and the development of more effective medical interventions (Carter et al., 2009: 25–26). However, the very possibility that societies could move in this direction makes some analysts reluctant to replace the moral model with a neurobiological perspective – both for the benefit of the addict and the protection of society.

The acceptance of the view of addiction as a disease could also have unintended negative consequences. Some worry that if addiction is viewed as primarily a genetic or brain disease it will contribute to negative perceptions of substance-use problems, much as it has in the case of mental illness (Buchman et al., 2010: 37). An uncritical acceptance of the brain disease model of addiction could encourage an overemphasis on pharmacological strategies to try to cure addiction rather than social-policy measures to reduce use of alcohol and drugs, which are more likely to be effective. In some circumstances it might also be interpreted as a warrant for the coercive treatment of addicts (Carter and Hall, 2007: 16).

An issue underlying much of this debate on the nature of addiction is the extent to which an addicted individual is in control of his or her actions, and concomitantly, the extent to which he or she should be held accountable by society. Specifically, how severely does addiction compromise the autonomous agency of the user and what are the implications? As Gideon Yaffe notes, there is both a legitimate moral and legal basis for distinguishing among: (1) those who pursue illegal or immoral courses of action freely; (2) those who do wrong out of compulsion – that is, unfreely; and (3) those who do wrong as a result of transitory powerful impulses (Yaffe, 2001: 179). The question is into which category addicts should be placed and whether the characterization applies to all addicts. This is a complex issue that has attracted much philosophical discussion too complex to recount adequately here.

To provide a simplified characterization, at one end of the spectrum there are those philosophers, psychologists, and medical doctors who believe that the autonomy or the capacity for self-determination of addicts is severely impaired. As noted, the two major medical classifications of dependence on psychoactive substances, one compiled by the WHO and the other by the American Psychiatric Association, cite a strong desire or sense of compulsion as one of the characteristics of addiction. Compulsion, which compromises the voluntary nature of choice, is one clinical defining feature of addiction that is usually taken to compromise decision-making capacity. Intoxication and withdrawal, which compromise the ability to comprehend choices, are two others (Charland, 2002: 40–41). Luis Charland argues that "the brain of a heroin addict has almost literally been hijacked by the drug" (Charland, 2002: 43). Although he acknowledges that the decisional impairments in heroin addiction fluctuate, he argues that their brain mechanisms and systems that govern evaluation have been disrupted and reoriented, thus entrenching the damage to their decision-making capacity (Charland, 2002: 43).

Charland's characterization, which comes in an article discussing whether heroin addicts are able to give consent to participating in clinical trials of heroin replacement therapy, is countered by other characterizations of addiction. Neil Levy argues that although addicts have impaired autonomy, the evidence available demonstrates that their actual behavior is sensitive to moderate incentives, both positive and negative in nature – for example, price increases in the drugs consumed – indicating they are not subject to irresistible desires. Levy argues that autonomy comes in degrees: it is not an all-or-nothing phenomenon. Addicts are subject to oscillations in preferences and suffer from diminished autonomy, but they are still capable of choice and are able to resist taking the substance to which they are addicted at least some of the time (Levy, 2011). Although Steven Hyman acknowledges that addiction impairs the capacity to make decisions about drug use, he, like Levy, maintains that this "loss of control is not complete or simple" (Hyman, 2007: 8). Similarly, Adrian Carter and Wayne Hall stress that "the fact that individuals with an addiction retain some control over their decisions about drug use and that the impulse to use drugs is resistible must be stated clearly" (Carter and Hall, 2007: 16).

Regardless of perspectives about the nature of addiction, most ethicists, even those who acknowledge at least a partial impairment of decision-making capacity, still argue that addicts should be held responsible. A (US) National Bioethics Advisory Commission Report concluded that the disease of addiction is not an excuse for behavior *per se*, because drug-dependent individuals are not always devoid of rational decision-making capacity (National Bioethics Advisory Commission, 1998: 8). Similarly, Stephen Morse points out that although an addict's rationality is often severely compromised at the time of drug seeking and using, it is not compromised at all times for most addicts. Therefore he or she is capable of and responsible for taking steps when not in a strongly driven state to prevent the maladaptive behavior that the addict knows will result when the craving returns (Morse, 2007: 13). Steven

Hyman cautions that some apparently voluntary behaviors of addicts may not be as freely planned and executed as they first appear (Hyman, 2007: 8), but he nonetheless still believes that it may be wise for societies to err on the side of holding addicted individuals responsible for their behavior – but "with a view to the rehabilitation of the addicted person and protection of society rather than moral opprobrium" (Hyman, 2007: 10). Likewise, Thomas Cochrane argues that fully replacing the moral model with a neurobiological perspective would be counterproductive because some demonstrations of moral judgment actually work to control addictive behavior. He goes on to say that "Even proof that addicts lack *all* control would not obviate the need for a moral stance on the part of others, as long as it can be shown that such a moral stance alters the addictive behavior" (Cochrane, 2007: 25).

Further complicating this whole issue, empirical studies of dependence symptoms indicate that the severity of dependence varies along a continuum from light to moderate and then severe. The cutoff point or threshold for addiction or dependence is somewhat arbitrary. Many people who use drugs and alcohol experience problems but do not meet criteria for dependence. To engage in genetic research it is important to have a good measure of the phenotype, but current diagnostic criteria for dependence and/or substance use are often highly correlated with a variety of other possible causes and consequences, including personality traits, demographic characteristics, and psychopathology. The complicated nature of addiction makes it unlikely that single causes and simple diagnostic criteria are likely to provide clear guidance on how best to define and diagnose the phenotype (T. Babor, personal communication, 2011).

Types of genetic research on addiction

The increasing evidence that addiction to alcohol and opioid substances has a genetic contribution has given rise to research to improve our understanding of addiction and thereby to be able to more effectively treat those afflicted and possibly improve our ability to prevent at least some addictive disorders. Genetic research on addiction seeks to identify the genes associated with a predisposition or vulnerability toward dependence and addiction. Qualitative family-based research designed to examine patterns of inheritance has been a cornerstone of this research. There are several types of family studies. Classical twin studies evaluate genetic inheritance by comparing data on a trait under study from identical/monozygotic and fraternal/dizygotic twin pairs. Additive genetic influences are shared 100% between members of monozygotic twin pairs, whereas dizygotic twin pairs on average share 50% of their genes, the same degree of genetic similarity as non-twin siblings. Adoption studies of biologically related people reared apart in presumably different environments help to separate genetic and environmental influences on variation in vulnerability to substance disorders. Some researchers have also pooled data from the various types of family studies to conduct a range of meta-analyses (Baker, 2004: 42–45).

Family, twin, and adoption studies provide robust evidence for a significant, but not exclusive, genetic contribution to the development of substance use and dependence. Environmental factors and individual experiences play an important role in shaping use patterns and dependence. Twin studies strongly indicate the existence of genetic risk factors for multiple aspects of smoking and AD, including initiation, continuation, amount consumed, and cessation (WHO, 2004: 151–152). Depending on the diagnostic criteria used, heritability estimates of AD range from 52 to 63% (WHO, 2004: 132). Heritability of opioid dependence is estimated to be even higher, at almost 70% (WHO, 2004: 136). However, the various types of family designs, with the exception perhaps of adoption studies, cannot identify the relative contribution of genetic and environmental factors (Agrawal and Lynskey, 2008). Nor can they identify which genes or chromosomes are involved.

Technological advances spurred by the Human Genome Project have made molecular approaches more readily available to investigate regions of DNA that may be involved in the susceptibility to AD and other forms of addiction. Linkage analysis, which examines genetic samples to try to identify the correlation of a trait and genetic markers among related individuals who have the phenotype in question (e.g., AD), has been an important tool for identifying the approximate chromosomal region in which some of the major genes contributing to the trait are located. Another technique, association studies, focuses on a single gene that has already been isolated, referred to as the candidate gene, to identify whether variation in this gene's alleles (alternate forms of the gene) might be statistically associated with variations in its expression by comparing people with and without the phenotype. The development of microarray analysis has accelerated the process by enabling scientists to examine thousands of genes simultaneously (Baker, 2004: 45–49; WHO, 2004: 127–128).

It should be emphasized that we are still a long way from identifying the individual genetic differences that contribute to the development of any form of substance dependence. Despite good evidence that genes contribute to addiction susceptibility, the results of qualitative family studies and molecular approaches to addiction disorders have been fairly modest thus far. The lack of commonly occurring susceptibility alleles that strongly predict addiction risk has been a major challenge to this research. The complexity of unraveling the genetic contributions to AD and other addictions precludes any likelihood that genetic research can contribute to predictive genetic screening or pharmacogenetic testing to inform treatment selection of addictive disorders in the near future. After reviewing the scientific evidence, the next chapter in this volume, contributed by Rebecca Mathews, Adrian Carter, and Wayne Hall, concludes that genetic testing is not ready for use to predict AD liability, especially for population screening, but shows that the evidence linking genetic variants with differential responses to treatment appears to be more robust for some population groups.

The complexity of the task is a major challenge to the application of genetics in the field of addiction. Contrary to the popular view of human genetics, which assumes a simple or direct relationship between a mutation or a variant form of a single gene and the development of a specific disorder, single gene or Mendelian disorders, such as Huntington's chorea, are very rare. Predisposition toward alcohol and/or drug dependence is a complex disorder, and like other complex disorders it appears to be shaped by multiple alleles (variant forms of a gene), each contributing a small effect, that dynamically interact with each other and with environmental factors. Gene/environmental interactions are key to determining outcomes. As a recent WHO review of evidence on genetic vulnerability to substance dependence explains, "while individual genetic differences contribute to the development of substance dependence, genetic factors are but one contributor to the complex interplay of physiological, social, cultural and personal factors that are involved" (WHO, 2004: 125).

There are several implications of this understanding of genetic heterogeneity. Multiple risk alleles in different combinations can contribute to genetic risk in individual cases. It is unlikely, therefore, that everyone with a particular "risk gene" for substance use or dependence will become dependent. Conversely, some of those who become dependent may not carry a specific genetic risk factor being researched (WHO, 2004: 125). Or to put the matter another way, patients diagnosed with a clinical condition labeled as alcohol dependency or another form of addiction presenting with similar symptoms can arrive at this phenotype through very different trajectories of genetic risk factors and exposure to environmental risk factors (Heilig et al., 2011: 671).

Ethical issues in conducting and translating genetic research on addiction

Like other areas of behavioral genetics, research on addiction touches on sensitive questions about the determinants of human behavior, the balance between freedom and determinism, and the extent and ways in which we share our genetic identity with other members of our family and our broader social community. The research raises ethical issues that fall under two broad categories: the ethical issues that arise in conducting the genetic research on addiction; and the broader social and ethical implications of interpreting the research and translating it into prevention and treatment programs and social policy. The decision of the directors of the Human Genome Project, funded by the National Institutes of Health, to devote 3–5% of their total research budget to ethical, legal, and social issues related to the science attests to the significance of these issues. It is hoped that this volume will contribute to the sensitization of genetics researchers to the ethical requirements of this research and will help to inform policymakers to be cautious in interpreting and applying the research findings.

Ethical issues in human genetic research on addiction

There is an international consensus that biomedical research should conform to a series of foundational ethical principles. Informed consent to protect a subject's right to make an autonomous choice is arguably the most important of these. The informed consent process requires that potential subjects be accurately informed of the purpose, methods, risks, benefits, and alternatives to the research; that they understand this information and be able to apply it to their own situation; and also that they make a voluntary and uncoerced decision as to whether to participate in the research (Emanuel et al., 2000). Genetic research on addiction pushes the limits of the protection typically accorded by informed consent when it seeks to obtain consent from addicted individuals, who may have reduced decision-making capacity or competence. Given this concern and the complexity of understanding the implications of genetic research, it is important that genetic research on addiction take special precautions to assess whether the requirements for informed consent can be met.

Concern with vulnerability, understood in terms of the ability to give or withhold informed consent or otherwise be taken advantage of in research, has been central to the development of the Common Rule, the portion of the Code of Federal Regulations that governs much of the human research conducted in the United States. The Common Rule restricts the research that may be conducted on a number of groups – which do not include persons suffering from addiction *per se*, but also notes that others may also be vulnerable. It also requires that research protocols include protections for those who might be vulnerable but does not specify what those should be. In recent years the association of vulnerability with membership in a specific group, such as children or prisoners, has been supplemented or in some cases reconceptualized to apply to the characteristics of individual persons or the factors or conditions that may render individuals vulnerable in a specific research setting (Iltis, 2009). The potential vulnerability of subjects in research on the genetics of addiction suggests the need for appropriate protections to be designed.

Obligations to protect the privacy and confidentiality of the research data collected constitute another ethical challenge for genetic research on addiction. The right to privacy and confidentiality has special salience for genetic research for several reasons. Genetic information may be seen by individuals as central to their personal identities in ways that other medical information is not. This reflects the genetic essentialism conveyed by images and narratives found in popular culture and the media that equates human beings with their genes. Some analysts even suggest that DNA functions in many respects as a secular equivalent of the medieval Christian conception of the immortal soul (Nelkin and Lindee, 1995: 2). In addition, genetic information carries implications not just for individuals but for their families as well. Therefore the release of that information can adversely affect relationships among family members. Also the predictive nature of genetic information has the potential to adversely affect people's lives. For example, it may foster a sense of determinism that causes depression or reduces the inclination to take precautionary measures. Yet another factor is that genetic information has the potential to be used for discriminatory purposes by employers and insurance companies. Like some other areas of behavioral genetics research, a known predisposition to addiction is also likely to be a stigmatizing health condition. Protection of the confidentiality of genetic data is more complex than for other forms of medical information, because genetic data are intrinsically identifiable – that is, traceable back to the individual – and cannot be easily de-identified. The development of genomic databases and biobanks that store large amounts of genetic data and make them available to researchers, although central to the advancement of biomedical research, complicates protection of the confidentiality of research participants.

Ethical issues in translating and applying genetic research

The need to guard against genetic research being misunderstood or misused is underscored by the early history of genetic research. In the first half of the twentieth century human genetics as a program of research was intertwined with the early eugenics movement, which sought to improve the physical, mental, and behavioral qualities of the human race through selective breeding. As a result, belief in the heritability of addiction translated into negative eugenic programs to prevent the reproduction of those persons considered to be genetically defective. This latter category often had more to do with cultural beliefs and prejudices at the time than with scientific findings.

Charles Davenport, the founding director in 1909 of Cold Spring Harbor Laboratory, a facility that played an important role in early genetics research, was also a leading figure in the American eugenics movement. Davenport argued that patterns of human heritability acting through physiological and anatomical mechanisms were evident in a wide range of mental deficiencies. The mental deficiencies he identified and sought to eliminate included alcoholism as well as insanity, epilepsy, pauperism, criminality, and feeblemindedness – a catchall used for a wide range of mental problems (Kevles, 1995: 46). Davenport's interest in fostering the development of good human stock led him to advocate for a selective immigration policy that would deny entry to individuals and families with what he viewed as a poor hereditary history. He also supported the introduction of state-enforced sterilization to prevent the reproduction of the genetically defective (Kevles, 1995: 47).

Several states enacted components of the eugenics movement's program into public policies. In 1907, Indiana became the first state to adopt a law mandating compulsory sterilization of the mentally deficient. Eventually 30 US states passed such laws. Until the repeal of these laws in the 1960s and 1970s, more than 60 000 sterilizations were performed. Alcoholism was a ground for compulsory sterilization in many of these states (Stern, 2005: 84, 144).

The much reviled Nazi eugenics program was modeled in part on American policies, especially the draconian California law. Going far beyond the American statutes, the Nazi Eugenic Sterilization Law was compulsory with respect to all people, institutionalized or not, who suffered from allegedly hereditary disabilities, including severe drug or alcohol addiction (Kevles, 1995: 116).

Although contemporary state-supported eugenic applications of genetic research on addiction seem unlikely, there are other concerns that should be noted. In a population that is inclined toward assumptions about genetic determinism, there is a need for careful and precise interpretation of the research findings to prevent them from being misunderstood as providing evidence for a direct causal relationship between genes and addiction. It is also important to guard against genetic research on addiction influencing public policy in the direction of supporting simple-minded policies that attempt to identify the minority of the community who are genetically vulnerable to addiction in order to treat them, while neglecting broader and more effective social policy options directed at the whole community to discourage substance and alcohol use and make these substances less available. A related concern expressed in Jonathan Kaplan's chapter (Chapter 14) in this volume is that genetic research into addiction susceptibility might result in an increased focus on the individual as the proper locus of research and less attention to the contribution of the social environment in explaining individual variations in addiction and in developing interventions. Some researchers have also expressed the concern that the development of more effective pharmacological and immunological treatments for addiction might lead to the coerced treatment of addicts, particularly for drug-dependent people who commit criminal offences (Hall et al., 2002: 1486–1467).

Another issue is the appropriate role of investments in genetic research in setting priorities for scarce public resources devoted to addiction disorders. The challenges of applying genetic research to complex disorders, such as addictions, and the limited progress in doing so have led some scientists to question substantial investment in high-cost molecular genomic profiling for this purpose. Arpana Agrawal and Michael Lynskey (2008) recommend focusing addiction research on less-expensive twin studies, especially designs with the power to examine genetic–environmental interaction. Kathleen Merikangas and Neil Risch (2003) propose according priority to a select number of complex diseases that appear to have the strongest genetic contribution, limited ability to modify exposure or risk factors, and high public health impact. They conclude that public health approaches may ultimately lead to far more effective prevention and intervention initiatives than genomics tools. Many public health specialists and policymakers would concur.

Overview of volume

This volume has four sections. The first of these, the introductory section, contains three chapters. The current "Introduction" chapter is followed by the chapter on "The implications of genetic research on alcohol dependence for prevention and treatment" written by Rebecca Mathews, Adrian Carter, and Wayne Hall, which assesses the current status of the evidence on the genetics of AD and its application to treatment programs. The chapter considers the research about susceptibility alleles for AD and its implications for the feasibility of undertaking population-level predictive genetic screening for AD. The chapter also reviews the potential application of research on pharmacogenetics to improve AD treatment efficacy. Prospective participants in genetic studies of risk for alcohol, drug, or nicotine disorders must decide if the benefits of participation outweigh the risks. Whereas the risks are largely (although not entirely) personal, the benefits are largely not personal, but rather societal in nature, and involve future scientific developments that build on genetics studies as one step in the process toward better prevention and treatment. The third chapter, coauthored by Carl Erik Fisher, Deborah Hasin, and Paul Appelbaum with the title "Promises and risks for participants in studies of genetic risk for alcohol or drug dependence," identifies the trade-offs between these risks and benefits.

Section 2 of the volume, on research ethics, contains seven chapters dealing with human subject protection issues in conducting genetic research on AD and addiction research more generally. Despite the centrality of informed consent to the protection of research partici-pants and the poor levels of consent comprehension and retention reported in the literature, few have empirically examined studies for improving understanding of consent information or reducing perceptions of coercion to inter-research studies, particularly among vulnerable populations, such as substance abusers. David S. Festinger's and Karen L. Dugosh's chapter "Improving the informed consent process in research with substance-abusing participants" addresses these issues. They also examine a number of novel and effective consent strategies that have been developed over the past two decades and evaluate the potential of apply-ing these methods to research with addicted subjects. Using ethical principles, empirical data, and practice guidelines, Thomas McMahon's chapter, "Ethical considerations in gen-etic research with children affected by parental substance abuse," explores challenges associ-ated with the enrolment of minor asymptomatic children living in high-risk family systems in developmental research designed to clarify genetic risk for chronic addictive disorders that do not typically emerge until sometime during late adolescence or early adulthood. Researchers in many areas of addiction research collect sensitive information about the behavior, health status, and associations of human subjects. Because disclosure of that infor-mation could expose research subjects to a variety of harms, maintaining the confidentiality of this sensitive research data is critical to the relationship of trust between research sub-jects and researchers as well as protecting the subjects. Zita Lazzarini's chapter, "Certificates of Confidentiality: Uses and limitations as protection for genetic research on addiction," describes the scope of protections provided by federal Certificates of Confidentiality, their limitations, and their uses in research on addiction.

One of the most significant recent trends in biomedical research with human subjects is the development of large databases and biobanks to study associations between genetic or genomic variation and diseases. The chapter "Protecting privacy in genetic research on alcohol dependence and other addictions" by Mark A. Rothstein covers two main issues: first, privacy issues raised by large-scale research studies and sources including biobanks, electronic health records, and intervention research with human subjects; and second, the efficacy of different strategies to protect subjects' privacy, particularly when dealing with research on vulnerable populations, such as de-identification, sequestration of sensitive health information, and certificates of confidentiality. This section also contains David B. Resnik's chapter, "Ethical issues in genomic databases in addiction research," which consid-ers additional ethical issues related to genomic databases and biobanks, such as informed consent for the future use of biological samples and data, safeguarding the privacy and con-fidentiality of human subjects, sharing samples and data, returning study results and inci-dental findings to individuals, protecting communities and third parties from harm, and intellectual property and benefit sharing.

The rest of this section has two chapters that address the ethical issues in seeking or accepting support for addiction research from industry. Some of the sizable profits generated from the sale of tobacco, alcohol, and gambling are made available in various ways to support research into addiction. Public interest and academic researchers are in a sensitive position relative to such profits, as their research efforts often set out to reduce the harm associated with consumption of these products. Peter J. Adams' chapter "Should addiction researchers accept funding derived from the profits of addictive consumptions?" identifies five of the main risks researchers need to consider and provides indicators of risk to estimate the moral jeopardy faced by addiction researchers in three quite different contexts. Thomas Babor and Katherine Robaina's chapter "Ethical issues related to receiving research funding from the alcohol industry and other commercial interests" evaluates the ethical challenges that have emerged from industry involvement in alcohol science research, including: industry involvement in sponsorship of research funding organizations; direct financing of university-based scientists and centers; efforts to influence public perceptions of research, research findings, and alcohol policies; publication of scientific documents and support of scientific journals; and sponsorship of scientific conferences and presentations at conferences.

Section 3 of the volume has four chapters addressing ethical and policy issues in translating addiction research. The first of these chapters, written by Rebecca Mathews, Wayne Hall, and Adrian Carter, "The public health implications of genetic research on addiction" focuses on the public health policy implications of genetic research on AD. The chapter outlines both the potential benefits of the research in improving public health and the risks that the research may be misused and misinterpreted in ways that harm individual and population health. It also provides an overview of the implications of the research for population-level policies that aim to reduce alcohol consumption, stigmatization, and discrimination against alcohol-dependent persons and individuals at increased genetic risk of developing these disorders, and priorities for research on alcohol as a public policy issue. In the next chapter, "Genetics, addiction, and stigma," Jo C. Phelan and Bruce G. Link explore the implications of genetic research for stigma related to addictions. They first discuss concepts related to stigma and then apply those concepts to the particular case of genetics, addiction, and stigma.

Using data from a 2006 survey of 193 Americans residing in the Midwest, the chapter "Lay beliefs about genetic influences on the development of alcoholism: Implications for prevention," written by Toby Jayaratne, Alicia Giordimaina, and Amy Gaviglio, examines the association between the lay public's genetic explanations for alcoholism and the belief that alcoholism cannot be prevented or controlled. It also discusses the implications of these findings for prevention and treatment of alcoholism. The fourth chapter in this section, by Jonathan M. Kaplan, "Personalizing risk: How behavior genetics research into addiction makes the political personal" addresses the problem that research into the genetic correlates of differences in individual susceptibility to addiction and/or addictive behaviors may tend to shift the focus of both research and policy discussions away from the social determinants of addiction/addictive behavior rates and toward treating addiction as primarily a problem of individual risk, susceptibility, and decisions. It raises the warning that these individual approaches fail to deal with the serious social consequences of addiction and addictive behavior and avoid the difficult but likely far more effective social interventions that are known to have real impacts on addictive behaviors and the harms caused by addiction.

In the concluding chapter, which constitutes Section 4, Jonathan Kaplan, Adrian Carter, and I draw conclusions from the essays in the volume and propose a set of research and policy guidelines.

References

Agrawal, A. and Lynskey, M. T. (2008). Are there genetic influences on addiction: Evidence from family, adoption and twin studies. *Addiction*, 103, 1069–1081.

American Psychiatric Association. (1994). *Diagnostic and Statistical Manual of Mental Disorders*, 4th ed. (DSM-IV). Washington, DC: American Psychiatric Association.

Baker, C. (2004). *Behavioral Genetics*. Washington, DC: American Association for the Advancement of Science.

Buchman, D. Z., Skinner, W., and Illes, J. (2010). Negotiating the relationship between addiction, ethics, and brain science. *AJOB Neuroscience*, 1, 36–45.

Carter, A. and Hall, W. (2007). The social implications of neurobiological explanations of resistible compulsions. *American Journal of Bioethics*, 7, 15–17.

Carter, A., Hall, W., and Copps, B. (2009). What is addiction? In A. Carter, B. Copps, and W. Hall (eds), *Addiction Neurobiology: Ethical and Social Implications*. Luxembourg: European Monitoring Centre for Drugs and Drug Addiction.

Charland, L. C. (2002). Cynthia's dilemma: Consenting to heroin prescription. *American Journal of Bioethics*, 2, 37–41.

Cochrane, T. J. (2007). Brain disease or moral condition? Wrong question. *American Journal of Bioethics*, 7, 24–25.

Emanuel, E. J., Wendler, D., and Grady, C. (2000). What makes clinical research ethical? *JAMA*, 283, 2701–2711.

Foddy, B. and Savulescu, J. (2007). Addiction is not an affliction: Addictive desires are merely pleasure-oriented desires. *American Journal of Bioethics*, 7, 29–32.

Foddy, B. and Savalescu, J. (2010). A liberal account of addiction. *Philosophy, Psychiatry, & Psychology*, 17, 1–22.

Hall, W., Carter, L., and Morley, K. I. (2002). *Ethical Implications of Advances in Neuroscience Research on the Addictions*. NDARC Technical Report No. 143. Sydney, Australia: Office of Public Policy and Ethics, Institute for Molecular Bioscience, University of Queensland and National Drug and Alcohol Research Centre, University of New South Wales.

Heilig, M., Goldman, D., Berrettini, W., and O'Brien, C. P. (2011). Pharmacogenetic approaches to the treatment of alcohol addiction. *Nature Reviews Neuroscience*, 12, 670–684, available at www.nature.com/reviews/neuro [accessed April 10, 2012].

Hyman, S. E. (2007). The neurobiology of addiction: Implications for voluntary control of behavior. *American Journal of Bioethics*, 7, 8–11.

Iltis, A. S. (2009). Introduction: Vulnerability in biomedical research. *Journal of Law, Medicine & Ethics*, 37, 6–11.

Kevles, D. J. (1995). *In the Name of Eugenics: Genetics and the Uses of Human Heredity*. Cambridge, MA: Harvard University Press.

Leshner, A. (1997). Addiction is a brain disease, and it matters. *Science*, 278, 46–47.

Levy, N. (2011). Autonomy, responsibility and the oscillation of preference. In A. Carter, W. Hall, and J. Illes (eds), *Addiction Neuroethics: The Ethics of Addiction Neuroscience Research and Treatment*, London: Elsevier, pp. 139–152.

Merikangas, K. R. and Risch, N. (2003). Genomic priorities and public health. *Science*, 302, 599–601.

Merriam-Webster Dictionary (n.d.) Available online at: www.merriam-webster.com/dictionary/addiction [accessed March 14, 2012].

Morse, S. J. (2007). Voluntary control of behavior and responsibility. *American Journal of Bioethics*, 7, 12–13.

National Bioethics Advisory Commission (1998). *Research Involving Subjects with Mental Disorders that May Affect Decision-making Capacity: Report and Recommendations of the National Bioethics Advisory Commission*. Rockville, MD: National Bioethics Advisory Commission.

Nelkin, D. and Lindee, M. S. (1995). *The DNA Mystique: The Gene as a Cultural Icon*. New York: W.H. Freeman.

Peele, S. (1990). Cures depend on attitude, not programs. *Los Angeles Times*, quoted on The Stanton Peele Addiction Website.

Available online at: www.peele.net/ philosophy/ [accessed February 29, 2012].

Peele, S. (2004). The suprising truth about addiction. *Psychology Today* (May–June): 43–46. Available online at: www. psychologytoday.com/articles/200405/the-surprising-truth-about-addiction [accessed February 29, 2012].

Sellman, D. (2009). The 10 most important things known about addiction. *Addiction*, 105, 6–13.

Stern, A. (2005). *Eugenic Nation: Faults and Frontiers of Better Breeding in Modern America*. Berkeley and Los Angeles: University of California Press.

World Health Organization (2004). *Neuroscience of Psychoactive Substance Use and Dependence*. Geneva: World Health Organization.

World Health Organization (2011). *Global Status Report on Alcohol and Health*. Geneva: World Health Organization.

Yaffe, G. (2001). Recent work on addiction and responsible agency. *Philosophy & Public Affairs*, 30, 178–221.

Chapter

The implications of genetic research on alcohol dependence for prevention and treatment

Rebecca Mathews, Adrian Carter, and Wayne Hall

Introduction

Alcohol dependence is a disorder that causes significant harm, not only to the health of affected individuals, but also through the significant social and economic costs borne by society. About 4% of the global burden of disease (measured by disability-adjusted life years; DALY) has been attributed to alcohol consumption and 1.6% to alcohol-use disorders specifically (WHO, 2008). In high-income countries such as the United States, alcohol-use disorders cause 3.4% of total disease burden (WHO, 2008).

Alcohol dependence (AD) may manifest in tolerance, withdrawal symptoms, or the use of alcohol to avoid or relieve withdrawal, drinking more than intended, unsuccessful attempts to cut down use, excessive time related to alcohol consumption (including alcohol seeking), impaired social or work activities, and continued use despite physical or psychological consequences. AD may increase a person's risk of other forms of substance abuse, psychiatric disorders, and physical illnesses, such as heart disease and cancers, and lead to unemployment, relationship breakdowns, accidents, and imprisonment due to crimes committed as a result of alcohol abuse.

The existence of a genetic component of AD has long been suggested by the observation that the disorder runs in families. The substantial genetic contribution has subsequently been confirmed by twin and adoption studies that estimate the heritability of AD to range from 50 to 60% (Agrawal and Lynskey, 2008). Approximately 56% of the variance in AD is caused by genetic factors, whereas 44% is as a result of specific environmental factors not shared by family members, including peer influences and experiences after leaving the home environment (Kendler and Prescott, 2006). Shared environmental factors such as social class, parental rearing styles, familial attitudes to drinking, parental drinking practices, and – in the case of twins – intrauterine environment, make little contribution to AD itself (Kendler and Prescott, 2006) but explain about 15% of the variance in initiation of alcohol use (Sartor et al., 2009).

Recent genetic research has identified a number of genetic variants thought to be involved in the development and persistence of AD. Researchers and clinicians hope that these discoveries will lead to reductions in the harms caused by alcohol, including in the numbers of people developing dependence, as well as more effective treatments of AD.

Advancements in genetic technology arising from the mapping of the human genome have reduced the costs of genome-wide scans and heralded optimistic predictions about the potential use of genetic information to personalize medicine and improve health (Collins

Genetic Research on Addiction, ed. Audrey R. Chapman. Published by Cambridge University Press.
© Cambridge University Press 2012.

et al., 2003). Proponents of this personalized genomic medicine have proposed that genetic research could be used preventively in the form of predictive genetic screening to identify healthy persons at a greater risk of developing AD and prevent them from doing so. It could also be used therapeutically through pharmacogenetic approaches to allow clinicians to better match alcohol-dependent individuals to more effective treatments. Given the significant challenges in effectively intervening to help persons with AD and in reducing harmful alcohol consumption, such proposals have great appeal.

Despite over a decade of research on the genetic basis of complex disorders, these optimistic predictions have yet to be realized (Williams, 2010). Although genetic research for some pseudo-Mendelian disorders has yielded clinically relevant genetic tests (e.g., for the neurodegenerative Canavan disease), for complex diseases such as diabetes, obesity, AD, and other mental illnesses that are shaped by multiple biological, social, and cultural factors, such reasearch has been less fruitful.

This chapter reviews the current evidence regarding the genetics of AD. It then assesses the feasibility of clinical applications arising from this research, such as predictive genetic screening for AD and pharmacogenetics for AD treatment.

Candidate genes for alcohol dependence: A summary

Candidate genes for AD have been identified primarily via linkage studies and genome-wide association studies (GWAS). Linkage studies examine the inheritance of a disorder through family members or pedigrees to try to identify coinheritance between a genetic marker and the disorder of interest. Typically, when linkage is found, it implicates a gene in a broader chromosomal region around the genetic marker in the development of the disorder. Linkage mapping projects, in particular the Collaborative Study on the Genetics of Alcoholism (COGA), have identified promising chromosomal regions for AD susceptibility loci, some of which have led to the identification of disease-influencing loci (Edenberg, 2002; Edenberg and Foroud, 2006). Linkage studies are best suited to conditions for which genes have a major effect on disease risk and typically identify large chromosomal regions that may be implicated in the development of a disorder (Ball, 2008). As we shall illustrate later in this chapter, the genes contributing to alcoholism do not appear to meet these criteria.

GWAS typically examine the differences in the distribution of a genetic variant in a sample of unrelated persons affected with a disorder compared to matched controls. These studies examine variants across the entire human genome and are designed to analyze whether certain alleles (alternative forms) of a gene are associated with a disease, trait, or symptom. Unlike linkage studies, association studies have the potential to identify genes of smaller effect sizes. However, false positives are common in association studies (Ball, 2008). See Buckland (2001) for an analysis of the impact of false positives on association studies investigating the genetics of AD.

Candidate gene association studies examine genetic markers in genes whose functions are related to the pathophysiology of the disease or genes that lie in a chromosomal region linked to disease through linkage studies. Candidate gene studies have identified multiple susceptibility alleles for AD that are only weakly predictive of disease liability. This suggests that AD is a polygenic disorder in which multiple genes of weak individual effect size predict disease risk, rather than a quasi-Mendelian disorder in which a small number of genes predict risk. Two broad groups of susceptibility alleles have been identified: (1) those that impact on alcohol metabolism; and (2) those that impact on the rewarding, reinforcing, and other cognitive effects of alcohol (e.g., impact on learning and memory) by regulating the activity of various neurotransmitter systems of the brain.

In the next section we highlight the genetic variants that have been most reliably associated with AD to illustrate the challenges in understanding and applying genetic research on dependence on alcohol. We do not provide an exhaustive review of all potential genetic variants associated with AD, as this is beyond the scope of this chapter, and comprehensive reviews of this already exist (see Kohnke, 2008; Gelernter and Kranzler, 2009; Kalsi et al., 2009).

Genes that impact on alcohol metabolism

Genes that regulate alcohol metabolism are the most significantly and reliably associated with alcohol dependence (Ball, 2008; Kohnke, 2008; Gelernter and Kranzler, 2009). These include genes that influence the enzymatic activity of alcohol dehydrogenase (ADH) and aldehyde dehydrogenase (ALDH). ADH converts ethanol to the toxin acetaldehyde, which is further broken down into acetate by ALDH. Seven genes encoding ADH isoforms have been identified (ADH1–7) and two encoding ALDH (ALDH1A1 and ALDH2) (Edenberg, 2007).

Alleles that increase ADH or decrease ALDH activity cause an accumulation of acetaldehyde in the body. Acetaldehyde produces unpleasant facial flushing, sweating, and mild headaches. In more severe cases, it can result in cardiovascular collapse, arrhythmias, unconsciousness, and convulsions. These aversive symptoms reduce alcohol consumption and protect against developing AD.

Three alleles that encode high-activity ADH enzymes, ADH1B*2, ADH1B*3, and ADH1C*1, are thought to protect against AD: individuals carrying these alleles are likely to have higher levels of acetaldehyde (Chen et al., 1999; Osier et al., 1999; Choi et al., 2005). ADH1B*2 and ADH1B*3 are thought to alter the enzymatic activity of ADH by more than 30-fold (Bosron et al., 1983), and both have been shown to protect against alcohol-related birth defects and fetal alcohol syndrome (McCarver et al., 1997; Viljoen et al., 2001; Warren and Li, 2005). A meta-analysis found that one copy of ADH1B*2 reduced AD risk fourfold, whereas two copies reduced risk fivefold (Luczak et al., 2006; Eng et al., 2007). Because ADH1C*1 is in linkage disequilibrium with ADH1B*2 and thus is usually coinherited with it, it remains unclear whether it exerts a protective effect independently of ADH1B*2 (Chen et al., 1999; Osier et al., 1999; Choi et al., 2005).

The prevalence of these alleles varies by ethnicity. ADH1B*2 is common in East Asian populations (around 60% prevalence) (Crabb et al., 2004), shows moderate frequency in Jewish populations (Neumark et al., 1998), and is associated with a lower risk of alcoholism in both (Hasin et al., 2002; Luczak et al., 2002; Luczak et al., 2006). ADH1B*3 is common in African Americans (over 15% prevalence), in whom it has been shown to have protective effects against alcoholism (Edenberg and Foroud, 2006). Protective effects of ADH1B*3 have also been reported in Native American populations (Wall et al., 2003). Both ADH1B*2 and ADH1B*3 are rare in Caucasians and have lower protective effects in them than in Asian and African populations, respectively (Whitfield, 2002). ADH1C*1 is very common in Han Chinese populations (about 90% prevalence) and is prevalent in about 55 to 60% of Caucasians (Osier et al., 1999).

Variants in the ALDH1A1 and ALDH2 genes (ALDH1A1*2, ALDH1A1*3, and ALDH2*2), have also been shown to protect against alcoholism (Thomasson et al., 1991; Chen et al., 1999; Ehlers et al., 2004b; Luczak et al., 2006). However, the protective effects of ALDH2*2 are the strongest and most well replicated. Low ALDH2 activity prevents the conversion of toxic acetaldehyde to acetate. Persons with two copies of ALDH2*2 (homozygotes) produce an inactive ALDH enzyme and are thought to have a ten times lower risk of AD, although such homozygotes are rare (Luczak et al., 2006). Persons with only one copy (heterozygotes) retain between 30 and 50% enzyme activity, which confers a fivefold reduction in risk of AD (Luczak et al., 2006). *ALDH2*2* is common in East Asians (as high as 30% prevalence) (Oota et al., 2004) but virtually non-existent in Caucasian and African populations. It is particularly protective against AD in Han Chinese, who also possess the *ADH1B*2* allele (Chen et al., 1999). Both *ALDH1A1*2* and *ALDH1A1*3* have been shown to protect against AD in African Americans (Spence et al., 2003). *ALDH1A1*2* also has protective effects in Native Americans (Ehlers et al., 2004a).

Genes that code for lower activity variants of ADH (e.g., *ADH4*, *ADH5*, *ADH6*, and *ADH7*) increase the risk of AD because they result in lower levels of the aversive acetaldehyde. Twelve single nucleotide polymorphisms (SNP) associated with the *ADH4* gene have been correlated with a greater risk for AD in European Americans (Edenberg and Foroud, 2006). Variants in *ADH4* have also been shown to be associated with AD in Brazilian populations (Guindalini et al., 2005), and in case–control studies of European American and African American families (Luo et al., 2005), as well as in European American families only (Luo et al., 2006).

Genes that influence neurotransmission

Several neurotransmitter systems have been implicated in AD including the dopaminergic, opioidergic, GABAergic, serotonergic, cholinergic, and glutamatergic systems (Heinz et al., 2009). These neurotransmitter signaling systems are central to neural circuits for a range of cognitions and behaviors involved in AD, such as reward and reinforcement, learning and memory, emotion and affect regulation, stress, impulse inhibition, and executive control (Koob and Le Moal, 2006). The neural circuits responsible for these cognitive behaviors are referred to as the mesolimbic reward pathway. A full discussion about the neuropsychology of AD is beyond the scope of this report. See Heilig et al. (2010) for a more detailed review.

A number of candidate genes have been identified that are thought to increase AD liability through their influence on these neurotransmitter systems. However, our understanding of the actual physiological mechanisms through which genetic variants in neurotransmission increase liability is much more limited than our understanding of genetic impacts on alcohol metabolism. Also, little is known about how these different neurotransmitter systems interact in causing dependence on alcohol (Heinz et al., 2009).

The gamma-aminobutyric acid system: GABRA2

Gamma-aminobutyric acid (GABA) is the brain's main inhibitory neurotransmitter whose activity is mediated by a family of two receptors (GABA-A and GABA-B). Alcohol is believed to activate the GABAergic system, inhibiting the activity of related neural circuits. Recent reviews (Gelernter and Kranzler, 2009) have confirmed *GABRA2* as a risk locus for AD. *GABRA2* is a gene that encodes for the alpha-2 subunit of the GABA-A receptor (the GABA-A receptor consists of five subunits in total). GABA-A mediates several important effects of alcohol, including sedation, anxiolysis, impairment of motor coordination, and withdrawal symptoms (Soyka and Rosner, 2008). The association between AD and *GABRA2* has been replicated with three different populations (Covault et al., 2008; Enoch et al., 2009; Gelernter and Kranzler, 2009). *GABRA2* has also been associated with subjective response to alcohol in healthy controls (Pierucci-Lagha et al., 2005). No specific causal (i.e., functional) variant in *GABRA2* has been identified, nor is a precise mechanism of action known (Gelernter and Kranzler, 2009). Given this, it is difficult to know how prevalent the association between *GABRA2* and AD is. It is also possible that associations between *GABRA2* and AD are in part driven by variants in *GABRG1*, an adjacent location on the gene that codes for the GABA-A gamma subunit receptor that has also been repeatedly associated with AD, and has been shown to be in linkage disequilibrium with *GABRA2* (Gelernter and Kranzler, 2009).

The dopaminergic system: The Taq1A polymorphism of DRD2

It is well known that consumption of alcohol activates dopamine receptors in the brain, stimulating the release of dopamine. This causes rewarding effects, leading to craving for alcohol and alcohol-seeking behavior (Heinz et al., 2009). Consequently, changes in the activity of dopamine receptors, particularly dopamine 1 and dopamine 2 receptors, are thought to increase the reward caused by alcohol and its resultant desirability (Kohnke, 2008), and have therefore been implicated in AD.

Variants in *DRD2*, the gene encoding the dopamine 2 receptor, have been the most extensively studied in AD (Le Foll et al., 2009). However, their role in AD is still controversial because of conflicting findings and nonreplication of associations. The Taq1A polymorphism of *DRD2* has been most consistently linked to AD, with meta-analyses showing that persons with the allele are 1.3 times more likely to have AD than those without (Munafò et al., 2007b; Smith et al., 2008). Recent evidence suggests Taq1A may not directly map onto *DRD2* but rather an adjacent gene (*ANKK1*) (Gelernter and Kranzler, 2009), leading researchers to question whether Taq1A directly impacts on AD risk or is a marker of a region of multiple co-located alleles involved in AD risk. Meta-analyses of the association between the A1 allele of Taq1A and AD revealed publication bias may have influenced initial optimism about the links (Munafò et al., 2007b). It also showed that the significance of the association varied for different population groups.

The opioid system: OPRM1

Intake of alcohol also stimulates the endogenous opioid system in the brain through activating various opioid receptors, including the mu opioid receptor. This is thought to release endorphins, which indirectly activate the dopaminergic reward system (Kohnke, 2008) leading to feelings of euphoria, analgesia, and withdrawal associated with alcohol use (Bond et al., 1998; Gianoulakis, 2001). Consequently, individual differences in the activity of the mu opioid receptor have been associated with the rewarding effects and desirability of alcohol and therefore AD liability.

Evidence suggests that differences in the activity of the mu opioid receptor may be genetically mediated. Specifically, genetic variants in *OPRM1* (the gene that encodes the mu opioid receptor) have been linked to AD, but their role is unclear because some studies have shown variants to be more prevalent in alcoholics (Kohnke, 2008), whereas others have shown the opposite (Szeto et al., 2001; Kim et al., 2004) or no association at all (van der Zwaluw et al., 2007).

More robust evidence exists for the association between variants in *OPRM1* and differential responses to opioid antagonist treatments (namely naltrexone) for AD (e.g., Anton et al., 2008). However, cases of nonreplication of this association have been reported (Gelernter et al., 2007). We discuss its impacts on treatment response in more detail in the section on clinical applications of genetic research.

Many other genes linked with AD risk include, but are not limited to, *CHRM2* (the gene that encodes the muscarinic acetylcholine receptor in the brain), variants of the *NMDAR* (glutamatergic N-methyl-D-aspartate receptor) gene, variants in the promoter region of the serotonin transporter gene (*SLC6A4*), as well as genes encoding dopamine-metabolizing enzymes [dopamine beta hydroxylase (DBH); catechol-*O*-methyltransferase (COMT) and monoamine oxidase A (MAOA)] and variants in genes encoding the dopamine transporter (DAT). However, the evidence regarding these associations is unclear because of conflicting results and nonreplications.

The serotonergic system: 5-HTTLPR

The serotonin, or 5-HT, transporter (5-HTT) regulates the reuptake of serotonin following synaptic release. The presence of long versus short alleles in the promoter region (*5-HTTLPR*) of the gene *SLC6A4*, which encodes 5-HTT, has been linked with compulsive craving (e.g., Heinz et al., 2004; Huang, 2010) and relapse (e.g., Pinto et al., 2008) in AD. However, some attempts to replicate these associations have failed (e.g., Kohnke et al., 2006) and gene–environment interactions have also been implicated in association with the *5-HTTLPR* genetic variation in alcohol use (e.g., Nilsson et al., 2005). To try to resolve these inconsistencies, McHugh et al. (2010) recently conducted a meta-analysis of the association between having a clinical diagnosis of AD and variants in the *5-HTTLPR* allele. They found that of the 22 case–control studies examined, 15 showed a significant association between the presence of a short allele in the *5-HTTLPR* gene and having a clinical diagnosis of AD. The results were consistent across age and cultural groups. However, analyses indicated that the results were moderated by sample size and publication bias, suggesting that they must be interpreted with caution (Feinn et al., 2005; McHugh et al., 2010).

Endophenotypes

In attempting to tie together these explanations of genetic mechanisms of alcohol metabolism and neurotransmission, researchers have argued that the alleles that influence susceptibility to alcoholism do so through individuals' subjective responses to the pharmacological and neurobiological effects of alcohol (Ray et al., 2010). These subjective responses are one example of an intermediate behavioral manifestation of alcoholism that is genetically mediated, commonly referred to as an "endophenotype." Subjective response to alcohol has been shown to be heritable (e.g., 60% heritability in twin studies; Viken et al., 2003) and affected by family history of alcoholism (Conrod et al., 1997). This supports its classification as an endophenotype. Genetic variations in an individual's stress response system caused by exposure to different substances (e.g., alcohol, opioids, nicotine, etc.) is another example of an endophenotype that is thought to be linked to an individual's susceptibility to various addictive behaviors (Zhou et al., 2010).

Examining endophenotypes can help to increase the power to detect genes implicated in risk of AD (e.g., Ray et al., 2010). They can also be useful in the prevention and treatment of alcoholism. In secondary prevention, they can be used as a marker of alcoholism risk and improve detection and subsequent prevention efforts. In treatment, they can be used as targets of pharmacological and psychological interventions such that measurable changes in the endophenotype indicate a positive treatment response.

Challenges in establishing a genetic basis for AD

The susceptibility alleles for AD identified to date account for only a fraction of the heritability estimated from twin and adoption studies. Identifying alleles that reliably predict AD liability is challenging for a number of reasons. First, with the exception of genetic variants related to ADH and ALDH activity, the AD-associated alleles identified to date only weakly predict risk of AD, have not been well replicated, and, for some markers, are of low prevalence in the population. ADH and ALDH variants that protect against AD are highly prevalent, particularly in Asian populations, but those that increase risk of AD are less prevalent in other racial groups, with estimates of their frequency in the COGA sample of Caucasians ranging from 8 to 30% (Edenberg, 2007).

Second, for non-Mendelian disorders such as AD, many alleles will only result in disease when combined with certain environmental factors or other genes, irrespective of the effect size and population prevalence of these alleles. For instance, polymorphisms in the promoter region of the serotonin transporter gene, i.e., 5-HTTLPR, have been associated with increased alcohol use in the presence of maltreatment (Rose and Dick, 2005), poor family relations (Nilsson et al., 2005), and multiple negative life events (Covault et al., 2007). Similarly, the promoter region of the MAOA gene has also been shown to interact with maltreatment, quality of family relations, and child sexual abuse in predicting alcoholism (Nilsson et al., 2007; Ducci et al., 2008). Both the A1 allele of the Taq1A polymorphism and variants in the CRF (corticotropin releasing factor 1) gene have also been linked to AD when combined with stressful life events (Clarke and Schumann, 2009; van der Zwaluw and Engels, 2009).

Because gene–environment interaction studies vary significantly in the measures, methods, and sample sizes used, it is difficult to draw clear conclusions or to replicate them. Indeed, most of the gene–environment interactions mentioned above have not been replicated. Also, because most gene–environment studies use small samples, some have questioned whether their findings are anything more than false positives (Flint and Munafò, 2008). Consequently, a degree of caution is needed in interpreting evidence from gene–environment interaction studies, including those pertaining to AD.

Third, genetic research on AD is revealing that multiple alleles, either from the same group or different groups of genes, predict disease risk via their interactions with other alleles. Associations between a low-activity variant of ADH1C*1 and reduced AD risk have been attributed to its interactions with ADH1B*1 (Kohnke, 2008). More recently, interactions between serotonin-related genes and ADH genes (Huang, 2010), and MAOA and ALDH2, have also been implicated in liability for AD (Lee et al., 2010). The number and complexity of gene–gene and gene–environment interactions involved in AD would be a major obstacle to the reliability and validity of predictive screening for susceptibility genes.

Fourth, advances in epigenetics may potentially complicate our understanding of the genetics of AD and the relative predictive strength of any genetic variations. Epigenetic mechanisms are cellular processes that integrate diverse environmental stimuli to modulate gene expression through the regulation of the chromatin structure (Renthal and Nestler, 2008). In more simple terms, they cause changes to gene expression without changing the underlying sequence of nucleotides that comprises DNA. Epigenetic modifications may mean that carrying a particular allele that confers disease risk does not necessarily translate to expression of that allele exemplified in manifestation of disease symptoms.

Alcohol is one environmental stimulus that could cause epigenetic modifications that modulate or even silence the expression of certain genes. Epigenetic modifications may be transferred from the carrier to their offspring, such as in cases of exposure to alcohol in utero (Kaminen-Ahola et al., 2010). A recent study found chromatin remodeling could be a plausible mechanism for AD itself (Pandey et al., 2008). To date such epigenetic research has largely been confined to rats; it is unclear how translatable these findings will be to humans. Further research is needed to better understand the epigenetic effects of alcohol and the implications of any such changes for the feasibility of predictive genetic screening for AD.

Applications of genomic medicine for AD

Prevention: Predictive screening for susceptibility to AD

On the basis of the available evidence about susceptibility alleles for AD, the feasibility of population-level predictive genetic screening for AD remains elusive. Because the candidate alleles have small effect sizes and lack replication, any attempts to use these in predictive genetic screening are likely to have limited specificity (the number of negative cases of disorder that are correctly identified) and sensitivity (the number of positive cases of disorder that are correctly identified). Moreover, until the gene–gene and gene–environment interactions and epigenetic modifications influencing AD liability are better understood, it seems highly unlikely that results from genetic research on AD could be applied with much confidence in the near term to clinical practice to ascertain an individual's risk for the disorder.

Single susceptibility alleles are thought to predict disease risk poorly unless the lifetime risk of the disease is 5% or more and the genotype is either very rare or increases disease risk by 20 or more times (Wald et al., 1999; Holtzman and Marteau, 2000; Khoury et al., 2004). The susceptibility alleles for AD identified thus far do not meet these criteria. Therefore any attempts to screen whole populations for these alleles would be prohibitively expensive (and not cost-effective) for the health-care system to implement because the number of subjects that would need to be screened to prevent one case of disease would be extremely high (Vineis et al., 2001).

Restricting genetic screening to persons with a family history of AD would substantially reduce the number of people tested and the associated costs of testing. Estimates of the recurrence risks of alcohol disorder in families have shown that between 20 and 30% of people with a family history of AD (exemplified by having at least one parent and one or two siblings with the disorder) will also be affected (Faraone, 1999). The predictive performance of genetic tests for AD is likely to be better for those who are at increased risk of disorder owing to a positive history of the disorder among first-degree relatives because they are also likely to possess the genetic and/or environmental factors that have predisposed their relatives to the disorder.

However, the costs of genetic screening, even if applied to a smaller and more select group, would only be justified if the addition of genetic information improved upon predictions based on family history. For smoking, the evidence suggests it does not. Gartner et al. (2009) found that screening for five alleles performed marginally better than chance and no better than the smoking history of the person's parents in predicting the likelihood of smoking. It is unclear whether genetic risk information for AD would improve upon predictions based on family history. More direct evaluations are needed.

It has been argued that the future prediction of risk for complex polygenic disorders would improve if we were able to identify between 200 and 400 susceptibility alleles (Janssens et al., 2006; Kraft and Hunter, 2009). Multiple alleles would be tested simultaneously to produce a combined disease risk score (Pharoah et al., 2002; Khoury et al., 2004). However, modeling of this approach has shown that it provides little useful information because most consumers find themselves in the middle of log-normal distributions with an "average" genetic risk (Hall, 2004). So even if more than 200 alleles for AD liability were identified, the information gleaned from them about genetic risk is likely to be of minimal use preventively over and above standard health advice to drink in moderation.

Personalized treatment of AD: Pharmacogenetics

Human responses to medications and to other therapeutic interventions vary widely; genetic variation is likely to explain some of this variation. This is also true for responses to pharmacological treatment for AD. Pharmacogenetics, the use of genetic information for the selection of treatments, is thought to have some promise in more effectively tailoring alcoholism treatments to individual patients' needs and improving treatment outcomes.

The potential application of pharmacogenetics to improve AD treatment efficacy is important because the pharmacological and psychological interventions commonly used have modest efficacy at best. Meta-analyses have shown that 12-month abstinence rates ranged from 17 to 35% for treatments of AD such as naltrexone, 12-step programs, motivational enhancement therapy, and cognitive behavior therapy (Miller et al., 2001). In addition, rates of relapse following treatment are high. According to the Combined Pharmacotherapies and Behavioral Interventions for Alcohol Dependence Study (COMBINE), one of the largest, most carefully controlled clinical trials for AD, approximately 80% of all AD patients will have a heavy drinking day during the 12 months following treatment (Anton et al., 2006). It is hoped that targeting specific treatments to those who are most responsive may increase the effectiveness of these drugs and reduce relapse.

Multiple studies have demonstrated that the *Asp40* allele of the gene encoding the mu opioid type 1 receptor in the brain (*OPRM1*) moderates alcohol-dependent individuals' response to treatment with naltrexone, a drug that inhibits alcohol-induced opioid activity (e.g., Ray and Hutchison, 2007). One study demonstrated that variants in *GABRA2/GABRA6* predicted responses to acamprosate (Ooteman et al., 2009), although the sample size for this study was small and the result has not been replicated. A single nucleotide polymorphism (SNP) in intron 9 of the glutamate receptor 5 (GluR5) gene (*GRIK1*) has also been shown to be a marker for side effects in cases of alcohol dependence treated by topiramate, an anticonvulsant drug that reduces alcohol craving by stimulating GABA activity and inhibiting glutamatergic activity (Ray et al., 2009). There is evidence that genetic variants may also predict responses to psychological therapies for AD, such as motivational enhancement therapy (Feldstein Ewing et al., 2009).

Using pharmacogenetics to personalize treatment for AD is contingent on the existence of highly prevalent genes that are strongly predictive of treatment response. On this basis, the *Asp40* allele of the *OPRM1* gene appears to be the most promising candidate for a pharmacogenetic test for naltrexone response for the treatment of AD. *Asp40* is found in 15 to 18% of Caucasian Americans (Kuehn, 2009). Clinical trials have shown persons with the *Asp40* allele are three times more likely to respond to naltrexone therapy for AD than those homozygous for the *Asn40* allele (Oslin et al., 2003; Anton et al., 2006; Ray and Hutchison, 2007).

However, a degree of caution is still required in interpreting this association. One study failed to replicate the association between *Asp40* and improved response to naltrexone (Gelernter et al., 2007), although its sample size was small. In addition, the findings of Anton and colleagues (2006) may be less promising than they seem. The association between *Asp40* and positive naltrexone response was only found in patients who received medical management alone, and not in patients who were also receiving a combined behavioral intervention (Mattes, 2009). Mattes (2009) argues that if the association between *Asp40* and naltrexone response is robust it should have been demonstrated in both patient groups. It also needs to be established whether the effect sizes for *Asp40* provide a sufficient gain in treatment response to justify the cost of the genetic test (Flowers and Veenstra, 2004). Further effectiveness and cost-effectiveness analyses are needed to resolve these issues.

OPRM1 has also been examined in pharmacogenetic studies of smoking cessation, although the results have been contradictory (Lerman et al., 2004; Munafò et al., 2007a). Other genetic variants examined in pharmacogenetic studies of smoking cessation have yielded small effect sizes that weaken over time, and most of the findings have not been replicated (Hall et al., 2008). The strength of the findings to date on the pharmacogenetics of smoking cessation does not encourage optimism regarding the likely success of pharmacogenetic applications to AD or to addiction more broadly, although further research is warranted.

Conclusion

Although genetic research has the potential to reduce AD and the harms associated with alcohol use, these hopes are yet to be borne out in research. Overall, genetic testing is not ready for use in the prediction of AD liability.

As we have shown, AD is a complex, multifactorial, polygenic disorder and the evidence to date shows that it is unlikely that one or even a small number of genes will be identified that explain all the variance in its heritability. As well as being a product of interactions between multiple genes, AD is also a product of interactions between genes and the environment. New epigenetic research on AD has revealed that external stimuli may influence the expression of genes, meaning that having a gene associated with disease risk does not necessarily translate to having that disease. Consequently, such genetic screening has minimal preventive use over and above advice to drink alcohol in moderation or abstain from alcohol completely and may be no more effective in predicting disease risk than family history.

Pharmacogenetic testing for naltrexone response may have more clinical utility than genetic tests for AD liability, because it can be used to inform treatment selection and improve treatment outcomes for alcohol-dependent persons. The evidence linking genetic variants with differential response to treatment, especially to naltrexone treatment, appears to be more robust than that for predictive genetic testing. Given this, pharmacogenetic testing for AD appears to be a more promising prospect than predictive genetic screening for AD. There are, however, some caveats to this. Because the gene that influences naltrexone response is prevalent in some population groups but virtually nonexistent in others, the potential positive impacts of such pharmacogenetic testing will be restricted to certain population groups. More research is required to demonstrate the utility and cost-effectiveness of pharmacogenetic testing for AD in the population who possess the relevant allele, before it is routinely applied in clinical practice.

References

Agrawal, A. and Lynskey, M. T. (2008). Are there genetic influences on addiction: evidence from family, adoption and twin studies. *Addiction*, 103, 1069–1081.

Anton, R. F., O'Malley, S. S., Ciraulo, D. A., et al. (2006). Combined pharmacotherapies and behavioral interventions for alcohol dependence: the COMBINE study: a randomized controlled trial. *JAMA*, 295, 2003–2017.

Anton, R. F., Oroszi, G., O'Malley, S., et al. (2008). An evaluation of mu-opioid receptor (OPRM1) as a predictor of naltrexone response in the treatment of alcohol dependence: results from the Combined Pharmacotherapies and Behavioral Interventions for Alcohol Dependence (COMBINE) study. *Archives of General Psychiatry*, 65, 135–144.

Ball, D. (2008). Addiction science and its genetics. *Addiction*, 103, 360–367.

Bond, C., Laforge, K. S., Tian, M., et al. (1998). Single-nucleotide polymorphism in the human mu opioid receptor gene alters beta-endorphin binding and activity: possible implications for opiate addiction. *Proceedings of the National Academy of Sciences USA*, 95, 9608–9613.

Bosron, W. F., Magnes, L. J., and Li, T. K. (1983). Kinetic and electrophoretic properties of native and recombined isoenzymes of human liver alcohol dehydrogenase. *Biochemistry*, 22, 1852–1857.

Buckland, P. R. (2001). Genetic association studies of alcoholism: problems with the candidate gene approach. *Alcohol and Alcoholism*, 36, 99–103.

Chen, C. C., Lu, R. B., Chen, Y. C., et al. (1999). Interaction between the functional polymorphisms of the alcohol-metabolism genes in protection against alcoholism. *American Journal of Human Genetics*, 65, 795–807.

Choi, I. G., Son, H. G., Yang, B. H., et al. (2005). Scanning of genetic effects of alcohol metabolism gene (*ADH1B* and *ADH1C*) polymorphisms on the risk of alcoholism. *Human Mutation*, 26, 224–234.

Clarke, T. K. and Schumann, G. (2009). Gene-environment interactions resulting in risky alcohol drinking behaviour are mediated by CRF and CRF1. *Pharmacology, Biochemistry and Behavior*, 93, 230–236.

Collins, F. S., Green, E. D., Guttmacher, A. E., and Guyer, M. S. (2003). A vision for the future of genomics research. *Nature*, 422, 835–847.

Conrod, P. J., Peterson, J. B., Pihl, R. O., and Mankowski, S. (1997). Biphasic effects of alcohol on heart rate are influenced by alcoholic family history and rate of alcohol ingestion. *Alcoholism, Clinical and Experimental Research*, 21, 140–149.

Covault, J., Tennen, H., Armell, S., et al. (2007). Interactive effects of the serotonin transporter 5-HTTLPR polymorphism and stressful life events on college student drinking and drug use. *Biological Psychiatry*, 61, 609–616.

Covault, J., Gelerenter, J., Jensen, K., Anton, R., and Kranzler, H. R. (2008). Markers in the 5'-region of *GABRG1* associate to alcohol dependence and are in linkage disequilibrium with markers in the adjacent *GABRA2* gene. *Neuropsychopharmacology*, 33, 837–848.

Crabb, D. W., Matsumoto, M., Chang, D., and You, M. (2004). Overview of the role of alcohol dehydrogenase and aldehyde dehydrogenase and their variants in the genesis of alcohol-related pathology. *The Proceedings of the Nutrition Society*, 63, 49–63.

Ducci, F., Enoch, M. A., Hodgkinson, C., et al. (2008). Interaction between a functional MAOA locus and childhood sexual abuse predicts alcoholism and antisocial personality disorder in adult women. *Molecular Psychiatry*, 13, 334–347.

Edenberg, H. J. (2002). The collaborative study on the genetics of alcoholism: an update. *Alcohol Research and Health*, 26, 214–218.

Edenberg, H. J. (2007). The genetics of alcohol metabolism: role of alcohol dehydrogenase and aldehyde dehydrogenase variants. *Alcohol Research and Health*, 30, 5–13.

Edenberg, H. J. and Foroud, T. (2006). The genetics of alcoholism: identifying specific genes through family studies. *Addiction Biology*, 11, 386–396.

Ehlers, C. L., Gilder, D. A., Wall, T. L., et al. (2004a). Genomic screen for loci associated with alcohol dependence in Mission Indians. *American Journal of Medical Genetics. Part B, Neuropsychiatric Genetics*, 129B, 110–115.

Ehlers, C. L., Spence, J. P., Wall, T. L., Gilder, D. A., and Carr, L. G. (2004b). Association of ALDH1 promoter polymorphisms with alcohol-related phenotypes in southwest

California Indians. *Alcoholism, Clinical and Experimental Research*, 28, 1481–1486.

Eng, M. Y., Luczak, S. E., and Wall, T. L. (2007). *ALDH2, ADH1B*, and *ADH1C* genotypes in Asians: a literature review. *Alcohol Research and Health*, 30, 22–27.

Enoch, M. A., Hodgkinson, C. A., Yuan, Q., et al. (2009). *GABRG1* and *GABRA2* as independent predictors for alcoholism in two populations. *Neuropsychopharmacology*, 34, 1245–1254.

Faraone, S. V. (ed.) (1999). *Genetics of Mental Disorders*. New York: Guilford Press.

Feinn, R., Nellissery, M., and Kranzler, H. R. (2005). Meta-analysis of the association of a functional serotonin transporter promoter polymorphism with alcohol dependence. *American Journal of Medical Genetics. Part B, Neuropsychiatric Genetics*, 133B, 79–84.

Feldstein Ewing, S. W., Lachance, H. A., Bryan, A., and Hutchison, K. E. (2009). Do genetic and individual risk factors moderate the efficacy of motivational enhancement therapy? Drinking outcomes with an emerging adult sample. *Addiction Biology*, 14, 356–365.

Flint, J. and Munafò, M. R. (2008). Forum: Interactions between gene and environment. *Current Opinion in Psychiatry*, 21, 315–317.

Flowers, C. R. and Veenstra, D. (2004). The role of cost-effectiveness analysis in the era of pharmacogenomics. *Pharmacoeconomics*, 22, 481–493.

Gartner, C. E., Barendregt, J. J., and Hall, W. D. (2009). Multiple genetic tests for susceptibility to smoking do not outperform simple family history. *Addiction*, 104, 118–1126.

Gelernter, J. and Kranzler, H. R. (2009). Genetics of alcohol dependence. *Human Genetics*, 126, 91–99.

Gelernter, J., Gueorguieva, R., Kranzler, H. R., et al. (2007). Opioid receptor gene (*OPRM1, OPRK1*, and *OPRD1*) variants and response to naltrexone treatment for alcohol dependence: results from the VA Cooperative Study. *Alcoholism, Clinical and Experimental Research*, 31, 555–563.

Gianoulakis, C. (2001). Influence of the endogenous opioid system on high alcohol consumption and genetic predisposition to alcoholism. *Journal of Psychiatry and Neuroscience*, 26, 304–318.

Guindalini, C., Scivoletto, S., Ferreira, R. G. M., et al. (2005). Association of genetic variants in alcohol dehydrogenase 4 with alcohol dependence in Brazilian patients. *American Journal of Psychiatry*, 162, 1005–1007.

Hall, W. (2004). Feeling 'better than well'. *EMBO Reports*, 5, 1105–1109.

Hall, W. D., Gartner, C. E., and Carter, A. (2008). The genetics of nicotine addiction liability: ethical and social policy implications. *Addiction*, 103, 350–359.

Hasin, D., Aharonovich, E., Liu, X., et al. (2002). Alcohol and *ADH2* in Israel: Ashkenazis, Sephardics, and recent Russian immigrants. *American Journal of Psychiatry*, 159, 1432–1434.

Heilig, M., Thorsell, A., Sommer, W. H., et al. (2010). Translating the neuroscience of alcoholism into clinical treatments: from blocking the buzz to curing the blues. *Neuroscience and Biobehavioral Reviews*, 35, 334–344.

Heinz, A., Goldman, D., Gallinat, J., Schumann, G., and Puls, I. (2004). Pharmacogenetic insights to monoaminergic dysfunction in alcohol dependence. *Psychopharmacology*, 174, 561–570.

Heinz, A., Beck, A., Wrase, J., et al. (2009). Neurotransmitter systems in alcohol dependence. *Pharmacopsychiatry*, 42 Suppl 1, S95–S101.

Holtzman, N. A. and Marteau, T. M. (2000). Will genetics revolutionize medicine? *New England Journal of Medicine*, 343, 141–144.

Huang, C. L. C. (2010). The role of serotonin and possible interaction of serotonin-related genes with alcohol dehydrogenase and aldehyde dehydrogenase genes in alcohol dependence: a review. *American Journal of Translational Research*, 2, 190–199.

Janssens, A. C. J. W., Aulchenko, Y. S., Elefante, S., et al. (2006). Predictive testing for complex diseases using multiple genes: fact or fiction? *Genetics in Medicine*, 8, 395–400.

Kalsi, G., Prescott, C. A., Kendler, K. S., and Riley, B. P. (2009). Unraveling the molecular mechanisms of alcohol dependence. *Trends in Genetics*, 25, 49–55.

Kaminen-Ahola, N., Ahola, A., Maga, M., et al. (2010). Maternal ethanol consumption alters the epigenotype and the phenotype of offspring in a mouse model. *PLoS Genetics*, 6, e1000811.

Kendler, K. S. and Prescott, C. A. (eds.) (2006). *Genes, Environment and Psychopathology*. New York: Guilford Press.

Khoury, M. J., Yang, Q., Gwinn, M., Little, J., and Dana, F. W. (2004). An epidemiologic assessment of genomic profiling for measuring susceptibility to common diseases and targeting interventions. *Genetics in Medicine*, 6, 38–47.

Kim, S. G., Kim, C. M., Kang, D. H., et al. (2004). Association of functional opioid receptor genotypes with alcohol dependence in Koreans. *Alcoholism, Clinical and Experimental Research*, 28, 986–990.

Kohnke, M. D. (2008). Approach to the genetics of alcoholism: a review based on pathophysiology. *Biochemical Pharmacology*, 75, 160–177.

Kohnke, M. D., Kolb, W., Lutz, U., Maurer, S., and Batra, A. (2006). The serotonin transporter promotor polymorphism *5-HTTLPR* is not associated with alcoholism or severe forms of alcohol withdrawal in a German sample. *Psychiatric Genetics*, 16, 227–228.

Koob, G. F. and Le Moal, M. (eds.) (2006). *Neurobiology of Addiction*. New York: Academic Press.

Kraft, P. and Hunter, D. J. (2009). Genetic risk prediction – are we there yet? *New England Journal of Medicine*, 360, 1701–1703.

Kuehn, B. M. (2009). Findings on alcohol dependence point to promising avenues for targeted therapies. *The Journal of the American Medical Association*, 301, 1643–1645.

Le Foll, B., Gallo, A., Le Strat, Y., Lu, L., and Gorwood, P. (2009). Genetics of dopamine receptors and drug addiction: a comprehensive review. *Behavioural Pharmacology*, 20, 1–17.

Lee, S. Y., Hahan, C.Y., Lee, J. F., et al. (2010). MAOA interacts with the *ALDH2* gene in anxiety-depression alcohol dependence. *Alcoholism, Clinical and Experimental Research*, 34, 1212–1218.

Lerman, C., Wileyto, E. P., Patterson, F., et al. (2004). The functional mu opioid receptor (*OPRM1*) *Asn40Asp* variant predicts short-term response to nicotine replacement therapy in a clinical trial. *Pharmacogenomics Journal*, 4, 184–192.

Luczak, S. E., Shea, S. H., Carr, L. G., Li, T. K., and Wall, T. L. (2002). Binge drinking in Jewish and non-Jewish white college students. *Alcoholism, Clinical and Experimental Research*, 26, 1773–1778.

Luczak, S. E., Glatt, S. J., and Wall, T. L. (2006). Meta-analyses of *ALDH2* and *ADH1B* with alcohol dependence in Asians. *Psychological Bulletin*, 132, 607–621.

Luo, X., Kranzler, H. R., Zuo, L., et al. (2005). *ADH4* gene variation is associated with alcohol and drug dependence: results from family controlled and population-structured association studies. *Pharmacogenetics and Genomics*, 15, 755–768.

Luo, X., Kranzler, H. R., Zuo, L., et al. (2006). *ADH4* gene variation is associated with alcohol dependence and drug dependence in European Americans: results from HWD tests and case-control association studies. *Neuropsychopharmacology*, 31, 1085–1095.

Mattes, J. A. (2009). Questionable efficacy for naltrexone in patients with *Asp40*. *Archives of General Psychiatry*, 66, 796; author reply 796–797.

McCarver, D. G., Thomasson, H. R., Martier, S. S., Sokol, R. J., and Li, T. K. (1997). Alcohol dehydrogenase-2*3 allele protects against alcohol-related birth defects among African Americans. *Journal of Pharmacology and Experimental Therapeutics*, 283, 1095–1101.

McHugh, R. K., Hofmann, S. G., Asnaani, A., Sawyer, A. T., and Otto, M. W. (2010). The serotonin transporter gene and risk for alcohol dependence: a meta-analytic review. *Drug and Alcohol Dependence*, 108, 1–6.

Miller, W. R., Walters, S. T., and Bennett, M. E. (2001). How effective is alcoholism treatment in the United States? *Journal of Studies on Alcohol*, 62, 211–220.

Munafò, M. R., Elliot, K. M., Murphy, M. F. G., Walton, R. T., and Johnstone, E. C. (2007a). Association of the mu-opioid receptor gene with smoking cessation. *Pharmacogenomics Journal*, 7, 353–361.

Munafò, M. R., Matheson, I. J., and Flint, J. (2007b). Association of the *DRD2* gene Taq1A polymorphism and alcoholism: a meta-analysis of case-control studies and evidence of publication bias. *Molecular Psychiatry*, 12, 454–461.

Neumark, Y. D., Friedlander, Y., Thomasson, H. R., and Li, T. K. (1998). Association of the *ADH2*2* allele with reduced ethanol consumption in Jewish men in Israel: a pilot study. *Journal of Studies on Alcohol*, 59, 133–139.

Nilsson, K. W., Sjoberg, R. L., Damberg, M., et al. (2005). Role of the serotonin transporter gene and family function in adolescent alcohol consumption. *Alcoholism, Clinical and Experimental Research*, 29, 564–570.

Nilsson, K. W., Sjoberg, R. L., Wargelius, H. L., et al. (2007). The monoamine oxidase A (MAO-A) gene, family function and maltreatment as predictors of destructive behaviour during male adolescent alcohol consumption. *Addiction*, 102, 389–398.

Oota, H., Pakstis, A. J., Bonne-Tamir, B., et al. (2004). The evolution and population genetics of the *ALDH2* locus: random genetic drift, selection, and low levels of recombination. *Annals of Human Genetics*, 68, 93–109.

Ooteman, W., Naassila, M., Koeter, M. W. J., et al. (2009). Predicting the effect of naltrexone and acamprosate in alcohol-dependent patients using genetic indicators. *Addiction Biology*, 14, 328–337.

Osier, M., Pakstis, A. J., Kidd, J. R., et al. (1999). Linkage disequilibrium at the *ADH2* and *ADH3* loci and risk of alcoholism. *American Journal of Human Genetics*, 64, 1147–1157.

Oslin, D. W., Berettini, W., Kranzler, H. R., et al. (2003). A functional polymorphism of the mu-opioid receptor gene is associated with naltrexone response in alcohol-dependent patients. *Neuropsychopharmacology*, 28, 1546–1552.

Pandey, S., Ugale, R., Zhang, H., Tang, L., and Prakash, A. (2008). Brain chromatin remodeling: a novel mechanism of alcoholism. *Journal of Neuroscience*, 28, 3729–3737.

Pharoah, P. D. P., Antoniou, A., Bobrow, M., et al. (2002). Polygenic susceptibility to breast cancer and implications for prevention. *Nature Genetics*, 31, 33–36.

Pierucci-Lagha, A., Covault, J., Feinn, R., et al. (2005). *GABRA2* alleles moderate the subjective effects of alcohol, which are attenuated by finasteride. *Neuropsychopharmacology*, 30, 1193–1203.

Pinto, E., Reggers, J., Gorwood, P., et al. (2008). The short allele of the serotonin transporter promoter polymorphism influences relapse in alcohol dependence. *Alcohol and Alcoholism*, 43, 398–400.

Ray, L. A. and Hutchison, K. E. (2007). Effects of naltrexone on alcohol sensitivity and genetic moderators of medication response: a double-blind placebo-controlled study. *Archives of General Psychiatry*, 64, 1069–1077.

Ray, L. A., Miranda Jr., R. MacKillop. J., et al. (2009). A preliminary pharmacogenetic investigation of adverse events from topiramate in heavy drinkers. *Experimental and Clinical Psychopharmacology*, 17, 122–129.

Ray, L. A., Mackillop, J., and Monti, P. M. (2010). Subjective responses to alcohol consumption as endophenotypes: advancing behavioral genetics in etiological and treatment models of alcoholism. *Substance Use and Misuse*, 45, 1742–1765.

Renthal, W. and Nestler, E. J. (2008). Epigenetic mechanisms in drug addiction. *Trends in Molecular Medicine*, 14, 341–350.

Rose, R. J. and Dick, D. M. (2005). Gene-environment interplay in adolescent drinking behaviour. *Alcohol Research and Health*, 28, 222–229.

Sartor, C. E., Lynskey, M. T., Bucholz, K. K., et al. (2009). Timing of first alcohol use and alcohol dependence: evidence of common genetic influences. *Addiction*, 104, 1512–1518.

Smith, L., Watson, M., Gates, S., Ball, D., and Foxcroft, D. (2008). Meta-analysis of the association of the Taq1A polymorphism with the risk of alcohol dependency: a HuGE gene-disease association review. *American Journal of Epidemiology*, 167, 125–138.

Soyka, M. and Rosner, S. (2008). Opioid antagonists for pharmacological treatment of alcohol dependence – a critical review. *Current Drug Abuse Reviews*, 1, 280–291.

Spence, J. P., Liang, T., Eriksson, C. J. P., et al. (2003). Evaluation of aldehyde dehydrogenase 1 promoter polymorphisms identified in human populations. *Alcoholism, Clinical and Experimental Research*, 27, 1389–1394.

Szeto, C. Y., Tang, N. L., Lee, D. T., and Stadlin, A. (2001). Association between mu opioid receptor gene polymorphisms and Chinese heroin addicts. *Neuroreport*, 12, 1103–1106.

Thomasson, H. R., Edenberg, H. J., Crabb, D. W., et al. (1991). Alcohol and aldehyde dehydrogenase genotypes and alcoholism in Chinese men. *American Journal of Human Genetics*, 48, 677–681.

Van der Zwaluw, C. S. and Engels, R. C. M. E. (2009). Gene-environment interactions and alcohol use and dependence: current status and future challenges. *Addiction*, 104, 907–914.

Van der Zwaluw, C. S., Van den Wildenberg, E., Wiers, R. W., et al. (2007). Polymorphisms in the mu-opioid receptor gene (*OPRM1*) and the implications for alcohol dependence in humans. *Pharmacogenomics*, 8, 1427–1436.

Viken, R. J., Rose, R. J., Morzorati, S. L., Christian, J. C., and Li, T. K. (2003). Subjective intoxication in response to alcohol challenge: heritability and covariation with personality, breath alcohol level, and drinking history. *Alcoholism, Clinical and Experimental Research*, 27, 795–803.

Viljoen, D. L., Carr, L. G., Foroud, T. M., et al. (2001). Alcohol dehydrogenase-2*2 allele is associated with decreased prevalence of fetal alcohol syndrome in the mixed-ancestry population of the Western Cape Province, South Africa. *Alcoholism, Clinical and Experimental Research*, 25, 1719–1722.

Vineis, P., Schulte, P., and McMichael, A. J. (2001). Misconceptions about the use of genetic tests in populations. *Lancet*, 357, 709–712.

Wald, N. J., Hackshaw, A. K., and Frost, C. D. (1999). When can a risk factor be used as a worthwhile screening test? *British Medical Journal*, 319, 1562–1565.

Wall, T. L., Carr, L. G., and Ehlers, C. L. (2003). Protective association of genetic variation in alcohol dehydrogenase with alcohol dependence in Native American Mission Indians. *American Journal of Psychiatry*, 160, 41–46.

Warren, K. R. and Li, T. K. (2005). Genetic polymorphisms: impact on the risk of fetal alcohol spectrum disorders. *Birth Defects Research. Part A, Clinical and Molecular Teratology*, 73, 195–203.

Whitfield, J. B. (2002). Alcohol dehydrogenase and alcohol dependence: variation in genotype-associated risk between populations. *American Journal of Human Genetics*, 71, 1247–1250; author reply 1250–1251.

Williams, R. (2010). Genomics in our own hands. *Lancet Neurology*, 9, 656–657.

World Health Organization (2008). *The Global Burden of Disease: 2004 Update*. Geneva: World Health Organization.

Zhou, Y., Proudnikov, D., Yuferov, V., and Kreek, M. J. (2010). Drug-induced and genetic alterations in stress-responsive systems: Implications for specific addictive diseases. *Brain Research*, 1314, 235–252.

Promises and risks for participants in studies of genetic risk for alcohol or drug dependence

Carl Erik Fisher, Deborah Hasin, and Paul Appelbaum

The rapid progression of genetic research is uniting two areas of investigation that each face significant challenges in their own right: substance-use disorders[1] and psychiatric genetics. Research on the genetics of alcohol and drug dependence offers great promise for improving our understanding of these disorders and developing new therapies, but this line of research also requires careful consideration from an ethical standpoint. In this chapter, we discuss the potential ethical challenges arising from the genetics of substance-use disorders, ranging from concrete risks that could stem from research participation to more abstract considerations related to the social and legal implications of this work.

Introduction: Promises

Genetic factors have long been known to be important for the development of substance-use disorders, as established by traditional genetic epidemiology methods such as twin, family, and adoption studies (Gelernter and Kranzler, 2009: 91–99; Gelernter and Kranzler, 2010: 77–84). Heritability estimates for nicotine, alcohol, and drug addiction generally fall in the range of 50 to 60% (Bierut, 2011: 618–627). The popular understanding of this genetic risk, however, is commonly clouded by inaccurate "folk genetic" concepts, e.g., the quasi-Mendelian idea that there could exist a "gene for" alcoholism or drug dependence. In fact, despite recent advances in the field, a significant fraction of the variance of genetic influences on substance-use disorders remains unexplained; clearly, these disorders are polygenic and develop in response to a complex set of variables (Frazer et al., 2009: 241–251). With that said, research on the genetics of alcohol and drug dependence does carry several important promises.

Genetic research may help better categorize substance-use disorders and predict response to treatment. Clinical studies of alcohol dependence have already demonstrated that patients with alcohol-use disorders who have a certain phenomenological profile – for

---

Genetic Research on Addiction, ed. Audrey R. Chapman. Published by Cambridge University Press.
© Cambridge University Press 2012.

[1] The terminology used to describe substance-use disorders has been extensively debated. The current version of the American Psychiatric Association's *Diagnostic and Statistical Manual* (DSM), DSM-IV, draws a distinction between "abuse" and "dependence," but the next iteration of the DSM (DSM-5) will combine these two entities into a single disorder of graded clinical severity (see, e.g., the extensive discussion on the DSM-5 website at www.dsm5.org/ProposedRevision/Pages/proposedrevision.aspx?rid=452#, accessed 29 February 2012). Debate on the terminology is beyond the scope of this chapter, so we use "dependence," "addiction," "substance-use disorder," and similar terms interchangeably.

example, a strong family history, strong cravings, and earlier age of onset – may be more likely to respond to treatment with naltrexone (Monterosso et al., 2001: 258–268). Similarly, researchers have attempted to classify alcoholism into subtypes on the basis of such data, but these efforts have had mixed results (Johnson, 2010: 630–639). One hope of genetic research on addictions is to use molecular genetic markers to classify such subtypes and better predict treatment outcomes. Recent genetic studies have suggested that response to naltrexone treatment may be predicted by patients' genotypes at a specific opioid receptor (OPRM1) (Anton et al., 2008: 135–144), and similar findings have suggested that the genotype of the 5′-regulatory region of the serotonin transporter gene can predict response to treatment with ondansetron (Johnson et al., 2011: 265–275). In many researchers' eyes, the long-term aim of this work is not only to better describe substance-use disorders or predict their course but also to determine which treatments to use on the basis of genetic testing. In the words of one researcher, "It will tell you who the drug won't work for, so you don't have to waste your time giving it to patients who won't respond" (Kuehn, 2011: 984–985).

Several related possibilities are suggested by this work. Broadly speaking, if one could better categorize substance-use disorders on the basis of molecular genetics alone, individuals at risk could be identified earlier, perhaps before the development of maladaptive substance use, and receive preventive measures. These studies may also have "top-down" implications for basic science and drug development, as the identification of such genotypes might suggest new potential targets for the development of pharmacological treatments. Clearly, the speculative conclusions of these preliminary findings could be taken quite far. First, though, we discuss the concrete risks that might arise from this research.

Risks related to research conduct

In general, there are two groups of risks related to conducting genetic research on substance-use disorders: risks that arise by virtue of studying participants who have substance-use disorders; and risks that arise specifically from the study of genetic material.

Risks arising from research on participants with substance-use disorders

The two most frequently expressed concerns regarding research on participants with substance-use disorders relate to the decisional capacity of the participants and to the use of incentives to encourage research participation. Although most researchers and many members of the public would acknowledge that having a substance-use disorder (or, for that matter, any mental disorder) does not necessarily imply that a person lacks capacity to participate in research or consent to treatment, many may still consider people with alcohol or drug dependence "vulnerable" in some way. Impaired judgment is a central feature of the popular conception of addiction, and, arguably, of professional diagnosis as well. This idea is made explicit in the criteria for defining substance-use disorders, as one criterion is continued use despite persistent or recurrent problems (American Psychiatric Association, 2000: 303.90).

Of course, poor judgment with regard to use of substances does not necessarily interfere with an individual's ability to consent to research or treatment. However, the perception that those with substance-use disorders suffer from a type of "myopia" for the future may persist nonetheless (Jeste and Saks, 2006: 607–628), with one writer arguing that substance dependence is "inherently incompatible" with the ability to give informed consent to research protocols that give participants their drugs of choice (a rare design for genetic research in any case) (Charland, 2002: 37–47). This position might lead some to question the capacity of participants with substance-use disorders to consent to research in general. However, empirical research on individuals with addiction and the consent process, albeit limited, has not found any evidence that this population suffers from impairment in decision-making capacity related to giving informed consent (Jeste and Saks, 2006: 607–628; Carter and Hall, 2008: 209–225), and therefore individuals with substance-use disorders are generally considered to have the cognitive capacity to participate in research (Carter and Hall, 2008: 209–225). Along similar lines, the capacity of inpatients with psychiatric disorders to participate in research does not differ greatly from that of general hospital inpatients (Okai et al., 2007: 291–297). Ultimately, there is no clear reason to suspect that those with substance-use disorders would be incapable of consenting to genetic research.

Ethical concerns have also been raised regarding the provision of incentives to participants in research. Participants who abuse drugs and alcohol are sometimes portrayed as particularly vulnerable to undue influence (often mistakenly referred to as "coercion") from incentives, on the assumption that they will use these cash incentives to buy alcohol or drugs (Dickert and Grady, 1999: 198–203). Similarly, concerns have been raised that incentives, by making cash immediately available, might precipitate or exacerbate drug use (Fry and Dwyer, 2001: 1319–1325). In practice, this concern is usually addressed by compensating participants with gift cards and other nonmonetary items or services. The broader issue is similar to the questions raised regarding decision making above; namely, do individuals with substance-use disorders have a specific type of vulnerability, a priori? Of note, one study directly assessed the effects of providing cash incentives of different values to substance-abusing participants and found that higher rewards correlated with better follow-up with no effect on substance use and no perception of having been coerced (Festinger et al., 2005: 275–281).

In summary, although concerns have been raised about research studies involving participants with substance-use disorders, no clear, inherent vulnerability appears to preclude their participation in research studies, including genetic studies, as long as standard research protections (i.e., thorough informed consent, reasonable incentives, and institutional oversight) are in place. Indeed, no evidence indicates that the judgment of patients with substance-use disorders with regard to research participation is any more impaired than the judgment of research participants with other disorders. Concerns about some unique "vulnerability" may be more a manifestation of the considerable stigma associated with substance-use disorders than a reflection of any real impairment in participants' autonomy (Crisp et al., 2005: 106–113; Keyes et al., 2010: 1364–1372; Pescosolido et al., 2010: 1321–1330).

Risks arising from the study of genetic material

There are certain risks common to all studies involving genetic material. For example, "biobanking" genetic samples raises concerns regarding risks to the autonomy and privacy of participants that may emerge from provision of broad consent for later unspecified uses of personal genetic information – risks that may not be covered by traditional ethical safeguards (Widdows and Cordell, 2011: 207–219). Also, the possibility of discrimination from genetic information is often cited as a general risk, e.g., insurers may learn of the results of genetic testing and deny coverage of at-risk persons, or employers may make decisions about hiring or firing on a similar basis. These concerns regarding discrimination have been addressed in part in the United States by the federal Genetic Information Nondiscrimination Act (GINA) of 2008, which bars health insurers from using genetic information to make underwriting decisions and prohibits employers from obtaining or using genetic information for a range of employment-related decisions (Appelbaum, 2010: 338–340). However, the scope of GINA does not extend to other forms of insurance, such as life, disability, or long-term care insurance, and it does not apply to the military (Hudson et al., 2008: 2661–2663). Furthermore, regardless of federal protections against such discrimination and complementary state laws, public fears about misuse may still exert a practical impact, as demonstrated by studies showing that patients and clinicians underuse genetic tests because of such concerns (Lowstuter et al., 2008: 691–698).

GINA also highlights the fact that genetic information is by no means limited to the results of genetic tests, as the definition in GINA extends to information about a family history of an illness or disorder. The importance of this protection is made clear by a recent example from Hong Kong in which the local government rejected two young men and terminated a third from the civil services because each had family histories of schizophrenia, based on a rule excluding persons with first-degree relatives with mental disorders from employment in law enforcement, fire, and ambulance services (ultimately, though, the courts found this discrimination to be unlawful) (Appelbaum, 2010: 338–340).

A definition of genetic information that includes family history also has important implications for research conduct, as illustrated by a recent, highly publicized case. A father of twins participating in a genetic twin study at Virginia Commonwealth University intercepted a questionnaire sent to his daughter that asked sensitive questions about other family members, e.g., whether any had mental disorders or abnormal genitalia. The father, upset that his daughter could be asked to provide personal information about him without his consent and apparently unable to get a response to his concerns from the researchers, filed a complaint with the federal Office of Protection from Research Risks (OPRR; now the Office of Human Research Protections, OHRP). Ultimately, OPRR ruled that the consent of third parties was needed before participants were asked to provide personal information about them or the requirement for consent had to be waived by an institutional review board (IRB) (Appelbaum, 2004: 343–351). Although the decision initially caused a good deal of consternation in the field, most IRBs appear to have responded by waiving the requirement on the grounds that obtaining consent is impractical in most genetic epidemiologic studies.

In the case of substance-use disorders, which are highly stigmatized, issues related to information about third parties may be particularly charged. Although it is relatively straightforward for research participants to report whether their family members had a discrete medical disorder, such as a heritable neoplasm or neurological condition, participants may find it more difficult to report whether their parents or siblings suffered from substance-use problems, and family members may be more sensitive to the disclosure of such information.

There has also been some debate over whether individual genetic information generated in a research study should be provided to participants. This has become a particular issue for the growing number of studies involving whole genome or whole exome sequencing, as these techniques can generate large amounts of data that may be relevant to participants' vulnerability to a variety of physical and mental disorders. Studies of participants' preferences have found consistent interest in knowing the results of these analyses (Kaufman et al., 2008: 831–839), and an emerging consensus of bioethicists states that at least some of these data should be made available to participants (Wolf et al., 2008: 219–248). However, others have argued that participants should not be given any results of tests performed on their genetic material for research purposes because the probabilistic nature of this information is difficult for nonscientists to understand (Hall et al., 2004: 1481–1495). This is particularly applicable to findings from genome-wide association studies (GWAS) that have large enough samples to generate significant findings for genetic variants with very weak effects. Authors have also raised concerns that individuals who receive their genetic test results may disclose them to third parties and suffer unforeseen negative consequences (Hall et al., 2004: 1481–1495).

Recent consensus guidelines make recommendations that may help in considering the specific relevance of these concerns to genetic studies of substance-use disorders (Wolf et al., 2008: 219–248). First, with regard to incidental findings, relevant discoveries should be anticipated and a plan should be articulated for dealing with them. Researchers should consult with one or more experts to determine which incidental findings are likely to have enough importance to participants to warrant disclosure. The reporting of incidental findings should be considered in light of the predicted net benefits. In other words, conditions that are not of serious health or reproductive importance should not be disclosed to participants.

Although these guidelines are helpful regarding incidental findings unrelated to substance-use disorders, the situation is less clear regarding whether participants should receive information about their addiction risk or their predicted response to treatment based on genetic findings. At present, given the lack of precise knowledge about genetic contributions to substance-use disorders, even carefully crafted individual interpretations of such findings appear premature. Of note, other than genes directly related to the metabolism of substances of abuse, the currently known effects of genetic variants related to substance disorders are weak and their disclosure is therefore presumably of little benefit to most research participants. Even if the field achieves greater power to make individualized predictions in the future, researchers should proceed cautiously. If conclusions were oversimplified or stated too strongly, or if participants misunderstood the findings, the result could be a false sense of security regarding participants' vulnerability to addiction (e.g., leading participants to engage in reckless drug use) or a false sense of nihilism regarding the likely effectiveness of treatment (Ball, 2008: 360–367). For the moment, though, these concerns are beyond the scope of existing technology.

Broader implications

Several broader concerns have also been raised regarding genetic research on addictions. Many researchers have been hopeful that this research could play a beneficial role in the overall debate on substance-use disorders, whereas ethicists have expressed concern about the unforeseen consequences of disseminating these findings without adequate public understanding. There are also several ways these results could be translated into social policies – some more speculative than others. Commercial applications of genetic testing should also be considered, because commercial products may be the public's first exposure to these concepts and findings, and because the conclusions reached by commercial ventures (e.g., regarding one's probability of risk) may not be presented and discussed as cautiously as such findings tend to be presented in academia.

First, the generalizability of these findings to minority groups may be limited by the scope of studies to date, creating unequal access to the benefits of genetic tests. An unrealized goal of the field has been to increase the representation of non-Hispanic African-Americans in genetic studies of psychiatric disorders in general (Murphy et al., 2009: 186–194). Although efforts have been made to include minority populations in such studies, and there are many genetic studies of substance-use disorders in Asians, Native Americans, and some in African

Americans, the latter still remain underrepresented in family, twin, adoption, and genetic studies of several psychiatric disorders, probably because of mistrust, wariness, and stigma regarding such research. Further, GWAS, which systematically examine hundreds of thousands of sites on the genome for associations of genetic variants with an illness or disorder, have largely been performed in populations of European descent (Bierut, 2011: 618–627). The underlying biological mechanisms that lead to substance dependence are likely to be similar across populations, but the contribution of different allele frequencies and therefore the relative importance of different risk factors may vary across ethnic populations.

Genetic research on addiction also carries great promise to affect the public understanding of, and perhaps policies toward, addiction. Several authors have expressed hope that genetic and neuroscience research on addiction could transform the debate between moral and medical models by providing more direct support for the disease model of addiction (Ball, 2008: 360–367). Some experts who argue for the disease model hope that a scientific explanation would decrease the stigmatization of addicted people and increase their access to medical treatments (Hyman, 2007: 8–11), although that does not appear to have occurred in the case of substance-use disorders (Pescosolido et al., 2010: 1321–1330). However, others have stressed the need for caution regarding over-reductionism, concerned that a scientifically informed model of addiction could be misinterpreted to imply strict genetic determinism, leading to support for social policies that assume that only a minority of genetically and biologically vulnerable individuals should be exposed to preventive interventions or receive treatment, or that social policy options such as drug-control policies, minimum legal drinking age laws, and other environmental approaches should be neglected (Hall, 2006: 1529–1532). Another concern arising from the tobacco industry's support of research on the genetics of nicotine addiction is that genetically based explanations might be used to turn attention away from harmful substances and industries, i.e., arguing that because a crucial component of addiction is genetic, it is not the substance but the individual that creates the danger (Gundle et al., 2010: 974–983). In the case of cigarette smoking, for example, the industry's argument has sometimes been that there are only a small number of people who should not smoke, and the vast majority of people can use cigarettes in a responsible way. This argument is contradicted by the overwhelming evidence on the relationship between cancer mortality and smoking, which is inconsistent with the notion that most can smoke "responsibly" (MMWR, 2011: 1243–1247).

Some evidence from large-scale survey data suggests that public acceptance of neurobiological explanations of mental disorders may not necessarily decrease stigma as had been hoped (Pescosolido et al., 2010: 1321–1330). Using responses to disease-specific vignettes, researchers found that between 1996 and 2006 an increased proportion of the public attributed psychiatric disorders to neurobiological causes, and more people supported of psychiatric disorders by medical providers as well. For vignettes depicting alcohol dependence, there was a notable increase in the proportion endorsing the value of psychiatric treatment (from 61% in 1996 to 79% in 2006). However, the people surveyed still held stigmatizing views of individuals with mental disorders, including alcohol dependence, and holding a neurobiological conception of these disorders did not decrease stigma. Consonant with the concerns about oversimplified acceptance of genetic causal models noted above, an understanding of substance-use disorders based entirely on neurobiological and behavioral genetic explanations may not helpfully influence public understanding of these disorders. However, in this survey study, acceptance of neurobiological theories did increase support for treatment, and data from other surveys regarding substance-use disorders and stigma clearly indicate that stigmatization is associated with a lower likelihood of receiving treatment (Keyes et al., 2010: 1364–1372). Ultimately, stigma and public acceptance of neurobiological explanations may be influenced by different beliefs. Scientists should continue to promote accurate public understanding of the science underlying addiction research, but this approach should not be relied upon as the only means to address public attitudes about substance-use disorders, as the overall need to reduce stigma and ensure adequate services remains clear regardless of the arguments used to promote public awareness of these issues.

There have also been speculative concerns about how these findings might lead to the enactment of potentially problematic social policies. For example, population-based genetic screening might be used to identify those at highest risk of becoming dependent on substances, paralleling predictive genetic testing for better-understood medical disorders. Of course, there exist significant questions regarding the clinical utility of such measures, as screening would not be valuable in the absence of known genetic factors conferring a substantially higher risk of developing addiction, and, aside from the relatively obvious recommendation to abstain from the substance for which the person is at risk, the appropriate preventive interventions for such hypothetically high-risk individuals are not clear (Hall et al., 2004: 1481–1495). More broadly, questions also arise regarding the clinical utility of predictive genetic testing in general, such as how large an effect is sufficient to justify genetic testing or what the desired outcome is (Burke et al., 2010: 215–223). As a general example from behavioral health, if the main outcome of testing is to recommend a better diet or other lifestyle changes, some might question whether such testing is an appropriate use of health-care resources. The situation is similar in the case of substance-use disorder risk, in which the only preventive measures at present are behavioral in nature.

A related set of concerns is that whatever benefits might accrue from population-based screening for genetic risk factors for substance-use disorders would be outweighed by the resulting stigma and discrimination. Interestingly, survey findings have suggested that although researchers and ethicists express these general concerns, patients and their families are most concerned with the potential criminal justice uses of stored genetic information and enforced therapy for individuals at risk (Coors and Raymond, 2009: 83–90). Social scientists note that public disappointment with novel treatment strategies for addiction has led to calls for coerced treatment (Hall, 2006: 1529–1532). In the case of genetic information, the danger is that those identified as "at risk" for addiction may face stricter, and perhaps unnecessarily coercive, requirements for treatment.

Such information might also make its way into the criminal justice system. The nature of its likely impact there, however, is not entirely clear, i.e., whether courts would consider such genetic information aggravating or mitigating. In one widely discussed case of an attorney facing disbarment proceedings, the Supreme Court of California considered evidence that he had not been told of his "genetic predisposition to addiction" as a mitigating factor (although it is not clear how important this consideration was in the final decision) (Appelbaum, 2005: 25–27). In these and related cases, the limits of GINA become apparent. Although GINA puts restrictions on uses of genetic information by employers and some insurers, it does not restrict use of such information in other spheres. In the legal arena, individuals could still volunteer genetic information in the hopes that it would help their case, or it may surface in other ways, and as noted above GINA does not apply to members of the military. It is conceivable that genetic information could be considered or testing mandated for military or other governmental purposes, such as security clearances.

Finally, commercial applications such as personal genetics are developing rapidly. As recently as May 2010, one "personal genomics" startup, Pathway Genomics, announced its intent [subsequently thwarted by the Food and Drug Administration (FDA) intervention] to sell its DNA collection kits in Walgreens pharmacies (Technologyreview.com, 2010). Customers who purchased the kits and sent back a cheek swab would have been able to receive information on drug response and metabolism, pre-pregnancy planning regarding serious genetic diseases, or risk for a number of health conditions such as Alzheimer's disease and diabetes. Other companies currently offer similar services online, including 23andMe, deCODEme, and Navigenics. To date, these companies have escaped federal regulation, although the FDA is reconsidering its approach to regulation of these tests (GenomicsLawReport.com, 2011). It is notable that these companies are offering information related to addictions and even using folk-Mendelian concepts to communicate their results. For example, on a web page describing the genetic risk of heroin addiction, one company states that polymorphisms of the opiate receptor gene *OPRM1* confer "substantially higher odds of heroin addiction," and it goes so far as to use "Greg Mendel" as the participant's name on a sample report (23andme.com, 2011). These enterprises currently promise more than they can deliver in terms of accurate genetic information and contribute to popular misunderstandings about the degree to which genetic findings affect one's addiction risk. That said, with appropriate academic–industrial relationships and better overall understanding of the contribution of these genetic risk factors, this explosion of commercial products might yet be harnessed for clinically useful purposes. However, it is unlikely that these benefits will be realized without appropriate collaborations with medical professionals (Hunter et al., 2008: 105–107).

Conclusions

Analogous to the discussion of incidental genetic findings above, the net benefit of genetic approaches to understanding addiction must be determined by carefully weighing the concerns reviewed above against the potential promises of this technology. Although genetic studies of addiction may not yet be able to fulfill the extravagant promises made by some commercial ventures, the promise they hold to improve our understanding of substance-use disorders and develop new therapies is already being realized. Meanwhile, for participants participating in these studies, the importance of informed consent and responsible research conduct remains paramount.

Acknowledgments

Dr. Appelbaum's contribution to this chapter was supported in part by a grant from the National Human Genome Research Institute (1P20HG005535–01, Center for Research on Ethical, Legal, and Social Implication of Psychiatric, Neurologic, and Behavioral Genetics).

References

23andme.com (2011). Heroin addiction – sample report. Available online at: www.23andme.com/health/Heroin-Addiction/ [accessed February 21, 2012].

American Psychiatric Association, Task Force on DSM-IV (2000). *Diagnostic and Statistical Manual of Mental Disorders: DSM-IV-TR.* Washington, DC: American Psychiatric Association, 303.90.

Anton, R. F., Oroszi, G., O'Malley, S., et al. (2008). An evaluation of mu-opioid receptor (OPRM1) as a predictor of naltrexone response in the treatment of alcohol dependence: results from the Combined Pharmacotherapies and Behavioral Interventions for Alcohol Dependence (COMBINE) study. *Archives of General Psychiatry*, 65, 135–144.

Appelbaum, P. S. (2004). Ethical issues in psychiatric genetics. *Journal of Psychiatric Practice*, 10, 343–351.

Appelbaum, P. S. (2005). Behavioral genetics and the punishment of crime. *Psychiatric Services*, 56, 25–27.

Appelbaum, P. S. (2010). Law & psychiatry: Genetic discrimination in mental disorders: the impact of the genetic information nondiscrimination act. *Psychiatric Services*, 61, 338–340.

Ball, D. (2008). Addiction science and its genetics. *Addiction*, 103, 360–367.

Bierut, L. J. (2011). Genetic vulnerability and susceptibility to substance dependence. *Neuron*, 69, 618–627.

Burke, W., Laberge, A. M., and Press, N. (2010). Debating clinical utility. *Public Health Genomics*, 13, 215–223.

Carter, A. and Hall, W. (2008). The issue of consent in research that administers drugs of addiction to addicted persons. *Accountability in Research*, 15, 209–225.

Charland, L. C. (2002). Cynthia's dilemma: consenting to heroin prescription. *American Journal of Bioethics*, 2, 37–47.

Coors, M. E. and Raymond, K. M. (2009). Substance use disorder genetic research: investigators and participants grapple with the ethical issues. *Psychiatric Genetics*, 19, 83–90.

Crisp, A., Gelder, M., Goddard, E., and Meltzer, H. (2005). Stigmatization of people with mental illnesses: a follow-up study within the Changing Minds campaign of the Royal College of Psychiatrists. *World Psychiatry*, 4, 106–113.

Dickert, N. and Grady, C. (1999). What's the price of a research subject? Approaches to payment for research participation. *New England Journal of Medicine*, 341, 198–203.

Festinger, D. S., Marlowe, D. B., Croft, J. R., et al. (2005). Do research payments precipitate drug use or coerce participation? *Drug and Alcohol Dependence*, 78, 275–281.

Frazer, K. A., Murray, S. S., Schork, N. J., and Topol, E. J. (2009). Human genetic variation and its contribution to complex traits. *Nature Reviews Genetics*, 10, 241–251.

Fry, C. and Dwyer, R. (2001). For love or money? An exploratory study of why injecting drug users participate in research. *Addiction*, 96, 1319–1325.

Gelernter, J. and Kranzler, H. R. (2009). Genetics of alcohol dependence. *Human Genetics*, 126, 91–99.

Gelernter, J. and Kranzler, H. R. (2010). Genetics of drug dependence. *Dialogues in Clinical Neuroscience*, 12, 77–84.

GenomicsLawReport.com (2011). Personal genomics follows pathway to corner drugstore; Is regulation next? Available online at: www.genomicslawreport.com/index.php/2010/05/11/pathway-walgreens-and-dtc-regulation/ [accessed February 21, 2012].

Gundle, K. R., Dingel, M. J., and Koenig, B. A. (2010). "To prove this is the industry's best hope": big tobacco's support of research on the genetics of nicotine addiction. *Addiction*, 105, 974–983.

Hall, W. (2006). Avoiding potential misuses of addiction brain science. *Addiction*, 101, 1529–1532.

Hall, W., Carter, L., and Morley, K. I. (2004). Neuroscience research on the addictions: A prospectus for future ethical and policy analysis. *Addictive Behaviors*, 29, 1481–1495.

Hudson, K. L., Holohan, M. K., and Collins, F. S. (2008). Keeping pace with the times – the Genetic Information Nondiscrimination Act of 2008. *New England Journal of Medicine*, 358, 2661–2663.

Hunter, D. J., Khoury, M. J., and Drazen, J. M. (2008). Letting the genome out of the bottle – will we get our wish? *New England Journal of Medicine*, 358, 105–107.

Hyman, S. E. (2007). The neurobiology of addiction: Implications for voluntary control of behavior. *The American Journal of Bioethics*, 7, 8–11.

Jeste, D. V. and Saks, E. (2006). Decisional capacity in mental illness and substance use disorders: empirical database and policy implications. *Behavioral Sciences & The Law*, 24, 607–628.

Johnson, B. A. (2010). Medication treatment of different types of alcoholism. *American Journal of Psychiatry*, 167, 630–639.

Johnson, B. A., Ait-Daoud, N., Seneviratne, C., et al. (2011). Pharmacogenetic approach at the serotonin transporter gene as a method of reducing the severity of alcohol drinking. *American Journal of Psychiatry*, 168, 265–275.

Kaufman, D., Murphy, J., Scott, J., and Hudson, K. (2008). Subjects matter: a survey of public opinions about a large genetic cohort study. *Genetics in Medicine*, 10, 831–839.

Keyes, K. M., Hatzenbuehler, M. L., McLaughlin, K. A., et al. (2010). Stigma and treatment for alcohol disorders in the United States. *American Journal of Epidemiology*, 172, 1364–1372.

Kuehn, B. M. (2011). Study suggests gene may predict success of therapies for alcohol dependence. *JAMA*, 305, 984–985.

Lowstuter, K. J., Sand, S., Blazer, K. R., et al. (2008). Influence of genetic discrimination perceptions and knowledge on cancer genetics referral practice among clinicians. *Genetics in Medicine*, 10, 691–698.

Monterosso, J. R., Flannery, B. A., Pettinati, H. M., et al. (2001). Predicting treatment response to naltrexone: The influence of craving and family history. *American Journal on Addictions*, 10, 258–268.

MMWR. (2011). State-specific trends in lung cancer incidence and smoking – United States, 1999–2008. *Morbidity and Mortality Weekly Report*, 60, 1243–1247.

Murphy, E. J., Wickramaratne, P., and Weissman, M. M. (2009). Racial and ethnic differences in willingness to participate in psychiatric genetic research. *Psychiatric Genetics*, 19, 186–194.

Okai, D., Owen, G., McGuire, H., Singh, S., Churchill, R., and Hotopf, M. (2007). Mental capacity in psychiatric patients: Systematic review. *British Journal of Psychiatry*, 191, 291–297.

Pescosolido, B. A., Martin, J. K., Long, J. S., et al. (2010). "A disease like any other"? A decade of change in public reactions to schizophrenia, depression, and alcohol dependence. *American Journal of Psychiatry*, 167, 1321–1330.

Technologyreview.com (2010). Drugstore genomic testing. Available online at: www.technologyreview.com/blog/editors/25169/ [accessed February 21, 2012].

Widdows, H. and Cordell, S. (2011). The ethics of biobanking: Key issues and controversies. *Health Care Analysis*, 19, 207–219.

Wolf, S. M., Lawrenz, F. P., Nelson, C. A., et al. (2008). Managing incidental findings in human subjects research: analysis and recommendations. *American Society of Law, Medicine & Ethics*, 36, 219–248.

Chapter

4

Improving the informed consent process in research with substance-abusing participants

David S. Festinger and Karen L. Dugosh

History of informed consent

The most important medical and behavioral advances made in the last century, including vaccinations for diseases such as smallpox and polio, required years of testing, often with human participants. Unfortunately, many were made at the expense of marginal and highly vulnerable populations, including asylum inmates, prisoners, and non-institutionalized minorities. In fact, study participants were often involved in clinical trials without ever being informed. Revelations about the horrors of World War II and the medical experiments that were performed by the Nazis as well as unethical investigations conducted within the United States, including the Tuskegee syphilis study (Centers for Disease Control and Prevention, 2011), the Milgram experiment (Milgram, 1974), and the human radiation experiments (see Welsone, 1999, for a review), heightened public awareness of the potential for research misconduct.

For over 60 years, the international and US medical communities have taken numerous steps to protect people who take part in clinical research. The Nuremberg Code (1950) was the first major international document to provide guidelines on research ethics. It was developed in response to the Nuremberg Trials of Nazi doctors who performed unethical experimentation during World War II. The Nuremberg Code made voluntary consent a requirement in clinical research studies and outlined that consent can be voluntary only if: (1) the participants are able to consent; (2) they are free from coercion (i.e., outside pressure); and (3) they comprehend the risks and benefits involved. Furthermore, the Nuremberg Code states that researchers should minimize risk and harm, ensure that potential risks do not significantly outweigh potential benefits, use appropriate study designs, and guarantee the participants' freedom to withdraw at any time. It was adopted by the United Nations General Assembly in 1948.

In 1964, a second major development in human research protections, the Helsinki Declaration (World Medical Association, 1964), emerged from the 18th World Medical Assembly in Helsinki, Finland. With the establishment of the Helsinki Declaration, the World Medical Association adopted 12 principles to guide physicians on ethical considerations related to biomedical research. The Declaration emphasized the distinction between medical care (which is provided to directly benefit the patient) and research (which may or may not provide direct benefit to the individual). These guidelines were revised at subsequent meetings in 1975 (Tokyo, Japan), 1983 (Venice, Italy), and 1989 (Hong Kong).

Genetic Research on Addiction, ed. Audrey R. Chapman. Published by Cambridge University Press.
© Cambridge University Press 2012.

Largely in response to the Tuskegee syphilis study, the US Congress signed the National Research Act into law (Public Law 93–348) in 1974, creating the National Commission for the Protection of Human Subjects of Biomedical and Behavioral Research. The National Research Act prompted the establishment of Institutional Review Boards (IRBs) at the local level and required IRB review and approval of all federally funded research involving human participants. The Commission was charged with: (1) identifying the ethical principles that should govern research involving human subjects; and (2) recommending steps to improve the regulations for the protection of human subjects.

Shortly thereafter, the National Commission for the Protection of Human Subjects of Biomedical and Behavioral Research (1979) issued *The Belmont Report: Ethical Principles and Guidelines for the Protection of Human Subjects of Research*. The report sets forth three principles underlying the ethical conduct of research: (1) respect for persons; (2) beneficence; and (3) justice. The principle of respect for persons recognizes the autonomy and dignity of individuals and protects those with diminished autonomy (i.e., impaired decision-making skills), including children, elderly people, and disabled people. The principle of beneficence protects persons from harm and maximizes their benefits and minimizes their risks. Finally, the principle of justice provides the fair distribution of the benefits and burdens of research. *The Belmont Report* explains how these principles apply to research practice. For example, it identifies informed consent as a process that is essential to the principle of respect. In response to the report, both the US Department of Health and Human Services and the US Food and Drug Administration revised their regulations on research studies that involve human participants.

Since the 1974 formation of the National Commission for the Protection of Human Subjects of Biomedical and Behavioral Research and the resulting Belmont Report, the Federal Government has issued several guidelines to enhance protections for human research participants. These guidelines have dealt primarily with the two essential protections for human participants: (1) independent review of research to balance potential risks and benefits; and (2) the consent process, which is intended to provide participants with an opportunity to voluntarily and knowledgeably decide whether to participate in research protocols.

Through these post-Nuremberg efforts, the doctrine of informed consent emerged as the major foundation for all human subject research. Informed consent requires that individuals truly understand and freely decide to participate in most types of experiments and clinical interventions. Informed consent is a process that optimally occurs in the context of an investigator–participant relationship characterized by trust and honesty.

Elements of informed consent

The three basic elements of informed consent are that it must be: (1) competent (*Teague v. Louisiana*, 1980); (2) knowing (*Edwards v. Arizona*, 1981); and (3) voluntary (*Colorado v. Connelly*, 1986). Each of these elements may be conceptualized as having its own unique sources of vulnerability. In the context of research, these potential vulnerabilities may be conceptualized as stemming from sources that may be intrinsic, extrinsic, or relational (Roberts and Roberts, 1999).

1. *Intrinsic* vulnerabilities are attributes of an *individual* that limit his or her capacities or freedoms. For example, a person who is under the influence of drugs or cognitively impaired may be rendered incapable of attending to or processing consent information.

These types of vulnerabilities relate to the first element of informed consent – that of competence.

2. *Extrinsic* vulnerabilities are *situational* factors that may limit an individual's capacities or freedoms. For example, a person who has just been arrested may be too anxious, confused, or subject to implicit duress to provide voluntary and informed consent. Such extrinsic vulnerabilities may relate either to knowingness or to voluntariness to the degree that the situation, not individual attributes, prevents the individual from making an informed and autonomous decision.

3. *Relational* vulnerabilities occur as a result of a *relationship* with another individual or group. Certain relationships may be implicitly coercive or manipulative or be perceived as such, and they may ultimately unduly influence the individual's decision to participate in research. For example, a person receiving treatment for depression may not feel free to decline participation in a study when they are recruited by their therapist. Likewise, an elderly person who is recruited into a study by a caregiver may confuse the caregiving and research roles. Relational vulnerabilities typically relate to the voluntariness of consent.

Competence

As discussed above, competence in relation to informed consent refers to one's intrinsic capacity to understand, appreciate, and express a choice. According to *The Belmont Report*, "An injustice occurs when some benefit to which a person is entitled is denied without good reason or when some burden is imposed unduly." Historically, and understandably, the most central focus of this principle has been to prevent the exploitation of vulnerable groups of individuals who may be systematically selected simply because of their easy availability or coercible nature, rather than for reasons directly related to the problem being studied. Importantly, however, the principle of justice is also intended to ensure that such individuals are not systematically excluded from research and have an equal right to the potential benefits of such research. This means that there should be methods for ensuring that even individuals deemed incompetent (e.g., individuals with dementia or brain injury) have the opportunity to participate in research that may benefit them. Nevertheless, the ethical debate continues as to whether and how even research deemed beneficial can be conducted with decisionally impaired individuals. Potential solutions such as surrogate consent for decisionally impaired individuals continues to be a highly contested legal area and incapable subjects in the United States still lack clear regulatory protection (Kim et al., 2004).

Knowingness

To provide informed consent, an individual must make a knowledgeable decision about their research participation. This requires that investigators disclose study-related information to potential participants in a way that facilitates such decision making. Recently, Festinger and colleagues (Festinger et al., 2009; Festinger et al., 2010) identified three classes of study-related information that must be understood in order to make a knowing decision about study participation: (1) study procedures; (2) human subject protections that are in place; and (3) the possible risks and benefits associated with participation. Furthermore, they argue that, although knowingness is traditionally thought to be relevant at the time of consent, long-term recall of study-related information, particularly in reference to human subject protections and possible risks and benefits, may be critical to ensuring a participant's safety over a longer period of time. For example, it is important to understand and remember the potential side effects of an exploratory drug well beyond the period of the clinical trial, as they may occur after the study is over.

Voluntariness

According to *The Belmont Report*, consent to participate in research is valid and informed only if it is voluntarily given and free from coercion and undue influence. Coercion occurs when an individual is threatened with harm by another in the event that he or she chooses not to participate in the study. Undue influence occurs when an individual is offered an excessive, unwarranted, inappropriate, or improper reward for participation or when a person of authority, particularly one who controls sanctions, urges an individual to act in a particular way.

Regrettably, empirical data have contributed little to operationalizing the construct of coercion or refining the concept of voluntariness (Appelbaum et al., 2009). Constraints on decision-making ability are likely to be influenced by a range of factors. For example, although large-magnitude participant payments may have little influence on individuals with higher incomes, they may wield greater leverage on individuals with lower incomes. To further complicate this issue, money may have no undue influence even for individuals with lower incomes if they clearly understand and comprehend the risks of participation. Moreover, influences on decision making may be either actual or perceived. For example, individuals involved in the criminal justice system may decide to participate in a study because they perceive that it will be favorably viewed by their judge and ultimately help their court case, even if this is not the case.

The problem

The extent to which research subjects engage in informed decision making about their research involvement is still not clear. In fact, problems with understanding of research protocols have been widely reported (Dunn and Jeste, 2001). Studies indicate that research participants are often not aware that they are participants in a research study, have poor recall of study information, have inadequate recall of important risks of the procedures or treatments, lack understanding of randomization procedures and placebo treatments, lack awareness of the ability to withdraw from the research study at any time, and are often confused about the dual roles of clinician and researcher (Robinson and Merav, 1976; Muss et al., 1979; Cassileth et al., 1980; Appelbaum et al., 1982; Silva and Sorrell, 1988; Levine, 1992; Verheggen and van Wijmen, 1996; Edwards et al., 1998; Sugarman et al., 1998).

Several client-level variables have been identified as relating to the understanding of consent information. A number of studies have found education and vocabulary level to be significantly related to a participant's understanding of consent information, with those having lower education and vocabulary levels demonstrating deficits in understanding (Taub et al., 1986; Taub et al., 1987; Young et al., 1990; Sorrell, 1991; Agre et al., 1994; Aaronson et al., 1996; Neptune et al., 1996; Bjorn et al., 1999). Two studies that evaluated vocabulary using the Wechsler Adult Intelligence Scale (WAIS) found that both comprehension and recall of consent information were significantly correlated with vocabulary level (Taub et al., 1981; Taub and Baker, 1983). Although age alone has *not* been consistently associated with diminished performance on consent quizzes, it does appear to interact with education in that older individuals with less education display decreased understanding of consent information (Taub and Baker, 1983; Taub et al., 1987).

Does substance abuse contribute to poorer understanding, attention, and recall?

Although substance abusers have not been specifically identified as a vulnerable population, they may present a number of unique issues when obtaining informed consent, both because of factors unique to their substance abuse and because of the wide range of conditions that are comorbid to substance abuse (McCrady and Bux, 1999). Substance abusers may experience impaired attention, cognition, or retention of important information as a result of acute drug intoxication or withdrawal (Victor et al., 1989; Munro et al., 2000; Saxton et al., 2000; Tapert and Brown, 2000). Furthermore, limited educational opportunities, chronic brain changes resulting from long-term drug or alcohol use, poor nutrition, and comorbid health problems are common among substance abusers. These conditions may contribute to deficits in their ability to concentrate and limit their understanding during the informed consent process (McCrady and Bux, 1999; Festinger et al., 2007).

There is substantial evidence that substance abuse interferes with cognitive abilities; however, the amount and type of interference may depend on the substance used, pattern of use, length of use, and length of abstinence. For example, cocaine-dependent participants who had achieved 2 weeks of abstinence were found to have decreased performance on measures of attention, verbal memory, and learning compared with controls (Cunha et al., 2004). Even after 6 months of abstinence, cocaine users demonstrated cognitive deficits related to attention, new learning, and visual and verbal memory (Strickland et al., 1993). Similar cognitive impairments have been found in chronic methamphetamine users (Simon et al., 2000; Sim et al., 2002) and opiate users (e.g., Verdejo et al., 2005). There is also considerable support that heavy or long-term marijuana use has similar deleterious effects on cognitive functioning (e.g., Kouri et al., 1995; Pope and Yurgelun-Todd, 1996; Solowij et al., 2002), although these effects may not persist in the long term (Karila et al., 2005). Consistent with these findings, a meta-analysis indicated that chronic cannabis use might negatively affect the ability to learn and remember new information (Grant et al., 2003).

Several studies have examined immediate and delayed recall of consent information among substance abusers. Rounsaville et al. (2008) evaluated consent recall in adult marijuana users immediately following the presentation of consent information. Only 55% of participants were able to correctly answer all four multiple-choice questions related to the basic elements of the study, and 20% incorrectly answered a question that their participation was voluntary. Research suggests that immediate recall of consent information is related to cognitive factors including intelligence and attention as well as educational attainment (Kiluk et al., 2010). Studies examining the delayed recall of consent have yielded similar results. In two studies of adult drug court clients, Festinger and colleagues (2009, 2010) demonstrated that clients, on average, failed to recall about 60% of their consent information just 2 weeks following their initial date of consent. Importantly, intelligence, reading level, memory, and attention were significant predictors of delayed (i.e., 2-week) recall of consent information (Festinger et al., 2007).

Is the autonomy of substance abusers participating in research compromised?

In addition to issues related to competency and understanding, substance abusers have certain situational factors that may present issues related to the autonomy of their participation. This source of vulnerability is very different from competence or knowingness because even the most knowledgeable and capable individual may not be able to make a truly autonomous decision if he or she is exposed to a potentially coercive situation. Substance-abuse researchers often recruit participants from settings that are implicitly "coercible," including inpatient units, detoxification facilities, and prisons (McCrady and Bux, 1999). Indeed, a substantially large proportion of substance-abusing individuals are involved in the criminal justice system (National Center on Addiction and Substance Abuse, 2010), and criminal justice clients, by the nature of the system, may be regularly exposed to implicit and explicit threats of coercion that may compromise their autonomy. Such individuals may perceive, correctly or incorrectly, that their cooperation with authorities is essential to well-being. For example, a recent study (Dugosh et al., 2010) demonstrated that a substantial proportion of drug court clients who were participating in a clinical trial agreed to participate in the study because they thought it would please their judge or help their court case. Although unfounded, these perceptions may unduly influence a client's participation in the study.

Furthermore, many have argued that payment levels that are not ordinarily considered to be excessive may present undue influence in substance-abusing populations (Ritter et al., 2003). Specifically, the low levels of educational attainment, high rates of unemployment, low income levels, and generally lower socioeconomic status that are characteristic of many substance abusers may make them highly susceptible to monetary influences and compromise their autonomy to participate in research studies. However, research by Festinger and colleagues demonstrated that perceived coercion in substance abusers was not related to the amount of money they received for participation; specifically, participants who received a $10 payment for attending a research appointment reported no higher rates of perceived coercion than those who received a $70 payment for their attendance (Festinger et al., 2005). This same finding held in a follow-up study in which the study payments ranged from $70 to $160 (Festinger et al., 2008).

Finally, many individuals with substance-use disorders lack access to treatment for their disorder. Given that research-based treatment programs often provide free or low-cost treatment to participants, individuals may not fully consider the risks and benefits of the study because participation will provide them with the services that they need. Under these circumstances, the voluntariness of their research participation may be questioned (Ostini et al., 1993).

Strategies for improving informed consent

Three extensive reviews of techniques associated with improving the consent process have been published in the past decade (Dunn and Jeste, 2001; Flory and Emanuel, 2004; Cohn and Larson, 2007). Overall, these articles have identified a broad array of interventions that have been shown to improve participants' understanding or recall of consent information. The strategies that have proven most successful can be conceptualized into two general categories: (1) those focusing on the *structure* of the consent document; and (2) those focusing on the *process* of presenting consent information.

Modifying the structure of consent materials

Simplifying printed consent materials

Much of the work examining ways of improving participants' understanding of consent information has focused on revising the basic *form* of printed consent materials to improve their readability. Readability is sometimes addressed by ensuring that the materials are written at a grade level that is commensurate with that of the average citizen or, in the case of children, at their particular grade level. Improving the readability of consent documents is important given that 14% of US adults have marginal literacy skills and another 29% can perform only simple literacy activities (White and Dillow, 2005).

A number of other methods have been used to improve the readability of consent materials. These methods include, but are not limited to, summarizing key points, infusing headings and bulleted points, using larger font sizes, clustering similar content in one location within the document, using briefer and more simplistic sentence structures and lay language, infusing visual aids (e.g., illustrations, pictures and graphics), and presenting relevant consent information in a streamlined booklet form rather than on standard 8.5 × 11″ sheets of paper (Silva and Sorrell, 1988; Campbell et al., 2004; Jefford and Moore, 2008; Knapp et al., 2009; Rubright et al., 2010). Not unexpectedly, there is evidence to suggest that these form modifications may be most beneficial to individuals with lower levels of reading or basic comprehension abilities (Dunn et al., 2001; Campbell et al., 2004).

It is important to note that, taken as a whole, these strategies designed to improve readability have received mixed results regarding their efficacy in improving research participants' comprehension of consent information (Hochhauser, 2000; Flory and Emanuel, 2004; Jefford and Moore, 2008). These inconsistent results may be related to the timing of the comprehension evaluation, given that the amount of time between the initial exposure to the consent information and the comprehension evaluation may have an impact on recall of information. In addition, the format of the questions in the evaluation (i.e., true/false, multiple choice, free response) is likely to influence participants' recall of consent information.

Use of audiovisual technologies

Researchers have also examined the utility of using both passive and active audiovisual technology to improve consent comprehension. Passive techniques do not involve the participant in the interaction, whereas active techniques are more interactive and involving. Delivering consent information though a PowerPoint presentation or on a DVD are examples of passive techniques. Active techniques include the use of touchscreen computer applications, "speaking" books, or applications that allow the individual to control the pace at which the consent information is presented.

The extent to which audiovisual techniques improve comprehension of informed consent materials presently is not clear (Flory and Emanuel, 2004; Henry et al., 2009; Ryan et al., 2009). With regard to passive audiovisual methods, some studies have identified improvements in comprehension (e.g., Dunn et al., 2001), whereas other studies have found no improvement (e.g., Weston et al., 1997; Campbell et al., 2004; Wirshing et al., 2005). More favorable results have been found for active audiovisual techniques, including interactive computer presentations (Carpenter et al., 2000; Kass et al., 2009), interactive speaking books (Dhai et al., 2010), and interactive DVDs (Jeste et al., 2009). There is some indication that these audiovisual methods may be particularly useful for individuals with impaired decision-making ability (Jeste et al., 2009) or when study protocols are complex (Agre and Rapkin, 2003).

There is no doubt that multimedia, interactive, and web-based technologies will receive continued attention, given the digital age in which we live. However, at the present time it is difficult to estimate the true value of using audiovisual methods to enhance consent comprehension because of the inconsistent findings associated with this relatively small body of research (Ryan et al., 2009). The conflicting results associated with these techniques may be the result of variations in study design, video content and delivery, the population under investigation, and the outcome measures used (Ryan et al., 2009). As such, the utility of these methods is worthy of additional systematic investigation in high-quality randomized controlled clinical trials.

Modifying the consent process

Although efforts to enhance the readability of consent forms and related materials have proven to be beneficial, some suggest that these efforts fall short when attempting to ensure that individuals truly understand what their involvement entails (Hochhauser, 2000; Jefford and Moore, 2008; Ogloff and Otto, 1991). Researchers have begun to recognize the need to focus greater attention onto the consent *process* itself in order to improve recall and comprehension (e.g., Agre and Rapkin, 2003; Ness et al., 2009). In recent years, viable strategies to improve consent comprehension involving the consent *process* have begun to emerge from the research literature. These procedures are consistent with the philosophy that consent is an ongoing process and not a single event (Ellis, 1999). Two procedures that have received the largest amount of empirical support are corrected feedback and the use of intermediaries.

Corrected feedback

The corrected feedback procedure is the one intervention that has been consistently associated with improvements, both in initial comprehension and in longer-term retention of informed consent information (Taub et al., 1981; Taub and Baker, 1983; Wirshing et al., 1998). This procedure typically involves assessing an individual's knowledge and comprehension of the informed consent information following an initial presentation and review of the consent form and then providing participants with corrected feedback about their incorrect items. In general, studies have shown the efficacy of the procedure in both clinical and nonclinical samples.

A line of research by Taub and colleagues has examined the efficacy of the corrected feedback procedure among elderly participants. In the initial study (Taub et al., 1981), one group of participants read the consent form, answered multiple-choice questions covering the main points on the form, and were then provided with a *single trial* of feedback and corrected answers. The second group of participants read the consent form but did not receive a consent quiz or corrected feedback. The use of the corrected feedback procedure significantly improved memory of consent information at all age levels and vocabulary levels. In a follow-up to this study, Taub and Baker (1983) varied the number of trials of corrected feedback that elderly participants received. The *multi-trial* corrected-feedback approach improved comprehension scores at all vocabulary levels but had a more limited effect on retention of information 2 to 3 weeks later.

These results have been extended to other clinical and nonclinical samples. Several studies have examined the use of the corrected feedback among individuals diagnosed with schizophrenia. Wirshing et al. (1998) demonstrated that the procedure improved comprehension at the time of the initial consent and retention 1 week later. In fact, there is evidence (Carpenter et al., 2000; Moser et al., 2006) that the corrected feedback procedure is effective in increasing schizophrenic patients' comprehension to levels of non-patient samples. Gains in the comprehension of consent materials after repeated learning trials have also been reported among individuals diagnosed with bipolar disorder and more general community members (Palmer et al., 2007). To date, only one published study (Eyler et al., 2005) has failed to find support for using corrective feedback to improve knowledge about consent information, but the authors suggest that the lack of significant findings might be the result of a lack of statistical power. Overall, the corrected feedback procedure has demonstrated substantial efficacy in improving comprehension and recall of consent information.

Research intermediaries

It has been suggested that having an independent third party involved in the consent process may facilitate potential research participants' understanding of consent information. This third party has been described in the literature as a "research intermediary" (Reiser and Knudson, 1993), "neutral educator" (Benson et al., 1988), "consent auditor" (DeRenzo, 1994), "decision aid" (Juraskova et al., 2008), "third-party facilitator" (Stiles et al., 2001), "interpreter" (Kucia and Horowitz, 2000), "research liaison" (Salas et al., 2008), and "subject advocate" (Stroup and Appelbaum, 2003). Intermediaries may play an important role in helping potential participants understand what their research involvement entails. The role of the intermediary can include explaining relevant consent information, advocating on the behalf of participants, monitoring and reporting intentional and unintentional forms of coercion or adverse events that may occur during all stages of the participants' involvement in the study, and reporting adverse events. Several federally commissioned advisory panels have issued formal recommendations in favor of including third-party intermediaries to improve the informed consent process (e.g., World Medical Association, 1997; Bioethics Interest Group, National Institutes of Health, 1998; National Bioethics Advisory Committee, 1998).

Studies that have experimentally examined the effects of third-party intermediaries on understanding and recall of consent information have yielded mixed but promising results. Benson and his colleagues (1988) demonstrated that providing psychiatric patients with a neutral educator resulted in a significantly better understanding of the study and definition of randomization than those in a standard consent condition. However, there were no differences in overall understanding scores in the study. Coletti et al. (2003) evaluated the impact of an intermediary on knowledge of ten key concepts relevant to participating in a multi-site HIV vaccine clinical trial over an 18-month period. Participants in the experimental condition met with an intermediary at 6, 12, and 18 months following enrollment. Recall of study-relevant information improved over time and was better than that of the individuals who completed a standard consent procedure.

The ongoing use of an intermediary appears to be a useful method for improving the amount of research-relevant information that is remembered over both brief and extended periods of time. In a study conducted by Kucia and Horowitz (2000), an intermediary reviewed information about a clinical trial with cardiac patients on two occasions (i.e., approximately 10 and 24 hours after their enrollment into the study). Patients' ability to recall information improved over time, especially with regard to potential risks associated with the study. Similar results have been found in studies of other clinical populations. Aaronson et al. (1996) reported that cancer patients who received a single information-oriented telephone follow-up call from an oncology nurse 1 week after they enrolled in a clinical trial reported more knowledge about their study participation in comparison to their counterparts who did not receive a telephone call. Improvements in comprehension were also found among participants who received an enhanced consent procedure to participate in an HIV clinical trial (Fitzgerald et al., 2002). Those who completed three information sessions with a counselor who was independent from the research team before being approached by the investigator to complete their formal consent meeting were more knowledgeable about what research involvement would entail than their counterparts who completed a single, standard consent procedure. This same research team found similar improvements in comprehension using a two-stage educational program that involved mental health providers who were not associated with the study (Joseph et al., 2006). A social worker introduced the study, showed a videotape, and facilitated a question and answer session with prospective participants. One day later a counselor met individually with these persons to review key consent elements. A psychologist then administered a consent quiz using a corrected feedback strategy, and those who passed the quiz were then allowed to meet with the investigator to complete the consent process and enroll in the study.

Although the studies described above provide evidence for positive effects of the intermediary in improving understanding of the research protocol, Stiles et al. (2001) found that the use of a research intermediary did not improve understanding or memory of consent information among groups of depressed, schizophrenic, and healthy control participants. Importantly, these studies did not evaluate participants' perceptions of *voluntariness* in the consent process, which may be more strongly influenced by the presence of the third-party facilitator.

Results from both form- and process-oriented studies are meaningful because they begin to address concerns raised about the potential vulnerability and decision-making capabilities of certain types of individuals who are asked to participate in, and are sometimes excluded from, participating in research (e.g., National Bioethics Advisory Commission, 1998; Sugarman et al., 1998; Iacono and Murray, 2003). Certain types of modifications in the readability and format of the consent materials coupled with techniques such as corrected feedback and use of an intermediary can improve the degree of comprehension and decision-making ability to a level necessary to believe that consent is truly "informed."

Strategies for improving the informed consent process in substance-abuse research

As discussed, substance abusers may have inherent and situational vulnerabilities that may hinder their ability to provide informed consent to participate in research studies. Despite the fact that their knowingness, understanding, and autonomy may be compromised by these vulnerabilities, research examining the use of enhanced consent procedures in this population has been scarce. Fortunately, research conducted in our own and other laboratories has begun to examine ways of improving the consent process for individuals with substance-use disorders.

Increasing understanding

Fureman et al. (1997) examined the extent to which providing supplemental audiovisual materials regarding the procedures of an HIV prevention trial improved understanding of the protocol in a sample of intravenous drug users. In the study, protocol understanding was evaluated following the consent process. Participants then received supplemental educational training on the study procedures in which they either: (1) received a pamphlet detailing the study followed by a brief discussion; or (2) watched a videotape about the trial before receiving the pamphlet and discussion. Results indicated that participants in both groups displayed significantly higher protocol understanding scores immediately following the educational training, but that only participants in the videotape group maintained the improved level of understanding 1 month later. Findings from this study provide support for the use of supplemental audiovisual materials to improve protocol understanding in substance abusers participating in research.

Another technique that has been evaluated as a way to improve understanding and recall of consent information among substance abusers is corrected feedback. Festinger et al. (2010) evaluated the efficacy of using this procedure with substance abusers who were participating in a real-world clinical trial. Importantly, the study examined recall of study-related information throughout the course of a longitudinal study, rather than just at one time point immediately following the provision of consent. In the study, participants completed a consent quiz 2 weeks after consenting to the parent study and again at months 1, 2, and 3. Findings indicated that participants who received corrected feedback of their erroneous responses were able to recall significantly more consent information over the course of the study than clients who did not. This was true for the consent quiz items as a whole and for specific content areas (i.e., procedures, protections, and risks/benefits). Although the corrected feedback procedure was shown to improve the recall of consent information over the course of the study, it should be noted that these gains were modest, with recall rates of only 55% after several repetitions of the corrected feedback procedure.

Enhancing motivation

Strategies such as corrected feedback are essentially *remedial* in nature, as their goal is to simplify the cognitive tasks or compensate for participants' deficits. Although, as discussed, numerous studies have found cognitive variables including IQ, educational attainment, and neuropsychological measures of memory and attention to be positively correlated with recall of consent information (e.g., Taub et al., 1986), in statistical combination these variables account for less than half of the variance in recall (Festinger et al., 2007). This suggests that cognitive remediation strategies might be addressing only part of the problem and, perhaps, other relevant factors are being neglected. One such factor may be *motivation*. It is plausible that some research participants might be insufficiently interested in learning the elements of informed consent. They may not view it as worth the time or effort to attend to the information presented during the consent process and commit that information to memory.

Festinger et al. (2009) experimentally manipulated research participants' motivation to attend to and recall consent information through the use of incentives. At the time of consent, incentivized clients were told that they would receive $5 for every correct response they provided to a consent quiz administered 1 week later, whereas control group clients received the consent process as usual. Results indicated that incentivized participants recalled significantly more consent information the following week than participants in the consent as usual condition. Again, this was true for the consent quiz items as a whole and for specific content areas (i.e., procedures, protections, and risks/benefits). Findings from this study indicate that the provision of incentives may be a useful strategy to improve consent recall among substance abusers, particularly in studies that have potentially serious side effects. In addition, the results provide evidence that motivational strategies may be useful in improving the consent process in substance-abusing and other vulnerable populations.

Improving autonomy

An evaluation of NIH-funded research practices (McCrady and Bux, 1999) surveyed investigators who were currently recruiting participants from settings designated as implicitly "coercible." Investigators from over 90 studies were surveyed about the types of procedures they used to ensure that participants were free from coercion. The most commonly reported protections involved: (1) contacting the participant's primary clinician to verify that their participation was voluntary; (2) not recruiting the potential participant if the researcher was not convinced that he or she understood the research; (3) re-emphasizing the participant's rights; (4) accentuating the language in the consent form regarding the participant's right to decline or withdraw from the study; and (5) not telling the individual about research payment incentives until after he or she had already consented to the study. Although most of these responses certainly seem practical and reasonable, it is clear from this list that, despite the recommendations of several federal agencies and presidential commissions, there are few strategies currently in use to reduce the influence of coercion or to promote the autonomy of human research subjects.

A recent study (Festinger et al., 2010) examined the efficacy of using an independent research intermediary in reducing perceptions of coercion among drug court clients who were being recruited into a clinical trial. The intermediary met with the potential participant before he or she provided written consent. In this meeting, the intermediary provided the client with a handout explaining the intermediary's role, a business card with his contact information, and a schedule of times during which he could be contacted. Clients were told that in the event that they wished to drop out of the study at some future time the intermediary would communicate this information to research staff and that he would continue to monitor study procedures to ensure there was no retaliation against the participant. Results indicated that individuals who met with a research intermediary reported lower levels of perceived coercion to enter the study than those who did not. Specifically, clients who met with a research intermediary were less likely to misperceive that their decision to participate might influence how they were viewed by clinical and judicial staff than those who did not. Consistent with prior research conducted in non-substance-abusing populations, the presence of a research intermediary had no effect on recall of consent information. These findings provide preliminary evidence that the use of an intermediary may improve participant autonomy in clinical trials involving substance-abusing populations.

Conclusions

Research involving human participants has led and will undoubtedly continue to lead to incalculable advances that improve and even save human lives. The importance of ensuring continued human subject protections throughout these endeavors must not be taken lightly. Informed consent has become one of the central foci of human subject protections because it stands as the primary understanding agreement and contract between researchers and participants that the participants are engaging in research in a knowing, competent, and voluntary manner. Although these primary tenets may seem fairly straightforward, research has demonstrated that the process of ensuring that they are met is not as simple. As discussed in this chapter, research has shown unacceptable low levels of participant understanding and recall of their human research protections, even when well-intentioned measures are undertaken. Fortunately, continued research in this area has begun to uncover several novel and efficacious procedures for improving informed consent and ensuring research participants' protections. Continued efforts in this direction will allow human subject research to continue to make great advances without compromising human rights and without recreating our past mistakes. A number of important recommendations can be gleaned from the existing research on informed consent. These recommendations apply to substance-abuse research more generally as well as to genetics research on substance abuse more specifically. Although none of the studies discussed in this chapter focused specifically on genetics research, there is no reason to believe that the focus of the research would change the importance of understanding and recall of consent information. The basic tenets of informed consent (i.e., competence, knowingness, and voluntariness) and the protections they provide are universal regardless of the nature of the research.

Recommendations

Based on this extensive review of the literature, we have identified several practical strategies to help ensure that substance-abusing research participants are adequately informed about their research participation and that their autonomy is protected.

Accurate assessment: One recurring message that can be derived from the literature is that conducting the informed consent procedure in and of itself may be of little use, without adequate validation. Unless there is some way of determining whether the potential research participants actually heard, understood, and can recall what they were told, it is possible that they were never "informed" at all. This is why it is highly recommended to conduct some form of assessment with potential research participants following the informed consent procedure, but prior to them providing written consent.

A second related recommendation is to use as valid and reliable an assessment as is possible. In the past few years there has been an increased focus on conducting these types of consent assessments. However, it remains unclear to what degree these assessments were being used to truly gauge participants' understanding, competence, and voluntariness or merely to convince the researcher that proper ethical procedures were followed. A review of some of the consent quizzes and assessments, including 2–4 items, often leading, true and false, or simple multiple-choice instruments, would be unlikely to convince even the most novice researcher that they accurately assess participants' understanding, competence, or voluntariness. Unfortunately, to date there are few well-developed standardized assessments available. One that has received some attention is the MacArthur competence assessment tool for clinical research (MacCAT-CR) (Appelbaum and Grisso, 2001). However, even if this particular instrument is unavailable, researchers should make every effort to assess the participant's comprehensive understanding and appreciation of the study, its risks and benefits, and their human research protections.

Adding coercion measures into consent quizzes: Even when consent assessments or quizzes are used they often are focused almost entirely on participant understanding and competence, rather than voluntariness. Simply asking a client if he or she voluntarily consented to participate in a research study may be both inaccurate and insufficient. Although some measures may ask about the participant's voluntariness in a number of ways to better assess the autonomy of their decision, other measures (see Dugosh et al., 2010) also help to uncover potential sources of perceived coercion, which in turn can be addressed by the research staff before obtaining consent. In summary, it is critical to conduct quizzes to assess autonomy or build them into the consent quiz to more accurately ensure autonomy, and if necessary address sources of perceived or actual coercion.

Consent is a process: Although a great deal of policy proceedings and reports indicate that informed consent is a process rather than a single event, it is clear from a review of the methods sections of many substance-abuse publications that this prescription has not been widely adopted. Nevertheless, because most research with human participants lasts longer than a day and may have risks or benefits that extend well beyond the duration of the research study, it is critical for researchers to conceptualize consent as an ongoing process. As such, the basic tenets of informed consent (i.e., competence, knowingness, and voluntariness) should be ensured throughout the entire course of a research study. This may involve ongoing assessments or reminders, or some assurance that the most relevant issues, such as those related to risks and benefits and human subject protections, are retained. The point here is that, even if participants are aware of potential risks and means of addressing these risks when they first enter a study, this information will be of no use to them if it is not recalled when the event for which they were at risk occurs weeks or months later. Research participants must be protected continuously throughout the study.

Focusing on attention and motivation: As discussed, the lion's share of efforts focused on improving the consent process have centered on the use of remedial strategies. This stems from the fact that reading ability, visual processing, memory, and other cognitive processes are major contributors to the variance in participants' understanding and recall. An unfortunate result of this is that other contributing factors such as attention and motivation have been largely overlooked. For example, recent research on the use of incentives has indicated that participants' motivation to recall consent information should also be addressed. Moreover, combining strategies that address multiple factors such as remedial and motivational approaches may lead to greater mastery of consent information.

Standardizing and mandating procedures: Despite the unambiguous research demonstrating research participants' substandard understanding and recall of informed consent information, there are no federal requirements to assess and address these concerns. One of the clear obstacles to such requirements would be the absence of a well-validated consent assessment that could be used across a wide range of clinical trials. Nevertheless, it is clear that human subjects research must begin to require some level of comprehensive assessment that, at the very least, assesses potential participants' understanding of their responsibilities, their risks and needs, and their protections. Without some way of assessing the integrity of our informed consent procedures we cannot begin to adequately ensure our participants' protections. Standards must begin to be set for adequate assessments and levels of mastery necessary for individuals to be permitted to participate in research.

Further research is required: Advocates for informed consent research need to make a concerted effort to address the inconsistent findings that are present in this body of research. This goal would best be served by conducting randomized controlled trials that: (1) are designed to develop and identify interventions which increase the likelihood that individuals understand what their participation in research entails; (2) are longitudinal in nature; and (3) occur in both sham and realistic research contexts (Simel and Feussner, 1992; Lavori et al., 1999). Moreover, it is necessary to avoid a one-size-fits-all approach to identify which types of form and process methods work best for improving comprehension and recall among specific types of individuals (Stiles et al., 2001; Stroup and Appelbaum, 2006; Jeste et al., 2009).

References

Aaronson, N. K., Visser-Pol, E., Leenhouts, G. H., et al. (1996). Telephone-based nursing intervention improves the effectiveness of the informed consent process in cancer clinical trials. *Journal of Clinical Oncology*, 14, 984–996.

Agre, P. and Rapkin, B. (2003). Improving informed consent: A comparison of four consent tools. *IRB: Ethics and Human Research*, 25, 1–7.

Agre, P., Kurtz, R. C., and Krauss, B. J. (1994). A randomized trial using videotape to present consent information for colonoscopy. *Gastrointestinal Endoscopy*, 40, 271–276.

Appelbaum, P. S. and Grisso, T. (2001). *MacArthur Competence Assessment Tool for Clinical Research* (MacCAT-CR). Sarasota, FL: Professional Resource Press.

Appelbaum, P. S., Roth, L. H., and Lidz, C. (1982). The therapeutic misconception: Informed consent in psychiatric research. *International Journal of Law and Psychiatry*, 5, 319–329.

Appelbaum, P. S., Lidz, C. W., and Klitzman, R. (2009). Voluntariness of consent to research: A conceptual model. *Hastings Center Report*, 39, 30–39.

Benson, P. R., Roth, L. H., Appelbaum, P. S., Lidtz, C. W., and Winslade, W. J. (1988). Information disclosure, subject understanding, and informed consent in psychiatric research. *Law and Human Behavior*, 12, 455–475.

Bioethics Interest Group, National Institutes of Health (1998). Research involving individuals with questionable capacity to consent: Ethical issues and practical considerations for Institutional Review Boards (IRBs). Available online at: www.nih.gov/sigs/bioethics/reports/exec_sum.htm [accessed February 21, 2012].

Bjorn, E., Rossel, P., and Holm, S. (1999). Can the written information to research subjects be improved? An empirical study. *Journal of Medical Ethics*, 25, 263–267.

Campbell, F. A., Goldman, B. D., Boccia, M. L., and Skinner, M. (2004). The effect of format modifications and reading comprehension on recall of informed consent information by low-income parents: A comparison of print, video, and computer-based presentations. *Patient Education and Counseling*, 53, 205–216.

Carpenter, W. T., Gold, J. M., Lahti, A. C., et al. (2000). Decisional capacity for informed consent in schizophrenia research. *Archives of General Psychiatry*, 57, 533–538.

Cassileth, B. R., Zupkis, R. V., Sutton-Smith, K., and March, V. (1980). Informed consent: Why are its goals imperfectly realized? *New England Journal of Medicine*, 302, 869–900.

Centers for Disease Control and Prevention (2011). *U.S. Public Health Service syphilis study at Tuskegee: The Tuskegee timeline.* Available online at: www.cdc.gov/tuskegee/timeline.htm [accessed February 21, 2012].

Cohn, E. and Larson, E. (2007). Improving participant comprehension in the informed consent process. *Journal of Nursing Scholarship*, 39, 273–280.

Coletti, A. S., Heagerty, P., Sheon, A. R., et al. (2003). Randomized, controlled evaluation of a prototype informed consent process for HIV vaccine efficacy trials. *JAIDS: Journal of Acquired Immune Deficiency Syndromes*, 32, 161–169.

Cunha, P. J., Nicastri, S., Gomes, L. P., Moino, R. M., and Peluso, M. A. (2004). Neuropsychological impairments in crack cocaine-dependent inpatients: Preliminary findings. *Revista Brasileira de Psiquiatria*, 26, 103–106.

DeRenzo, E. G. (1994). The ethics of involving psychiatrically impaired persons in research. *IRB: Ethics and Human Research*, 16, 7–9, 11.

Dhai, A., Etheredge, H., and Cleaton-Jones, P. (2010). A pilot study evaluating an intervention designed to raise awareness of clinical trials among potential participants in the developing world. *Journal of Medical Ethics*, 36, 238–242.

Dugosh, K. L., Festinger, D. S., Croft, J. R., and Marlowe, D. B. (2010). Measuring coercion to participate in research within a double vulnerable population: Initial development of the Coercion Assessment Scale. *Journal of Empirical Research on Human Research Ethics*, 5, 93–102.

Dunn, L. B. and Jeste, D. V. (2001). Enhancing informed consent for research and treatment. *Neuropsychopharmacology*, 24, 595–607.

Dunn, L. B., Lindamer, L. A., Palmer, B. W., Schneiderman, L. J., and Jeste, D. V. (2001). Enhancing comprehension of consent for research in older patients with psychosis: A randomized study of a novel consent procedure. *American Journal of Psychiatry*, 158, 1911–1913.

Edwards, S. J., Lilford, R. J., Thornton J., and Hewison, J. (1998). Informed consent for clinical trials: In search of the "best" method. *Social Science and Medicine*, 47, 1825–1840.

Ellis, G. B. (1999). Protecting the rights and welfare of human research subjects. *Academic Medicine*, 74, 1008–1009.

Eyler, L. T., Mirzakhanian, H., and Jeste, D. V. (2005). A preliminary study of interactive questioning methods to assess and improve understanding of informed consent among patients with schizophrenia. *Schizophrenia Research*, 75, 193–198.

Festinger, D. S., Marlowe, D. B., Croft, J. R., et al. (2005). Do research payments precipitate drug use or coerce participation? *Drug and Alcohol Dependence*, 78, 275–281.

Festinger, D. S., Ratanadilok, K., Marlowe, D. B., et al. (2007). Neuropsychological functioning and recall of research consent information among drug court clients. *Ethics & Behavior*, 17, 163–186.

Festinger, D. S., Marlowe, D. B., Dugosh, K. L., Croft, J. R., and Arabia, P. L. (2008). Higher magnitude cash payments improve research follow-up rates without increasing drug use or perceived coercion. *Drug & Alcohol Dependence*, 96, 128–135.

Festinger, D. S., Marlowe, D. B., Croft, J. R., et al. (2009). Monetary incentives improve recall of research consent information: It pays to remember. *Experimental and Clinical Psychopharmacology*, 17, 99–104.

Festinger, D. S., Dugosh, K. L., Croft, J. R., Arabia, P. L., and Marlowe, D. B. (2010). Corrected feedback: A procedure to enhance recall of informed consent to research among substance abusing offenders. *Ethics & Behavior*, 20, 387–399.

Fitzgerald, D. W., Marotte, C., Verdier, R. I., Johnson, W. D., and Pape, J. W. (2002). Comprehension during informed consent in a less-developed country. *Lancet*, 360, 1301–1302.

Flory, J. and Emanuel, E. (2004). Interventions to improve research participants' understanding in informed consent for research: A systematic review. *JAMA: Journal of the American Medical Association*, 292, 1593–1601.

Fureman, I., Meyers, K., McLellan, A. T., Metzger, D., and Woody, G. (1997). Evaluation of a video-supplement to informed consent: Injection drug users and preventive HIV vaccine efficacy trials. *AIDS Education & Prevention*, 9, 330–341.

Grant, L., Gonzales, R., Carey, C. L., Natarajan, L., and Wolfson, T. (2003). Non-acute (residual) neurocognitive effects of cannabis use: a meta-analytic study. *Journal of the International Neuropsychological Society*, 9, 679–689.

Henry, J., Palmer, B. W., Palinka, L., et al. (2009). Reformed consent: Adapting to new media and research participant preferences. *IRB: Ethics and Human Research*, 31, 1–8.

Hochhauser, M. (2000). Informed consent and patient's rights documents: A right, a rite, or a rewrite? *Ethics and Behavior*, 9, 1–20.

Iacono, T. and Murray, V. (2003). Issues of informed consent in conducting medical research involving people with intellectual disability. *Journal of Applied Research in Intellectual Disabilities*, 16, 41–51.

Jefford, M. and Moore, R. (2008). Improvement of informed consent and the quality of consent documents. *Lancet Oncology*, 9, 485–493.

Jeste, D. V., Palmer, B. W., Golshan, S., et al. (2009). Multimedia consent for research in people with schizophrenia and normal subjects: A randomized controlled trial. *Schizophrenia Bulletin*, 35, 719–729.

Joseph, P., Schackman, B. R., Horwitz, R., et al. (2006). The use of an educational video during informed consent in an HIV clinical trial in Haiti. *Journal of Acquired Immune Deficiency Syndromes*, 42, 588–591.

Juraskova, I., Butow, P., Lopez, A., et al. (2008). Improving informed consent: Pilot of a decision aid for women invited to participate in a breast cancer prevention trial (IBIS-II DCIS). *Health Expectations*, 11, 252–262.

Karila, L., Vignau, J., Alter, C., and Reynaud, M. (2005). Acute and chronic cognitive disorders caused by cannabis use. *La Revue du Praticien*, 55, 27–29.

Kass, N. E., Sugarman, J., Medley, A. M., et al. (2009). An intervention to improve cancer patients' understanding of early-phase clinical trials. *IRB: Ethics and Human Research*, 31, 1–10.

Kiluk, B. D., Nich, C., and Carroll, K. M. (2010). Neurocognitive indicators predict results of an informed-consent quiz among substance-dependent treatment seekers entering a randomized clinical trial. *Journal of Studies on Alcohol and Drugs*, 71, 704–712.

Kim, S. Y. H., Appelbaum, P. S., Jeste, D. V., and Olin, J. T. (2004). Proxy and surrogate consent in geriatric neuropsychiatric research: Update and recommendations. *American Journal of Psychiatry*, 161, 787–806.

Knapp, P., Raynor, D. K., Silcock J., and Parkinson, B. (2009). Performanced-based readability testing of participant materials for a phase I trial: TGN1412. *Journal of Medical Ethics*, 35, 573–578.

Kouri, E. M., Lukas, S. E., Pope, H. G., Jr., and Olivia, P. S. (1995). Increased aggressive responding in male volunteers following the administration of gradually increasing doses of testosterone cypionate. *Drug and Alcohol Dependence*, 40, 73–79.

Kucia, A. M. and Horowitz, J. D. (2000). Is informed consent to clinical trials an "upside selective" process in acute coronary syndromes? *American Heart Journal*, 140, 94–97.

Lavori, P. W., Sugarman, J., Hays, M. T., and Feussner, J. R. (1999). Improving informed consent in clinical trials: A duty to experiment. *Controlled Clinical Trials*, 20, 187–193.

Levine, R. (1992). Clinical trials and physicians as double agents. *The Yale Journal of Biology and Medicine*, 65, 65–74.

McCrady, B. S. and Bux, D. A., Jr. (1999). Ethical issues in informed consent with substance abusers. *Journal of Consulting & Clinical Psychology*, 67, 186–193.

Milgram, S. (1974). *Obedience to Authority*. New York: Harper Collins.

Moser, D. J., Reese, R. L., Hey, C. T., et al. (2006). Using a brief intervention to improve decisional capacity in schizophrenia research. *Schizophrenia Bulletin*, 32, 116–120.

Munro, C. A., Saxton, J., and Butters, M. A. (2000). The neuropsychological consequences of abstinence among older alcoholics: a cross-sectional study. *Alcoholism: Clinical & Experimental Research*, 24, 1510–1516.

Muss, H. B., White, D. R., Michielutte, R., et al. (1979). Written informed consent in patients with breast cancer. *Cancer*, 43, 549–556.

National Bioethics Advisory Committee (1998). *Research Involving Persons with Mental Disorders That May Affect Decision-making Capacity*. Rockville, MD: National Bioethics Committee.

National Center on Addiction and Substance Abuse (2010). *Behind Bars II: Substance Abuse and America's Prison Population*. New York: National Center on Addiction and Substance Abuse.

National Commission for the Protection of Human Subjects of Biomedical and Behavioral Research (1979). *The Belmont Report: Ethical principles and guidelines for the protection of human subjects of research*. Available online at: http://ohsr.od.nih.gov/guidelines/belmont.html [accessed March 13, 2012].

Neptune, S. M., Hopper, K. D., Houts, P. S., et al. (1996). Take-home informed consent for intravenous contrast media. *Investigative Radiology*, 31, 109–113.

Ness, D. E., Kiesling, S. F., and Lidz, C. W. (2009). Why does informed consent fail? A discourse analytic approach. *Journal of the American Academy of Psychiatry and Law*, 37, 349–362.

Ogloff, J. R. P. and Otto, R. K. (1991). Are research participants truly informed? Readability of informed consent forms used in research. *Ethics and Behavior*, 1, 239–252.

Ostini, R., Bammer, G., Dance, P. R., and Goodwin, R. E. (1993). The ethics of experimental heroin maintenance. *Journal of Medical Ethics*, 19, 175–182.

Palmer, B. W., Dunn, L. B., Depp, C. A., Eyler, L. T., and Jeste, D. V. (2007). Decisional capacity to consent to research among patients with bipolar disorder: Comparison with schizophrenia patients and healthy subjects. *Journal of Clinical Psychiatry*, 68, 689–696.

Pope, H. J., and Yurgelun-Todd, D. (1996). The residual cognitive effects of heavy marijuana use in college students. *Journal of the American Medical Association*, 275, 521–527.

Reiser, S. J. and Knudson, P. (1993). Protecting research subjects after consent: The case for the "research intermediary." *IRB: A Review of Human Subjects Research*, 15, 10–11.

Ritter, A. J., Fry, C. L., and Swan, A. (2003). The ethics of reimbursing injecting drug users for public health research interviews: What price are we prepared to pay? *International Journal of Drug Policy*, 14, 1–3.

Roberts, L. and Roberts, B. (1999). Psychiatric research ethics: An overview of evolving guidelines and current ethical dilemmas in the study of mental illness. *Biological Psychiatry*, 46, 1025–1038.

Robinson, G. and Merav, A. (1976). Informed consent: Recall by patients tested post-operatively. *Annals of Thoracic Surgery*, 22, 209–212.

Rounsaville, D. B., Hunkele, K., Easton, C. J., Nich, C., and Carroll, K. M. (2008). Making consent more informed: preliminary results from a multiple-choice test among probation-referred marijuana users entering a randomized clinical trial. *Journal of the American Academy of Psychiatry and Law*, 36, 354–359.

Rubright, J., Sankar, P., Casarett, D. J., et al. (2010). A memory and organizational aid improves Alzheimer disease research consent capacity: Results of a randomized, controlled trial. *American Journal of Geriatric Psychiatry*, 18, 1124–1132.

Ryan, R., Prictor, M., and McLaughlin, K. J. (2009). Audio-visual presentation of informed consent for participation in clinical trials (review). *The Cochrane Library, Issue 3.*

Salas, H. S., Aziz, Z., Villareale, N., and Diekema, D. S. (2008). The research and family liaison: Enhancing informed consent. *IRB: Ethics and Human Research*, 50, 1–8.

Saxton, J., Munro, C. A., Butters, M. A., Schramke, C., and McNeil, M. A. (2000). Alcohol, dementia, and Alzheimer's disease: Comparison of neuropsychological profiles. *Journal of Geriatric Psychiatry & Neurology*, 13, 141–149.

Silva, M. C., and Sorrell, J. M. (1988). Enhancing comprehension of information for informed consent: A review of empirical research. *IRB: Ethics and Human Research*, 10, 1–5.

Sim, T., Simon, S. L., Domier, C. P., et al. (2002). Cognitive deficits among methamphetamine users with attention deficit hyperactivity disorder symptomatology. *Journal of Addictive Diseases*, 21, 75–89.

Simel, D. L. and Feussner, J. R. (1992). Suspended judgment: Clinical trials of informed consent. *Controlled Clinical Trials*, 13, 321–324.

Simon, S., Domier, C., Carnell, J. C., et al. (2000). Cognitive impairment in individuals currently using methamphetamine. *American Journal on Addictions*, 9, 222–231.

Solowij, N., Stephens, R. S., Roffman, R. A., et al. (2002). Cognitive functioning of long-term heavy cannabis users seeking treatment. *Journal of the American Medical Association*, 287, 1123–1131.

Sorrell, J. M. (1991). Effects of writing/speaking on comprehension of information for informed consent. *Western Journal of Nursing Research*, 13, 110–122.

Stiles, P. G., Poythress, N. G., Hall, A., Falkenbach, D., and Williams, R. (2001). Improving understanding of research consent disclosures among persons with mental illness. *Psychiatric Services*, 52, 780–785.

Strickland, T. L., Mena, I., Villanueva-Meyer, J., et al. (1993). Cerebral perfusion and neuropsychological consequences of chronic cocaine use. *Journal of Neuropsychiatry and Clinical Neurosciences*, 5, 419–427.

Stroup, S. and Appelbaum, P. (2003). The subject advocate: Protecting the interests of participants with fluctuating decisionmaking capacity. *IRB: Ethics and Human Research*, 25, 9–11.

Stroup, T. S. and Appelbaum, P. S. (2006). Evaluation of "subject advocate" procedures in the clinical antipsychotic trials of intervention effectiveness (CATIE) schizophrenia study. *Schizophrenia Bulletin*, 32, 147–152.

Sugarman, J., McCrory, D. C., and Hubal, R. C. (1998). Getting meaningful informed consent from older adults: A structured literature review of empirical research. *Journal of the American Geriatric Society*, 46, 517–524.

Tapert, S. F. and Brown, S. A. (2000). Substance dependence, family history of alcohol dependence and neuropsychological functioning in adolescence. *Addiction*, 95, 1043–1053.

Taub, H. A. and Baker, M. T. (1983). The effect of repeated testing upon comprehension of informed consent materials by elderly volunteers. *Experimental Aging Research*, 9, 135–138.

Taub, H. A., Kline, G. E., and Baker, M. T. (1981). The elderly and informed consent: Effects of vocabulary level and corrected feedback. *Experimental Aging Research*, 7, 137–146.

Taub, H. A., Baker, M. T., and Sturr, J. F. (1986). Informed consent for research: Effects of readability, patient age, and education. *Journal of the American Geriatric Society*, 34, 601–606.

Taub, H. A., Baker, M. T., Kline, G. E., and Sturr, J. F. (1987). Comprehension of informed consent information by young-old through old-old volunteers. *Experimental Aging Research*, 13, 173–178.

Verdejo, A., Toribio, I., Orozco, C., Puente, K. L., and Perez-Garcia, M. (2005). Neuropsychological functioning in methadone maintenance patients versus abstinent heroin abusers. *Drug and Alcohol Dependence*, 78, 283–288.

Verheggen, F. W. S. M., and van Wijmen, F. C. B. (1996). Informed consent in clinical trials. *Health Policy*, 36, 131–153.

Victor, M., Adams, R., and Collins, G. (1989). *The Wernicke-Korsakoff Syndrome and Related Neurologic Disorders Due to Alcoholism and Malnutrition,* 2nd edn. Philadelphia: FA Davis.

Welsone, E. (1999). *The Plutonium Files: America's Secret Medical Experiments in the Cold War*. New York: Dial Press.

Weston, J., Hannah, M., and Downes, J. (1997). Evaluating the benefits of a patient information video during the informed consent process. *Patient Education and Counseling*, 30, 239–245.

White, S. and Dillow, S. (2005). *Key Concepts and Features of the 2003 National Assessment of Adult Literacy*. Washington, DC: Institute of Educational Sciences, National Center for Educational Statistics, US Department of Education.

Wirshing, D. A., Wirshing, W. C., Marder, S. R., Liberman, R. P., and Mintz, J. (1998). Informed consent: Assessment of comprehension. *American Journal of Psychiatry*, 155, 1508–1511.

Wirshing, D. A., Sergi, M. J., and Mintz, J. (2005). A videotape intervention to enhance the informed consent process for medical and psychiatric treatment research. *American Journal of Psychiatry*, 162, 186–188.

World Medical Association (1964). Declaration of Helsinki: Ethical principles for medical research involving human subjects. Available online at: www.wma.net [accessed February 21, 2012].

World Medical Association (1997). Declaration of Helsinki: Recommendations Guiding Physicians in Biomedical Research Involving Human Subjects. [Reprinted in the] *Journal of the American Medical Association*, 277, 925–926.

Young, D. R., Hooker, D. T., and Freeberg, F. E. (1990). Informed consent documents: increasing comprehension by reducing reading level. *IRB: A Review of Human Subjects Research*, 12, 1–5.

Chapter 5

Ethical considerations in genetic research with children affected by parental substance abuse

Thomas J. McMahon

Research done from several different perspectives over more than 40 years indicates that children with a substance-abusing parent are at risk for an array of poor developmental outcomes. Investigations based on family-study methods have clearly documented the aggregation of substance use and psychiatric difficulty within family systems affected by substance abuse (e.g., see Rounsaville et al., 1991; Bierut et al., 1998; Merikangas et al., 1998). Comparative, longitudinal studies of children with a substance-abusing parent followed from early childhood through adolescence into early adulthood also document substantial risk for intergenerational transmission of substance abuse that seems to increase as the density of substance abuse within the family increases (e.g., see Chassin et al., 1996; Zhou et al., 2006). Moreover, research based on the principles of behavioral genetics has clearly documented genetic liability for problematic use of substances (e.g., see Tsuang et al., 1998; Hicks et al., 2004; Kendler et al., 2003; Rhee et al., 2003), and molecular research has begun to identify specific markers of that genetic risk (e.g., see Uhl et al., 2008; Bierut et al., 2010).

Given the empirical data documenting familial risk, researchers (e.g., see Tarter et al., 1999; Vanyukov et al., 2003) have begun to define conceptual models of intergenerational transmission that explain how genetic liability and psychosocial stress interact over time to promote the aggregation of substance abuse across generations. Because developmental precursors to chronic substance abuse are present surprisingly early in childhood, high-risk use of substances typically begins during early adolescence, and substance-use disorders often emerge during middle to late adolescence (Schulenberg and Maggs, 2008), research designed to untangle genetic influences on risk must include children. Given the current state of the science, complex questions about which children with a substance-abusing parent are affected across generations cannot be answered without examining the genetic liability and developmental trajectory of children known to be at risk.

Because children with a substance-abusing parent represent a particularly vulnerable population of participants, research on the intergenerational transmission of substance abuse raises a number of ethical questions about how to best protect this population of children as they enroll in research typically viewed as involving minimal risk with the potential to benefit this class of children but not the individual participant. The critical task for researchers exploring genetic liability is to balance the need to protect this vulnerable population of research participants from harm against the need to generate scientific knowledge

Genetic Research on Addiction, ed. Audrey R. Chapman. Published by Cambridge University Press. © Cambridge University Press 2012.

Support for preparation of this chapter was provided by the National Institute on Drug Abuse (R01 DA020619).

to inform prevention, early intervention, and treatment pursued with this population of children. Although *The Belmont Report* (National Commission for the Protection of Human Subjects of Biomedical and Behavioral Research, 1979) outlined the basic ethical principles of human subjects research and the *Regulations for the Protection of Human Subjects of Biomedical and Behavioral Research* (US Department of Health and Human Services, 2009) outlined special guidelines applicable to research being done with children, many ethicists (e.g., Gillam et al., 2006; Anderson and DuBois, 2007; Buchanan et al., 2009) believe that they only provide a broad, sometimes inadequate, conceptual framework within which to examine some of the very specific ethical issues related to the conduct of substance-abuse research with children and their parents.

Therefore, this review of the literature was pursued to outline ethical considerations likely to emerge in genetic research done with children at risk for poor developmental outcomes in the context of parental substance abuse. There were two broad considerations that guided development of the discussion. First, there was interest in examining ethical issues from both a conceptual and a practical perspective. That is, there was interest in identifying ethical issues that researchers are most likely to confront when planning genetic research with children affected by the substance abuse of their parents. Second, there was interest in using the results of ethics research, as Anderson and DuBois (2007) did, to inform consideration of ethical issues likely to emerge in this type of research. That is, there was interest in highlighting the results of research directly relevant to ethical issues likely to emerge in genetic research pursued with this population of children and their parents.

Ethical considerations related to community consultation

In their synthesis of major declarations, policy statements, and ethical guidelines, Emanuel et al. (2000) outlined seven broad ethical principles they believe should guide the development and evaluation of clinical research: (1) social value; (2) scientific validity; (3) fair subject selection; (4) favorable risk–benefit ratio; (5) independent review; (6) informed consent; and (7) respect for enrolled subjects. Emanuel et al. (2004) subsequently added the principle of community collaboration, arguing that the ethical conduct of clinical research requires consultation with the community in which the research will be done. When developed with respect for the concept of community consultation, the research process becomes a collaborative endeavor, in which the investigator provides expertise concerning the science of a proposed project and the community provides expertise concerning the values and concerns of potential participants (for further discussion, see Fisher, 1997, 1999, 2000). Practically, ethicists (e.g., Buchanan et al., 2009) have argued that community participation in the design of research can help: (1) ensure the goals of the research are valued by the community; (2) protect against exploitation of vulnerable populations; (3) ensure fair terms of cooperation; (4) minimize risk for misunderstandings about the nature of the research; and (5) promote use of research methods acceptable to potential participants.

Because genetic research may be controversial when pursued with a vulnerable population of children, researchers will, from the perspective of many ethicists (e.g., Fisher, 1997, 1999, 2000; Field and Behrman, 2004; Buchanan et al., 2009), enhance the quality of their work if they consult with the community when developing a research project designed to document genetic liability to substance abuse. How that is done will depend on the nature of the research design and initial plans for recruitment of specific segments of the community. However, several professional advisory groups (e.g., see Fisher et al., 2002; Field and

Behrman, 2004) have recommended that community collaboration for research involving minor children should, when indicated, include consultation with an ethnically diverse sampling of children, adolescents, parents, and other members of the community in a position to provide information about potential concerns of individuals likely to participate. Moreover, Fisher and her colleagues (Fisher and Masty, 2006a, 2006b; Fisher and Ragsdale, 2006; Masty and Fisher, 2008; Buchanan et al., 2009) have proposed a generic approach to research ethics that outlines a process for identifying and resolving ethical challenges likely to emerge in research done with populations of children at risk for poor developmental outcomes that is directly relevant to the ethical conduct of genetic research with this population of children.

Within this conceptual model, Fisher and her colleagues (Fisher and Masty, 2006a, 2006b; Fisher and Ragsdale, 2006; Buchanan et al., 2009) have outlined a research process whereby scientists and community representatives collaborate to develop research designs that are both scientifically valid and socially responsible. When considered from this perspective, ethical decision making is viewed as deficient if it does not involve a serious dialogue with the community. Emphasizing the importance of mutual respect, this conceptual model holds that researchers and community representatives should be collaborating experts in the development of ethically sound research procedures, such that researchers bring expertise about the scientific method to the process and community representatives bring expertise about community values and perceptions. Within this process, researchers can share their views on the importance of using scientific methods to examine crucial social questions, and they can share ethical questions related to the conduct of the research. Conversely, community representatives can share their perspective on the social and scientific value of the research. They can also provide comment on questions about the ethics of the research being proposed, and they can offer an opinion about the research procedures. When pursued within a framework of mutual respect, research procedures that emerge from the process accommodate both the values of science and the values of the community in which the work will be done.

Increasingly, genetic researchers (e.g., Gillam et al., 2006) are emphasizing the need to consult with potential participants about ethical issues of concern within a specific population of susceptible individuals. Building upon this position, Gillam et al. (2006) argued that a simple pilot study done with potential participants can inform the final design of a genetic research project, and the practice is becoming increasingly common. Consultation originally pursued largely with susceptible adults (e.g., see Kreiger et al., 2001) is now being extended to parents of susceptible children (e.g., see Gillam at al., 2006; Kaufman et al., 2008; Coors and Raymond, 2009) and children themselves (e.g., see Coors and Raymond, 2009).

Ethical considerations related to recruitment

As noted above, successful efforts to identify genetic markers of risk for chronic substance abuse rely upon the success of family-oriented research, and the success of family-oriented research is built, first and foremost, upon the successful recruitment of family members. When considering ethical questions concerning recruitment, it is important to note that adults considering enrollment of children in family-oriented research on genetic liability may be doing so for any number of reasons. They may be most interested in advancing knowledge of a disease process that has affected their family, but they may also be most interested in learning something about the susceptibility of their children (Biesecker and

Peay, 2003). Although the topic has not received much attention in the literature, the recruitment of family members raises a number of ethical considerations relevant to work being done with children at risk for substance abuse. Unfortunately, relatively little research has been done specifically on the topic of recruitment, and the research that has been conducted has been done almost exclusively with adult family members (for a review, see Beskow et al., 2004).

With support from the National Cancer Institute, the Cancer Genetics Network recently convened a special work group to examine the ethics of family-based recruitment of participants into genetic research. In the final report of an extensive dialogue about the ethics of recruitment, that work group (Beskow et al., 2004) highlighted two general strategies for the recruitment of family members: (1) participants already enrolled in a study, usually as a proband, provide family members with information about the study and information about how to enroll; or (2) participants already enrolled in a study, again usually as a proband, provide the research team with information about family members along with permission for the research team to contact them directly to discuss participation. Both strategies are likely to be appropriate in family-oriented research being done with children at risk for substance abuse.

When planning research projects involving this population of children, researchers should, as recommended by Beskow et al. (2004), distinguish risks associated with research recruitment from risks associated with research participation, and they should be aware that recruitment into family-based studies of genetic risk involves at least three potential sources of harm. First, if they did not express interest in the study or have prior knowledge of the study, some people, including some children and adolescents, might consider the recruitment process to be an invasion of their privacy. Second, recruitment procedures might lead to inadvertent disclosure of familial risk. This may be a particularly salient issue in research being pursued with children and caregivers who do not know about the substance abuse of a family member.

Third, whether approached by another family member or a research team, family members might feel, or actually be, pressured by others to participate. To ensure full participation, family members already enrolled in a study might pressure other family members to enroll, or they might allow the research team to contact family members who they know do not wish to participate. Moreover, if family members do not wish to participate, their reluctance might become a source of conflict within the family. Again, these issues may be particularly salient in research being pursued with children living in high-risk family situations, where there might be risk for the children to be pressured by adults to participate in family-oriented research, particularly if financial compensation offered to one family member is dependent on the participation of another or extra financial compensation is offered if the entire family completes the study.

· Therefore, when planning research designed to clarify genetic risk in children with a substance-abusing parent, researchers should consider how best to balance the need for research quality against the need to protect children and the adults in their lives from harm that might occur within the recruitment process (Beskow et al., 2004). As noted by Beskow and colleagues, the actual recruitment strategy selected by the research team determines the extent to which the privacy of family members is balanced against the need for representative samples to advance scientific understanding of risk. When participants recruit family members, the privacy of family members will be maximized, but recruitment may be compromised. When participants provide information about family members to the research team, the privacy of family members may be compromised, but recruitment will be maximized, albeit with the risk that family members may object to the process because the research team has collected information about them without their consent (Beskow et al., 2004).

Ethical issues related to inclusion of children in the custody of the child welfare system

Responding in part to risk for exploitation, federal regulations (US Department of Health and Human Services, 2009) include special provisions for the conduct of research with children in the custody of the child welfare system that may be an important consideration in research being done with this population, because parental substance abuse is clearly associated with risk for extended placement within the child welfare system (Child Welfare League of America, 2001). As noted by the Institute of Medicine's Committee on Clinical Research Involving Children (Field and Behrman, 2004), state policy on research participation with children in the custody of the child welfare system is rarely articulated in any detail in state statute, case law, or agency regulations. State to state, the child welfare system may not have clear, written guidelines concerning the participation of children in research. Varma and Wendler (2008) argued that the absence of clear safeguards may leave children in the custody of the child welfare system at risk of being inappropriately enrolled in research because they are more accessible to researchers. However, Field and Behrman (2004) suggested that some parts of the child welfare system may actively restrict access to children in the custody of the state such that researchers may find it more convenient to simply exclude these children from participation. Although the concern that children in the custody of the child welfare system may be exploited cannot be dismissed, it is important to note that exclusion of this class of children from research may also contribute to an injustice by denying them an opportunity to participate in research that may directly or indirectly affect their well-being. Exclusion may also unreasonably shift the burden of research participation to another class of affected children. As much as possible, samples of children enrolled in this type of research should represent the entire population of children at risk.

Consequently, researchers planning projects need to consider a number of ethical questions relevant to the enrollment of children in the custody of the child welfare system. Varma and Wendler (2008) argued that this class of children should not be enrolled in any research without scientific justification. Ensuring that children in the custody of the child welfare system are properly represented in a study directly relevant to their status as children with a substance-abusing parent could be offered as reasonable scientific justification. Moreover, representation of this class of children in relevant research is important because they may, by virtue of their custodial status, represent a subgroup of children with even greater genetic and environmental liability for poor developmental outcomes. However, researchers interested in ensuring that this class of children is properly represented in a sample of children with a substance-abusing parent should proceed with awareness that special safeguards may be needed (Varma and Wendler, 2008). Because they will not have parents directly involved to ensure that their best interests are adequately represented, Varma and Wendler (2008) argued that, even when the study involves minimal risk, it may be appropriate to appoint an independent advocate to help represent the interests of this particularly vulnerable class of children.

Ethical considerations related to parental permission, child consent, and child assent

Federal regulations (US Department of Health and Human Services, 2009) presently require that, under most circumstances, a legal guardian provide permission for a child to participate in research, and the regulations outline the elements that should be addressed by researchers when they seek parental permission. Federal regulations also require that, under most circumstances, children who have the developmental capacity to do so provide assent for their participation in research (US Department of Health and Human Services, 2009). Given these expectations, researchers planning genetic research in consultation with community representatives have to define a process for legal guardians to decide whether it is appropriate for children in their care to participate in the research, and a process for children to decide whether they would like to participate in the research as they understand it. Fisher and Goodman (2009) argued that researchers working with high-risk populations in which there may be more vulnerability need to minimize risk for misunderstanding when obtaining parental permission and child assent by carefully avoiding *a priori* assumptions about decisional capacity and realistically shaping the research procedures to accommodate the characteristics of potential participants. Although a thorough review of parental permission and child assent is beyond the scope of this discussion, there are some concerns for genetic researchers to consider in consultation with their community partners.

Motivation to grant parental permission

Empirical research on parental considerations when providing permission for research participation is limited and focused largely on considerations associated with participation in clinical trials (for a review, see Field and Behrman, 2004). The data that are available on parental considerations when they are asked to enroll children in research involving minimal risk without potential for direct benefit suggest that parents may agree to participate in research with expectations that they will learn more about the genetic susceptibility of their children (Kaufman et al., 2008), even when they have been told this will not happen (Gillam et al., 2006). Consequently, substance-abusing parents anxious about the genetic risk their children incur may be more likely to grant permission with unrealistic expectations about the potential benefits of participation.

Given that research on genetic susceptibility generally offers no direct benefit to the participant, researchers frequently emphasize ways in which participation will contribute to the generation of knowledge about risk that may inform prevention and treatment of the population under study. Interestingly, Biesecker and Peay (2003) suggested that researchers need to be careful about overstating the potential for any specific genetic study to have a dramatic impact on the assessment, prevention, and treatment of a complex disease process like substance abuse. Highlighting risk that parents may inflate the potential significance of participation in a specific study because of their own needs, they encourage researchers to be careful about exploiting the understandable interests parents may have in advancing knowledge of a disease process that may affect their children by providing parents with realistic information about the scientific contribution a specific study is likely to make.

Securing parental permission

Federal regulations (US Department of Health and Human Services, 2009) require that parents understand 11 key concepts relevant to the participation of children in research.

Although researchers often believe that procedures to secure permission for participation of children from parents help them understand these concepts, research done primarily with parents of children being recruited into clinical trials suggests that parents frequently do not (e.g., see Tait et al., 2003). Consistent with this, research has repeatedly shown that procedures to secure consent for research participation, including procedures used to secure parental permission for children to participate in research, usually require cognitive and reading skill far beyond that typically present in the study population (for a review, see Field and Behrman, 2004). Generally, parents tend to overestimate the extent to which they actually understand key concepts associated with participation (e.g., see Tait et al., 2003). Specific characteristics of parents may influence comprehension of presentations used to secure permission for children to participate (e.g., see Tait et al., 2003), and parents who more accurately comprehend key concepts may be more likely to grant permission for a child to participate (e.g., see Tait et al., 2003). For researchers interested in developing more effective procedures to secure parental permission, it is important to note that review committees (e.g., see Field and Behrman, 2004) have argued that the flow of ideas, the use of headings, the layout of pages, the size and style of the font, and the use of graphics may also influence comprehension of parental permission forms.

Securing child consent and child assent

Federal standards (US Department of Health and Human Services, 2009), professionals (Field and Behrman, 2004), parents (e.g., see Kaufman et al., 2008), and children (e.g., see Fisher, 2003; Geller et al., 2003) value the idea that children should somehow grant permission for their participation in research. Federal guidelines expect that researchers seek assent from children who can provide it. Assent is broadly defined as an affirmative agreement to participate in the research provided by the child that involves more than mere failure to object to participation. Despite agreement about the general right of children to provide permission for participation, there is no clear agreement about the circumstances under which children might provide consent for participation independent of their legal guardian. There is also no clear agreement about the circumstances under which children should provide assent, and there are surprisingly little empirical data on the nature of the assent process as it actually occurs (for a review, see Field and Behrman, 2004).

Despite the absence of empirical data, there is agreement that consent and assent procedures for a study of children with a substance-abusing parent involving minimal risk should be grounded, as Santelli et al. (2005) did for a study of pregnant minors, in a comprehensive review of the characteristics of the study population. If the research design involves case–control considerations, the characteristics of the comparison group must also be considered (Santelli et al., 2005). As illustrated by Santelli and colleagues, legal and ethical considerations might define situations where it could be appropriate for affected children younger than 18 years of age to provide consent for participation in genetic research independent of their legal guardian.

Research exploring the capacity of children to provide informed assent indicates that children younger than 9 or 10 years of age usually have limited ability to understand the purpose, risks, and potential benefits of research, especially more complex research (for a review, see Field and Behrman, 2004). Younger children are also less likely to fully understand abstract concepts, such as confidentiality of participation, and they are more likely to understand the practical aspects of research that focus on what they are expected to do (for a review, see Field and Behrman, 2004). This same research indicates that children more than

14 or 15 years of age differ very little from adults in terms of their ability to understand the key concepts associated with participation in research (for a review, see Field and Behrman, 2004). Although age is most frequently used as the criterion for obtaining assent, researchers should be aware that the empirical data that are available suggest that age alone may not be the best proxy for capacity to provide assent (Dorn et al., 1995).

As researchers plan assent procedures, they should do so with awareness that, consistent with research done on the nature of consent documents designed for use with adults, assent documents, including assent documents used in genetic research, often include concepts and language not likely to be understood by children (e.g., see Weir and Horton, 1995). This may be particularly true in genetic research, where children must have some capacity to understand the concept of genetic endowment. For example, Bernhardt et al. (2003) explored children's attitudes toward participation in a genetic susceptibility study and found that children 10 to 17 years of age frequently did not fully understand the potential risks and benefits of participation. Because there are relatively few data on the ways in which risk status may affect children's understanding of research participation, researchers should develop assent procedures with awareness that exposure to parental substance abuse may somehow affect children's understanding of the research process and their willingness to participate.

Assent procedures used in genetic research pursued with children affected by parental substance abuse must also protect children from being pressured by adults to participate. This is particularly important because empirical data suggest that, although children and adolescents have some capacity to understand, they may have difficulty comprehending their right to refuse even though a legal guardian has provided consent for participation (Abramovitch et al., 1995; Bruzzese and Fisher, 2003). Thompson (2000) argued that children may find it difficult to dissent because invitations to participate typically occur in a setting in which there is: (1) an institution familial to the child supporting the research; (2) a legal guardian providing permission for the child to participate; and (3) a researcher with an interest in the child participating. Because children have limited experience asserting their rights in response to requests from adults, the assent process should be designed to demonstrate, as much as possible, that participation is truly voluntary and dissent will really not be penalized.

Although some researchers (e.g., see Field and Behrman, 2004) have argued that parent–child discussion with a facilitator during the assent process may be appropriate, it is presently not clear if children are less likely to dissent when assent is requested in the presence of a legal guardian who has usually already agreed that the child can participate. Moreover, the Institute of Medicine's Committee on Clinical Research Involving Children (Field and Behrman, 2004) argued that it is acceptable for legal guardians to make an effort to persuade children to participate when they are reluctant to do so, but allowing parents to do so may make it difficult to determine when parental persuasion is becoming parental coercion. Ironically, the same review group suggested that investigators should be sensitive to non-verbal indicators of children's interest in research participation, particularly when children may be reluctant to distress their legal guardian by refusing to participate. Although rates of actual dissent within ongoing research are not widely reported, the data that are available suggest that, although altruistic and experiential considerations may motivate some children to participate in research with no potential for direct benefit, children are likely to be most concerned about the nature of the research procedures when making decisions about whether to participate in this type of research (Wolthers, 2006). Given that this research almost always involves minimal risk to children with no potential for direct benefit, federal regulations (US Department of Health and Human Services, 2009) imply that, when researchers make final decisions about participation, a child's dissent should always take precedence over parental permission.

Ethical considerations related to phenotyping

Research focusing on genetic risk for chronic substance abuse will, by definition, require careful phenotyping of children. Increasingly, investigation of genetic liability to substance abuse involves examination of phenotypes involving early substance use, concurrent clinical conditions, and related constructs such as impulsivity, risk taking, and stress reactivity (for further discussion, see Kreek et al., 2005). Whatever the primary construct, phenotyping will inevitably raise ethical questions about the presence of clinically significant emotional–behavioral disturbance in children for which clinical intervention may be indicated and readily available. Phenotyping that involves the assessment of early substance use will also raise ethical questions about what should be done when participants confirm early substance use, particularly when children at risk because of a positive family history confirm early substance use that represents risk for the development of substance abuse as an adult. Given this, researchers planning projects designed to clarify genetic risk in children with a substance-abusing parent will have to decide how to balance a number of critical issues involving the need for informed consent from legal guardians, informed assent from children, confidentiality of participation for children, and responsibility to advance the well-being of minor participants.

When considering whether to enroll their children in a genetic study of risk affected parents may, as noted above, be anxious about the risk status of the children and see the study as a way to somehow obtain information about the extent of that risk. Consequently, the consent process pursued with affected parents must make it clear that enrollment in the study is not a way to obtain information about the risk status of their children. Building upon the concept of therapeutic misconception first outlined by Appelbaum et al. (1982), a number of researchers (e.g., see Clayton and Ross, 2006) have argued that routinely providing research participants with information about their clinical status may create confusion about the difference between a clinical versus a research assessment, and they have argued that the difference should be clear to research participants.

Given the potential for confusion, researchers need to make it clear that the phenotyping process in genetic research is not a substitute for a clinical assessment by a licensed health-care professional with knowledge of risk and resilience among children with a family history of substance abuse. There are two simple ways to do this. First, researchers can be clear that, except under very specific circumstances, children have a right to confidentiality of participation and a legal guardian will not be provided with a summary of the phenotyping. Second, to the extent that consent forms require that researchers outline alternatives to participation, researchers can be clear that an alternative for legal guardians interested in an assessment of clinical risk is to seek a clinical assessment, and the research team can provide information about ways a legal guardian might do so.

Moreover, when enrolling children in a study of genetic risk, researchers need to establish clear procedures to deal with situations in which they may have a responsibility to take immediate action to protect the well-being of children, and they need to be clear about the extent to which they have an obligation to advance the well-being of children who may present with clinically significant emotional–behavioral difficulty. Inevitably, questions about responsibility to protect the well-being of children in this type of research are linked with questions about the limits of confidentiality, because ethical decisions about taking action designed to protect the well-being of minor participants will inevitably involve decisions about disclosure of information obtained during a research assessment.

Obviously, consent and assent procedures need to make it clear to children and their legal guardians what the limits to confidentiality of participation are (Field and Behrman, 2004). That is, children and their legal guardians need, as much as possible, to be clear under what circumstances the researcher will act on information provided during a research assessment, particularly research assessments designed to identify clinically meaningful phenotypes associated with risk for substance abuse. Although research suggests that substance-abuse researchers almost always establish procedures for disclosure of information (e.g., see McCrady and Bux, 1999), it is important to note that investigators have some authority to determine under what circumstances to disclose information about high-risk circumstances (Buchanan et al., 2009) and they do not consistently inform potential participants of the limits on confidentiality of participation (McCrady and Bux, 1999). Generally, there are three situations in which researchers incur a legal or ethical obligation to take action to protect the well-being of minor participants. When researchers also collect information from parents about themselves, these considerations typically also apply to parents.

First, state statute, case law, ethical considerations, and clinical standards of practice may create mandates for researchers to take appropriate steps to ensure the well-being of children and parents who provide information indicating that there is immediate risk for them to harm themselves or others (for further discussion, see Buchanan et al., 2009; Fisher and Goodman, 2009; Gable, 2009). Moreover, there are empirical data that suggest adolescents and their legal guardians expect that researchers will do so (Fisher et al., 1996; O'Sullivan and Fisher, 1997; Fisher, 2003). There are, however, also data suggesting that, although informing teens of ethical obligations to act on disclosures of risk of harm to self or others may not affect recruitment, doing so may affect disclosure of sensitive information involving risk of harm to self or others (Lothen-Kline et al., 2003).

Second, researchers may have a legal or ethical obligation to report to the child welfare system any potential child abuse or neglect that becomes evident during a research assessment. Although there has been extensive discussion about the question (e.g., see Steinberg et al., 1999; Allen, 2009), there is growing consensus that researchers have an ethical obligation to do so (for further discussion, see Allen, 2009). Furthermore, there are empirical data that suggest adolescents and their legal guardians believe that researchers should do so (e.g., see Fisher et al., 1996; O'Sullivan and Fisher, 1997), and the results of research done on the topic suggest that sensitive mandated reporting of potential child abuse or neglect does not threaten the integrity of recruitment or participation (Knight et al., 2006; Fuller et al., 2010). Assuming researchers decide to systematically report any situation that provokes reasonable concern that a child is being maltreated, the research team must develop clear procedures to effectively and sensitively manage the report to the child welfare system.

Finally, when children enrolled in genetic research present with evidence of serious emotional–behavioral difficulty, researchers may have an ethical obligation to take some reasonable action. The ethical obligation to do so may be even greater when children present with signs of serious emotional–behavioral difficulty for which they are not receiving clinical intervention. Unfortunately, there appears to be relatively little consensus among researchers, legal guardians, and minor participants about the circumstances under which researchers should do so (e.g., see Fisher et al., 1996; Fisher, 2003). Furthermore, even when there appears to be agreement that action should be taken, there does not appear to be agreement about how that should be done (e.g., see Fisher et al., 1996; Fisher, 2003), and depending on the circumstances, researchers may be able to choose among several different responses (for further discussion, see Wilfond and Carpenter, 2008).

Because children with a substance-abusing parent are at greater risk for both child abuse or neglect and clinically significant emotional–behavioral difficulty, researchers planning projects designed to characterize genetic risk must have clear procedures for responding to concerns about the well-being of children. Even if the research does not involve phenotyping of clinical syndromes or formal assessment of exposure to life events that may represent child abuse or neglect, researchers must be prepared to respond, because reports of threats to the well-being of children may become evident incidental to the research participation. That is, even if the research protocol does not involve formal assessment of clinical syndromes or exposure to psychological trauma, children may present with clinically significant signs and symptoms of emotional–behavioral difficulty or they may spontaneously make personal disclosures documenting exposure to potential child abuse or neglect.

When research focuses on genetic liability for substance abuse and phenotyping involves the systematic collection of information about early substance use, researchers will also have to consider how they will respond to reports of substance use that represents risk for lifelong problems with substance abuse. Because they will be pursuing the research with awareness of the long-term risk children with a substance-abusing parent incur, researchers working with this population have an ethical obligation to consider how best to respond to manifestations of that risk evident in the data they collect from children. Empirical data suggest that adolescents frequently believe researchers should not disclose substance use to parents or other adults (e.g., see Fisher et al., 1996; Fisher, 2003), and adolescents are typically afforded confidentiality concerning reports of substance use in epidemiologic research. However, the risk associated with substance use within this population is clearly not comparable to the risk associated with the same substance use within the general population. Consequently, researchers working with this population of children may have an ethical responsibility to respond to reports of substance use that represent early manifestations of that risk. When considering how best to respond, researchers should do so with awareness that substance use may be an emotionally laden issue within the family and adolescents frequently have a legal right to seek substance-abuse treatment without parental permission.

As research projects begin, researchers working with this high-risk population of children should, in consultation with community representatives, develop simple procedures to address ethical issues involving the disclosure of information provided during confidential participation. Fisher (1994, 2002; Fisher and Goodman, 2009) and others (e.g., Brooks-Gunn and Rotherham-Borus, 1994; Wilfond and Carpenter, 2008; Gable, 2009) have offered suggestions about a process to guide the development of research procedures that will govern the disclosure of confidential information provided by research participants. More specifically, Fisher and Goodman (2009) outlined a five-step process very relevant to genetic research being done with children affected by the substance abuse of their parents.

When examined from the perspective of Fisher and Goodman (2009), the first step in this process is to anticipate under what circumstances disclosures of information provided by children and their parents may be necessary and, as much as possible, define thresholds that will warrant a disclosure whether the information is provided in a spontaneous manner or within the structure of a research assessment. Some researchers (e.g., Wilfond and Carpenter, 2008) have suggested that only incidental findings with clear and proximate clinical importance warrant action. As outlined by Fisher and Goodman (2009), the second step in the process involves being clear about the legal dimensions of the potential need for disclosure, including disclosure of a concern to a legal guardian. State statutes and case law that afford minors of a certain age the right to seek health, mental-health, or substance-abuse services without permission from a legal guardian may be a consideration in the resolution of ethical questions concerning the clinical assessment of children participating in research, disclosure of clinical concerns to a legal guardian, and referral of children for further assessment. The next step involves generating ethical alternatives and selecting the best ethical position possible on disclosure. When considering alternatives, researchers need to be aware that some disclosures can place participants in social, psychological, economic, or legal jeopardy. They also need to recognize that procedures designed to protect the well-being of an individual participant may also threaten the social benefit of the study by compromising its scientific validity. Once the best ethical position has been defined, the research team needs to determine the resources necessary to implement the policy consistently.

As the study begins, researchers must, in the opinion of Fisher and Goodman (2009), establish clear procedures for the screening of data, and they must establish clear procedures for research assistants to secure immediate assistance from a licensed health-care professional when there are questions about situations that may warrant a response from the research team. The fourth step in this process involves clearly communicating the disclosure policy to: (1) the research team during training sessions; (2) parents when securing permission for their children to participate; and (3) children when securing their assent for participation. The final step requires that investigators monitor implementation of the disclosure policy, solicit feedback from the research team, consult with affected participants, and if indicated, modify the policy and procedures as the study evolves over time.

When a research assessment suggests the presence of serious emotional–behavioral difficulty, including serious substance use, Fisher (1993) has also outlined a procedure whereby a researcher who is qualified to do so asks the child and a legal guardian to participate in a clinical assessment. Depending on the situation, the clinical assessment might begin with the child alone and, if indicated, include a direct request for permission to discuss the concern with a legal guardian. If that assessment confirms the presence of serious difficulty, the need for clinical intervention should be reviewed and an appropriate referral should be made. *A priori*, the research team should, as much as possible, be clear under what circumstances the concern will and will not be disclosed to a legal guardian, particularly if the child does not provide permission for the research team to do so. Again, children and their legal guardians should be advised of these procedures when providing permission, consent, or assent for participation in the study.

Ethical considerations related to genotyping

Genetic research pursued with children affected by parental substance abuse will also raise ethical issues specific to the genotyping. Historically, genetic testing has been viewed differently from other medical testing because of the risk of social and psychological harm to the individual undergoing testing that can extend to family members. Within this type of research, the critical ethical questions involve concern about balancing the right to disclosure of information about genetic liability against the potential for harm associated with disclosure of information about genetic liability for disease. When children participate in genetic research, the ethical questions become more complex, because children do not provide consent for their participation. Consequently, the burden to protect minors participating in genetic research is high because children typically do not have the legal authority to make informed decisions on their own, and research suggests that neither children nor their legal guardians are likely to appreciate the risks associated with participation in this type of research (Gillam et al., 2006; Coors and Raymond, 2009).

Current guidelines dictate that, whether done for clinical or research purposes, genetic information provided to individuals must be derived from a genetic analysis done in a laboratory that meets Clinical Laboratory Improvement Amendments (CLIA) standards, and the genetic information must have some degree of reasonable medical certainty (for further discussion, see Bookman et al., 2006). Although there is presently no agreement about the disclosure of genetic results to research participants (e.g., see Clayton and Ross, 2006 versus Shalowitz and Miller, 2005, 2006; Meltzer, 2006 versus Ravitsky and Wilfond, 2006), professionals have generally argued against providing genetic information to parents or children participating in susceptibility research unless the results will inform preventive or clinical intervention for a disease process likely to begin during childhood or adolescence (for further discussion, see Elger, 2010). However, it is important to note that current practice may be at odds with the results of qualitative research that suggests most parents believe they should be able to receive information about genetic liability (e.g., see Gillam et al., 2006; Coors and Raymond, 2009).

Although there may presently be agreement that there is no sound ethical argument to provide research participants with ambiguous information about the genetic liability of children, ethical issues associated with genotyping of liability for substance abuse will become even more complicated as typing of genetic markers for phenotypes representing complex behavioral syndromes becomes more sophisticated. Looking to the near future, ethical questions about disclosure of genetic information to parents and children will also become increasingly complex as understanding of the ways in which phenotypes representing genetic liability interact with environmental exposure to moderate risk for the development of substance abuse and related problems. Moreover, ethical questions may be complicated by the fact that understanding of genetic liability will, as Biesecker and Peay (2003) suggested, probably precede the development of targeted prevention that can systematically mitigate risk. Although conceptual frameworks to guide decision making about disclosure of genetic information to individuals have been developed (e.g., see Ravitsky and Wilfond, 2006), there are not yet clear standards to guide decision making about the clinical significance of specific genetic profiles and the release of information concerning genetic liability (Biesecker and Peay, 2003).

Moreover, it is important to note that, regardless of professional standards, the potential benefit of having versus not having information concerning genetic liability is a highly personal matter. Although most parents indicate they want information about markers of genetic risk for their children, some parents may not want that information, even if it is of clinical importance (Swartling et al., 2007). It is also possible that a parent and child may not agree about receiving information about genetic risk. With time, the social and psychological consequences of providing information will undoubtedly become clearer (e.g., see McConkie-Rosell et al., 2008), and that information will have to be factored into ethical decisions about disclosure of genetic risk.

As the ethical considerations become more focused, questions regarding who decides about the release of information concerning the genetic liability of children under specific circumstances will become increasingly complex when the information may cause psychological, familial, and social changes with the potential to positively or negatively affect the psychosocial development of the children (for further discussion, see Elger, 2010). Considerations for younger children may also be different from those for adolescents entering the developmental period during which chronic substance use typically begins (for further discussion, see Elger, 2010). When science advances to the point that researchers may have an ethical obligation to offer participants information about genetic liability, there will have to be clear criteria and procedures that address a number of difficult ethical issues specific to genetic research being pursued with children (for further discussion, see Biesecker and Peay, 2003; Burke and Diekma, 2006; Elger, 2010).

While debate continues about the circumstances under which information about genetic risk generated by participation in research may be released to parents and children, it is important to note that there is similar controversy about disclosure of incidental findings (for further discussion, see Clayton, 2008; Van Ness, 2008). When genetic information is gathered from children and parents, one of the common incidental findings is misattributed parentage, particularly misattributed paternity. This is an important ethical issue involving complicated questions about competing interests within the family, reasons for disclosure, and potential harm about which clinicians and researchers do not agree (for further discussion, see Ross, 1996). Despite the concern within professional circles, parents considering participation in genetic research do not report being very concerned about the controversy (Gillam et al., 2006), and they believe parents should be informed about the potential for disclosure of misattributed paternity (Gillam et al., 2006). Like clinicians and researchers, they do not agree about what should be done when it is discovered (Turney, 2005).

Given the absence of clear ethical standards, most researchers have argued against disclosure of misattributed parentage, even if parents are interested in receiving the information. When proposing standards against disclosure, researchers have argued that, in the absence of clear and proximate clinical benefit to children, the social and psychological risks associated with disclosure of misattributed parentage may outweigh any potential benefit. Furthermore, even if one could argue that disclosure of genetic information might have clear and proximate clinical importance, parents and children may not want the information. For researchers considering procedures to address questions concerning misattributed parentage, it is important to note that, although parents and children may have an interest in confirming biological parentage while participating in genetic research, they can be told that this will not be done within a study of genetic risk, and they can be referred to a clinical service where clinicians are available to help the family cope with the psychosocial complexity surrounding misattributed parentage. Again, consultation with potential participants may help clarify procedures to deal with this complex issue in a sensitive, ethical manner.

Ethical considerations related to payment of parents and children

Wendler et al. (2002) distinguished four types of payment related to participation in research: (1) reimbursements for expenses related to participation; (2) gifts of appreciation; (3) compensation for the time devoted to participation; and (4) incentive payments. Unfortunately, there is relatively little systematic information concerning the use of different forms of compensation in research being done with children where there is no potential for direct benefit. What data are available suggest that institutional review boards vary significantly in their position on compensation for parents and children participating in research (e.g., see Weise et al., 2002), even when considering the same research protocol (e.g., see Whittle et al., 2004). Surveys of researchers also suggest tremendous variability in patterns of payment across research protocols that seems to be unrelated to the nature of the research (e.g., see Borzekowski et al., 2003; Iltis et al., 2006).

In policy statements, review groups (e.g., see Field and Behrman, 2004) usually take the position that it is appropriate for researchers to offer reimbursement for expenses directly related to participation in research. After that, there does not appear to be clear agreement about offering compensation to parents and children. Much of the disagreement centers on offering compensation and incentive payments to children (for further discussion, see Fernhoff, 2002 versus Wendler et al., 2002). If researchers choose to offer payment for time spent completing the research procedures, ethicists (e.g., see Wendler et al., 2002) consistently argue that compensation should not be structured in a way that unduly influences decisions about participation. Researchers should be particularly sensitive to questions about compensation and incentives when the study involves the recruitment of children living in family systems with limited economic resources. Although not supported by others (e.g., see Wendler et al., 2002; Field and Behrman, 2004), the American Academy of Pediatrics (1995) has suggested that compensation for participation should not be reviewed until after decisions about participation have been made. Federal guidelines (US Department of Health and Human Services, 1993) and recommendations by ethicists (e.g., see Wendler et al., 2002) suggest that compensation for research participation should never be listed as a potential benefit of participation.

Although it may be reasonable to compensate parents for the time they spend completing research procedures, incentive payments to parents to facilitate the participation of children is generally opposed because it may induce parents to exploit their position as decision-makers for children to benefit financially without having to incur any of the risks associated with participation (American Academy of Pediatrics, 1995; Wendler et al., 2002). Incentive payments to parents that are somehow tied to participation of children, such as a bonus payment to a parent if a parent–child dyad completes the study, may also be inappropriate because they may create a situation in which adults pressure children to participate (for further discussion, see Wendler et al., 2002; Field and Behrman, 2004). Although researchers and institutional review boards may be concerned about substance-abusing parents viewing research compensation as income to purchase alcohol or illicit drugs, Fry and Dwyer (2001) found that motivations to participate in research vary within populations of substance-abusing adults. Festinger et al. (2005) found that substance-abusing adults did not view research payments as coercive and such payments did not seem to contribute to any increase in substance use. In other research, Crider et al. (2006) noted that relatively small incentive payments increased participation in a genetic study of relative risk that involved collection of DNA samples from mothers and their infant children, particularly for ethnic minority mothers and their children, but the increase was not dramatic. Festinger et al. (2005) also found that incentive payments increased rates of follow-up in a short-term longitudinal study of substance abuse.

When research involves no potential for benefit and little burden beyond inconvenience, advisory groups (e.g., see Field and Behrman, 2004), ethicists (e.g., see Wendler et al., 2002), researchers (e.g., see Borzekowski et al., 2003), and many institutional review boards (e.g., see Whittle et al., 2004) believe that it is appropriate to offer children reasonable compensation for their participation, and some (e.g., see Bagley et al., 2007) believe that it is appropriate to compensate children in the same manner that researchers would compensate adults, as long as the compensation is not used to unduly influence parents and children. Although the data are somewhat inconsistent across investigations, empirical support for this position comes from research that suggests financial compensation may be a key reason that parents and children participate in research that holds no promise of direct benefit (for a review, see Field and Behrman, 2004). In a qualitative study of payment issues, Bagley et al. (2007) recently argued that payment for research participation should be informed by developmental research on age-related differences in the concepts of time and money, and they suggested that younger children should be offered an age-appropriate gift of appreciation for participation in research and older children should be offered reasonable financial compensation for time and effort devoted to participation in research. When offering financial compensation for participation in substance-abuse research, researchers should be aware that Fisher (2003) found evidence that there may be risk for potential participants to lie about eligibility to secure access to payment for participation.

Ethical considerations related to biodata banks

Over the past ten years, researchers have begun to systematically collect and bank biogenetic samples to support genetic epidemiological research. Many biobanks do not, by design, presently include biodata collected from children, in part because decisions concerning the use of human tissue in biodata banks are regarded as a right of the individual and it is not clear who provides consent for the use of human tissue collected from children (for further discussion, see Williams, 2005). However, exclusion of children from biodata banks may involve social and personal costs of importance to children as a class of individuals, and ethical issues relevant to the storage and use of human tissue collected from children need to be considered in the context of several large, longitudinal investigations being pursued around the world in an effort to clarify genetic and environmental liability for disease processes known to begin during childhood and adolescence (e.g., see Landrigan et al., 2006). To inform thinking about the ethical issues, Hens et al. (2009) recently did a systematic review of the existing literature on the participation of children in research involving the storage of biodata, and they distilled five clusters of ethical issues relevant to the use of biobanks.

As might be expected, the five clusters of questions outlined by Hens et al. (2009) involved issues pertaining to: (1) consent; (2) potential risks; (3) potential benefits; (4) disclosure; and (5) rights of ownership. For researchers considering the long-term storage of biogenetic samples it is important to note that, in addition to realizing the complexity of the ethical issues, Hens et al. (2009) concluded that there were considerations that made the ethical issues associated with the storage of biogenetic samples obtained from children different from the ethical issues associated with the storage of biogenetic samples obtained from adults. Given the focus of this discussion, researchers considering longer-term storage of genetic material should be aware that there are unresolved questions about parental permission, child assent, and child consent at age of majority. There are also ethical questions about the identifiability and confidentiality of genetic material entered into biodata banks, particularly as sequencing and matching of DNA samples becomes increasingly feasible, and there are questions about asking children, even with parental permission, to assume unforeseen risks largely for the benefit of others. When samples can be linked to individuals, there are difficult questions about the return of information to children and parents, particularly unexpected or incidental information about risk for other disease processes, and even when permission for long-term storage has been secured, there will be questions about ownership of the samples. It is also important to note that Hens et al. (2009) did not explore complex issues associated with commercial use of biogenetic samples banked for use in the study of relative risk.

Finally, it is interesting that, in the midst of ongoing debate about the long-term storage of genetic material for use in research, Gurwitz et al. (2009) recently distinguished between biodata banks established for cohorts of children with a specific disease and cohorts of children recruited to study relative risk. They argued that the balance of risks against benefits is different when genetic material is being used to advance research on a specific disease affecting the children. Under these circumstances, they believe that, with appropriate ethical and administrative oversight, it is appropriate for parents to grant permission for genetic and phenotypic data to be shared with researchers pursuing projects directly related to the diagnosis and treatment of the disease in question. From their perspective, participants should then be contacted at the age of majority to provide consent for continued use of their genetic and phenotypic data.

In contrast to this, Gurwitz et al. (2009) argued that the balance of risks against benefits is different when genetic material is collected from a cohort of children to document genetic liability within the general population. Under these circumstances, they believe that it is appropriate for parents to grant permission for genetic and phenotypic data to be banked, but they do not believe it is appropriate to release the data of any specific individual to researchers outside the biodata bank until participants reach the age of majority and can provide consent for the use of their data as an adult. Gurwitz et al. (2009) believe that, until participants reached the age of majority, biodata banks should be responsible to aggregate genetic data for publication, but they should not be able to release individual-level data to other researchers. Consistent with this, some large genetic investigations of relative risk in children have been limiting access to genetic information concerning individual participants to primary investigators protected by a Certificate of Confidentiality (e.g., see Jenkins et al., 2008).

Ethical considerations related to institutional review

Institutional review of genetic research being done with children affected by parental substance abuse may pose special challenges from the perspective of institutional review. Institutional review boards responsible for evaluating protocols involving clinical research being pursued with this population of children should have reviewers who can integrate expertise drawn from the fields of substance abuse, genetics, family process, and child development. Consistent with the value of community participation, institutional review boards may also want to consult with community representatives, substance-abusing parents, and affected children. Clear institutional policy and procedures on: (1) parental permission, (2) child assent, (3) mandated reporting of child abuse or neglect, (4) release of genetic information, (5) payment of children for research participation, and (6) banking of biogenetic samples will also facilitate systematic review of genetic research pursued with this particular population of children.

Conclusion

As genetic research continues to move beyond the study of relatively rare clinical syndromes associated with a single gene toward the study of complex behavioral syndromes involving the interaction of genetic risk with environmental exposure, family-oriented research on genetic liability for substance abuse will require that children at risk because of a positive family history participate in increasingly sophisticated, longitudinal research. Greater understanding of genetic risk will also spawn increasingly sophisticated investigations of prevention, early intervention, and treatment that incorporate information about genetic liability. As this work expands, researchers will be required to negotiate a complex array of ethical considerations involving the recruitment, enrollment, phenotyping, genotyping, and payment of children with a substance-abusing parent. Over time, the ethical challenges will involve questions about how to best balance the need to protect this vulnerable population of children participating in research from which they will probably not derive direct benefit against the need to generate scientific knowledge that will support the development of more effective approaches to prevention, early intervention, and ongoing treatment for other members of this vulnerable population of children.

References

Abramovitch, R., Freedman, J. L., Henry, K., and Van Brunschot, M. (1995). Children's capacity to agree to psychological research: Knowledge of risks and benefits and voluntariness. *Ethics and Behavior*, 5, 25–48.

Allen, B. (2009). Are researchers ethically obligated to report suspected child maltreatment? A critical analysis of opposing perspectives. *Ethics and Behavior*, 19, 15–24.

American Academy of Pediatrics (1995). Guidelines for the ethical conduct of studies to evaluate drugs in pediatric populations. *Pediatrics*, 95, 286–294.

Anderson, E. E. and DuBois, J. M. (2007). The need for evidence-based research ethics: A review of the substance abuse literature. *Drug and Alcohol Dependence*, 86, 95–105.

Appelbaum, P., Roth, L., and Lidz, C. (1982). The therapeutic misconception: Informed consent in psychiatric research. *International Journal of Law and Psychiatry*, 5, 319–329.

Bagley, S. J., Reynolds, W. W., and Nelson, R. M. (2007). Is a "wage-payment" model for research participation appropriate for children? *Pediatrics*, 119, 46–51.

Bernhardt, B. A., Tambor, E. S., Fraser, G., Wissow, L. S., and Geller, G. (2003). Parents' and children's attitudes toward the enrollment of minors in genetic susceptibility research: Implications for informed consent. *American Journal of Medical Genetics*, 116A, 315–323.

Beskow, L. M., Botkin, J. R., Daly, M., et al. (2004). Ethical issues in identifying and recruiting participants for familial genetic research. *American Journal of Medical Genetics*, 130A, 424–431.

Bierut, L. J., Dinwiddie, S. H., Begleiter, H., et al. (1998). Familial transmission of substance dependence: Alcohol, marijuana, cocaine, and habitual smoking. A report from the Collaborative Study on the Genetics of Alcoholism. *Archives of General Psychiatry*, 55, 982–988.

Bierut, L. J., Agrawal, A., Bucholz, K. K., et al. (2010). A genome-wide association study of alcohol dependence. *Proceedings of the National Academy of Sciences*, 107, 5082–5087.

Biesecker, B. B. and Peay, H. L. (2003). Ethical issues in psychiatric genetics research: Points to consider. *Psychopharmacology*, 171, 27–35.

Bookman, E. B., Langehorne, A. A., Eckfeldt, J. H., et al. (2006). Reporting genetic results in research studies: Summary and recommendations of an NHLBI working group. *American Journal of Medical Genetics*, 140A, 1033–1040.

Borzekowski, D. L. G., Rickert, V. I., Ipp, L., and Fortenberry, J. D. (2003). At what price? The current state of subject payment in adolescent research. *Journal of Adolescent Health*, 33, 378–384.

Brooks-Gunn, J. and Rotherham-Borus, M. J. (1994). Right to privacy in research: Adolescents versus parents. *Ethics and Behavior*, 4, 109–121.

Bruzzese, J. M. and Fisher, C. B. (2003). Assessing and enhancing the research consent capacity of children and youth. *Applied Developmental Research*, 7, 13–16.

Buchanan, D., Gable, L., and Fisher, C. B. (2009). Best practices for responding to threats of violence in research ethically and legally. In D. Buchanan, C. B. Fisher, and L. Gable (eds.), *Research with High-risk Populations: Balancing Science, Ethics, and Law*. Washington, DC: American Psychological Association, pp. 233–252.

Burke, W. and Diekma, D. S. (2006). Ethical issues arising from the participation of children in genetic research. *Journal of Pediatrics*, 149, S34–S38.

Chassin, L., Curran, P. J., Hussong, A. M., and Colder, C. R. (1996). The relation of parent alcoholism to adolescent substance use: A longitudinal follow-up study. *Journal of Abnormal Psychology*, 105, 70–80.

Child Welfare League of America (2001). *Alcohol, Other Drugs, and Child Welfare*. Washington, DC: Child Welfare League of America.

Clayton, E. W. (2008). Incidental findings in genetics research using archived DNA. *Journal of Law, Medicine, and Ethics*, 36, 286–291.

Clayton, E. W. and Ross, L. F. (2006). Implications of disclosing individual results of clinical research. *JAMA: The Journal of the American Medical Association*, 295, 37.

Coors, M. E. and Raymond, K. M. (2009). Substance use disorder genetic research: Investigators and participants grapple with the ethical issues. *Psychiatric Genetics*, 19, 83–90.

Crider, K. S., Reefhuis, J., Woomert, A., and Honein, M. A. (2006). Racial and ethnic disparity in participation in DNA collection at the Atlanta site of the National Birth Defects Prevention Study. *American Journal of Epidemiology*, 164, 805–812.

Dorn, L. D., Susman, E. J., and Fletcher, J. C. (1995). Informed consent in children and adolescents: Age, maturation and psychological state. *Journal of Adolescent Health*, 16, 185–190.

Elger, B. S. (2010). Ethical, legal, and social issues in the genetic testing of minors. In K.P. Tercyak (ed.), *Handbook of Genomics and the Family: Psychosocial Context for Children and Adolescents*. New York: Springer Science and Business Media, pp. 485–521.

Emanuel, E., Wendler, D., and Grady, C. (2000). What makes clinical research ethical? *JAMA: The Journal of the American Medical Association*, 283, 2701–2711.

Emanuel, E. J., Wendler, D., Killen, J., and Grady, C. (2004). What makes clinical research in developing countries ethical? The benchmarks of ethical research. *Journal of Infectious Diseases*, 189, 930–937.

Fernhoff, P. M. (2002). Paying for children to participate in research: A slippery slope or an enlightened stairway? *Journal of Pediatrics*, 141, 153–154.

Festinger, D., Marlowe, D., Croft, J., et al. (2005). Do research payments precipitate drug use or coerce participation? *Drug and Alcohol Dependence*, 78, 275–281.

Field, M. J. and Behrman, R. E. (eds.) (2004). *The Ethical Conduct of Research Involving Children*. Washington, DC: National Academies Press.

Fisher, C. B. (1993). Integrating science and ethics in research with high-risk children and youth. *SCRD Social Policy Report*, 7, 1–27.

Fisher, C. B. (1994). Reporting and referring research participants: Ethical challenges for investigators studying children and youth. *Ethics and Behavior*, 4, 87–95.

Fisher, C. B. (1997). A relational perspective on ethics-in-science decision making for research with vulnerable populations. *IRB: Review of Human Subjects Research*, 19, 1–4.

Fisher, C. B. (1999). Relational ethics and research with vulnerable populations. In National Bioethics Advisory Commission (eds.), *Research Involving Persons with Mental Disorders that May Affect Decision Making Capacity. Volume II: Commissioned Papers by the National Bioethics Advisory*

Commission. Rockville, MD: US Government Printing Office, pp. 29–49.

Fisher, C. B. (2000). Relational ethics in psychological research: One feminist's journey. In M. Brabeck (ed.), *Practicing Feminist Ethics in Psychology*. Washington, DC: American Psychological Association, pp. 125–142.

Fisher, C. B. (2002). Participant consultation: Ethical insights into parental permission and confidentiality procedures for policy relevant research with youth. In R. M. Lemer, F. Jacobs, and D. Wertlieb (eds.), *Handbook of Applied Developmental Science*, vol. 4. Thousand Oaks, CA: Sage Publications, pp. 371–396.

Fisher, C. B. (2003). Adolescent and parent perspectives on ethical issues in youth drug use and suicide survey research. *Ethics and Behavior*, 13, 303–332.

Fisher, C. B. and Goodman, S. J. (2009). Goodness-of-fit ethics for nonintervention research involving dangerous and illegal behavior. In D. Buchanan, C. B. Fisher, and L. Gable (eds.), *Research with High-risk Populations: Balancing Science, Ethics, and Law*. Washington, DC: American Psychological Association, pp. 25–46.

Fisher, C. B. and Masty, J. K. (2006a). A goodness-of-fit ethic for informed consent to pediatric cancer research. In R. T. Brown (ed.), *Comprehensive Handbook of Childhood Cancer and Sickle Cell Disease*. New York: Oxford University Press, pp. 205–217.

Fisher, C. B. and Masty, J. K. (2006b). Community perspectives on the ethics of adolescent risk research. In B. Leadbeater, T. Reicken, C. Benoit, M. Jansson, and A. Marshall (eds.), *Research Ethics in Community-based and Participatory Action Research with Youth*. Toronto: University of Toronto Press, pp. 22–41.

Fisher, C. B. and Ragsdale, K. (2006). A goodness-of-fit ethics for multicultural research. In J. Trimble and C. B. Fisher (eds.), *The Handbook of Ethical Research with Ethnocultural Populations and Communities*. Thousand Oaks, CA: Sage Publications, pp. 3–26.

Fisher, C. B., Higgins-D'Alessandro, A., Rau, J. B., Kuther, T. L., and Belnager, S. (1996). Referring and reporting research participants at risk: Views from urban adolescents. *Child Development*, 67, 2086–2100.

Fisher, C. B., Hoagwood, K., Boyce, C., et al. (2002). Research ethics for mental health science involving ethnic minority children and youths. *American Psychologist*, 57, 1024–1040.

Fry, C. and Dwyer, R. (2001). For love or money? An exploratory study of why injecting drug users participate in research. *Addiction*, 96, 1319–1325.

Fuller, K. J., Smith, K. R., Dolan, M., and Cohen, L. M. (2010). *Mandatory Reporting: Potential Effects on Retention Rates in a Longitudinal Survey*. Paper presented at the annual conference of the American Association of Public Opinion Research, Chicago, IL. Available online at: www.rti.org/publications/rtipress.cfm?pub=14879 [accessed February 21, 2012].

Gable, L. (2009). Legal challenges raised by non-intervention research conducted under high-risk circumstances. In D. Buchanan, C. B. Fisher, and L. Gable (eds.), *Research with High-risk Populations: Balancing Science, Ethics, and Law*. Washington, DC: American Psychological Association, pp. 47–74.

Geller, G., Tambor, E. S., Bernhardt, B. A., Fraser, G., and Wissow, L. S. (2003). Informed consent for enrolling minors in genetic susceptibility research: A qualitative study of at-risk children's and parents' views about children's role in decision-making. *Journal of Adolescent Health*, 32, 260–271.

Gillam, L., Poulakis, Z., Tobin, S., and Wake, M. (2006). Enhancing the ethical conduct of genetic research: Investigating views of parents on including their healthy children in a study of mild hearing loss. *Journal of Medical Ethics*, 32, 537–541.

Gurwitz, D., Fortier, I., Lunshof, J. E., and Knoppers, B. M. (2009). Research ethics: Children and population biobanks. *Science*, 325, 818–819.

Hens, K., Nys, H., Cassiman, J. J., and Dierickx, K. (2009). Genetic research on stored tissue samples from minors: A systematic review of the ethical literature. *American Journal of Medical Genetics*, 149A, 2346–2358.

Hicks, B. M., Krueger, R. F., Iacono, W. G., McGue, M., and Patrick, C. J. (2004). Family transmission and heritability of externalizing disorders: A twin-family study. *Archives of General Psychiatry*, 61, 922–928.

Iltis, A. S., DeVader, S., and Matsuo, H. (2006). Payments to children and adolescents enrolled in research: A pilot study. *Pediatircs*, 118, 1546–1552.

Jenkins, M. M., Rasmussen, S. A., Moore, C. A., and Honein, M. A. (2008). Ethical issues raised by incorporation of genetics into the National Birth Defects Prevention Study. *American Journal of Medical Genetics*, 148C, 40–46.

Kaufman, D., Geller, G., LeRoy, L., et al. (2008). Ethical implications of including children in a large biobank for genetic-epidemiologic research: A qualitative study of public opinion. *American Journal of Medical Genetics*, 148C, 31–39.

Kendler, K. S., Jacobson, K. C., Prescott, C. A., and Neale, M. C. (2003). Specificity of genetic and environmental risk factors for use and abuse/dependence of cannabis, cocaine, hallucinogens, sedatives, stimulants, and opiates in male twins. *American Journal of Psychiatry*, 160, 687–695.

Knight, E. D., Smith, J. B., Dubowitz, H., et al. (2006). Reporting participants in research studies to child protective services: Limited risk to attrition. *Child Maltreatment*, 11, 257–262.

Kreek, M. J., Neilson, D. A., Butelman, E. R., and LaForge, K. S. (2005). Genetic influences on impulsivity, risk-taking, and stress reactivity and vulnerability to drug abuse and addiction. *Nature Neuroscience*, 8, 1450–1457.

Kreiger, N., Ashbury, F., Cotterchio, M., and Macey, J. (2001). A qualitative study of subject recruitment for familial cancer research. *Annals of Epidemiology*, 11, 219–224.

Landrigan, P. J., Trasande, L., Thorpe, L. E., et al. (2006). The National Children's Study: A 21-year prospective study of 100,000 American children. *Pediatrics*, 118, 2173–2186.

Lothen-Kline, C., Howard, D. E., Hamburger, E. K., Worrell, K. D., and Boekeloo, B. O. (2003). Truth and consequences: Ethics, confidentiality, and disclosure in adolescent longitudinal prevention research. *Journal of Adolescent Health*, 33, 385–394.

Masty, J. and Fisher, C. B. (2008). A goodness of fit approach to parent permission and child assent pediatric intervention research. *Ethics and Behavior*, 13, 139–160.

McConkie-Rosell, A., Spiridigliozzi, G. A., Melvin, E., Dawson, D. V., and Lachiewicz, A. M. (2008). Living with genetic risk: Effect on adolescent self-concept. *American Journal of Medical Genetics*, 148C, 56–69.

McCrady, B. and Bux, D. J. (1999). Ethical issues in informed consent with substance abusers. *Journal of Consulting and Clinical Psychology*, 67, 186–193.

Meltzer, L A. (2006). Undesirable implications for disclosing individual genetic results to research participants. *American Journal of Bioethics*, 6, 28–30.

Merikangas, K. R., Stolar, M., Stevens, D. E., et al. (1998). Familial transmission of substance use disorders. *Archives of General Psychiatry*, 55, 973–979.

National Commission for the Protection of Human Subjects of Biomedical and Behavioral Research (1979). *The Belmont Report: Ethical Principles for the Protection of Human Subjects of Research* (GPO 887–809). Washington, DC: US Government Printing Office.

O'Sullivan, C. and Fisher, C. B. (1997). The effect of confidentiality and reporting procedures on parent-child agreement to participate in adolescent risk research. *Applied Developmental Science*, 1, 187–199.

Ravitsky, V. and Wilfond, B. S. (2006). Disclosing individual genetic results to research participants. *American Journal of Bioethics*, 6, 8–17.

Rhee, S. H., Hewitt, J. K., Young, S. E., et al. (2003). Genetic and environmental influences on substance initiation, use, and problem use in adolescents. *Archives of General Psychiatry*, 60, 1256–1264.

Ross, L. F. (1996). Disclosing misattributed paternity. *Bioethics*, 10, 114–130.

Rounsaville, B. J., Kosten, T. R., Weissman, M. M., et al. (1991). Psychiatric disorders in relatives of probands with opiate addiction. *Archives of General Psychiatry*, 48, 33–42.

Santelli, J., Geller, G., and Chen, D. T. (2005). Recruitment of pregnant, minor adolescents and minor adolescents at risk of pregnancy into longitudinal, observational research: The case of the National Children's Study. In E. Kodish (ed.), *Ethics and Research with Children*. New York: Oxford University Press, pp. 100–122.

Schulenberg, J. E. and Maggs, J. L. (eds.) (2008). Destiny matters: Childhood and adolescent prediction of adult alcohol use and abuse in six multi-decade longitudinal studies [Special Issue]. *Addiction*, 103 (Suppl. 1).

Shalowitz, D. I. and Miller, F. G. (2005). Disclosing individual results of clinical research: implications of respect for participants. *JAMA: The Journal of the American Medical Association*, 294, 737–740.

Shalowitz, D. I. and Miller, F. G. (2006). Implications of disclosing individual results of clinical research: Reply. *JAMA: The Journal of the American Medical Association*, 295, 37.

Steinberg, A. M., Pynoos, R. S., Goenjian, A. K., Sossanabadi, H., and Sherr, L. (1999). Are researchers bound by child abuse reporting laws? *Child Abuse and Neglect*, 23, 771–777.

Swartling, U., Eriksson, S., Ludvigsson, J., and Helgesson, G. (2007). Concern, pressure, and lack of knowledge affect choice of not wanting to know high-risk status. *European Journal of Human Genetics*, 15, 556–562.

Tait, A. R., Voepel-Lewis, T., and Malviya, S. (2003). Do they understand? Part I: Parental consent for children participating in clinical anesthesia and surgery research. *Anesthesiology*, 98, 603–608.

Tarter, R. E., Vanyukov, M. M., Giancola, P., et al. (1999). Etiology of early age onset substance use disorder: A maturational perspective. *Development and Psychopathology*, 11, 657–683.

Tsuang, M. T., Lyons, M. J., Meyer, J. M., et al. (1998). Co-occurrence of abuse of different drugs in men: The role of drug-specific and shared vulnerabilities. *Archives of General Psychiatry*, 55, 967–972.

Turney, L. (2005). The incidental discovery of nonpaternity through genetic carrier screening: An exploration of lay attitudes. *Qualitative Health Research*, 15, 620–634.

Uhl, G. R., Drgon, T., Liu, Q. R., et al. (2008). Genome-wide association for methamphetamine dependence: Convergent results from two samples. *Archives of General Psychiatry*, 65, 345–355.

US Department of Health and Human Services (2009). *Code of Federal Regulations, Title 45: Public Welfare, Part 46: Protection of Human Subjects*, 45 CFR § 46.101–46.505.

US Department of Health and Human Services, Office of Protection from Research Risks. (1993). *Protecting human research subjects: Institutional review board guidebook*. Washington, DC: US Government Printing Office.

Van Ness, B. (2008). Genomic research and incidental findings. *Journal of Law, Medicine, and Ethics*, 36, 92–97.

Vanyukov, M. M., Tarter, R. E., Kirisci, L., et al. (2003). Liability to substance use disorders: 1. Common mechanisms and manifestations. *Neuroscience and Biobehavioral Reviews*, 27, 507–515.

Varma, S. and Wendler, D. (2008). Research involving wards of the state: Protecting particularly vulnerable children. *Journal of Pediatrics*, 152, 9–14.

Weir, R. F. and Horton, J. R. (1995). Genetic research, adolescents, and informed consent. *Theoretical Medicine*, 16, 347–373.

Weise, K. L., Smith, M. L., Maschke, K. J., and Copeland, H. L. (2002). National practices regarding payment to research subjects for participating in pediatric research. *Pediatrics*, 110, 577–582.

Wendler, D., Rackoff, J., Emanuel, E. J., and Grady, C. (2002). The ethics of paying for children's research participation. *Journal of Pediatrics*, 141, 166–171.

Whittle, A., Shah, S., Wilfond, B., Gensler, G., and Wendler, D. (2004). Institutional review board practices regarding assent in pediatric research. *Pediatrics*, 113, 1747–1752.

Wilfond, B. W. and Carpenter, K. J. (2008). Incidental findings in pediatric research. *Journal of Law, Medicine, and Ethics*, 36, 332–340.

Williams, G. (2005). Bioethics and large-scale biobanking: Individualistic ethics and collective projects. *Genomics, Society, and Policy*, 1, 50–65.

Wolthers, O. D. (2006). A questionnaire on factors influencing children's assent and dissent to non-therapeutic research. *Journal of Medical Ethics*, 32, 292–297.

Zhou, Q., King, K. M., and Chassin, L. (2006). The roles of familial alcoholism and adolescent family harmony in young adults' substance dependence disorders: Mediated and moderated relations. *Journal of Abnormal Psychology*, 115, 320–331.

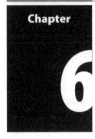

Protecting privacy in genetic research on alcohol dependence and other addictions

Mark A. Rothstein

Introduction

From the official beginning of the Human Genome Project in 1990 to the present, genomic and genetic research has been characterized by its enormous scale. Genome researchers often analyze and manipulate vast data sets derived from the 3.2 billion base-pair human genome. Other new "omics" fields, such as proteomics, transcriptomics, and metabonomics, also involve large-scale research undertakings. To facilitate these efforts, research biobanks containing many thousands of biological specimens are used to provide statistically significant numbers of even rare genomic variants. Genome research also requires sophisticated, high-speed computational technology for genome-wide association studies and other analytical techniques. The phenotypic data for researchers increasingly come from electronic health records (EHR), another automated and large-scale contribution to the scientific enterprise.

Some areas of genome research involve especially sensitive or stigmatizing health conditions, such as behavioral health. For example, substantial genetic research has established correlations between certain genes and a propensity to addictive behavior, including gambling and the use of alcohol, tobacco, and various licit and illicit substances (Blum et al., 2000; Caron et al., 2005; Goldman et al., 2005). When large-scale biomedical research and powerful computational technologies are combined and applied to research involving sensitive health conditions, a range of important privacy issues are raised. These issues include: the consent needed for using biological specimens and health records, even if de-identified; the tangible and intangible harms, including group-based harms, that can flow from disclosure of genetic information; and the autonomy interests of individuals in controlling the uses of their specimens and health records.

Privacy issues raised by different research methods

Biobanks

Biobanks are repositories of human biological materials collected for biomedical research. As of 2011, there were in excess of 500 million stored specimens in hundreds of biobanks in the United States, and the number grows by at least 20 million per year (Eiseman and Haga, 1999).[1] Biobanks are an integral part of large-scale, high-throughput genetic research,

---

Genetic Research on Addiction, ed. Audrey R. Chapman. Published by Cambridge University Press. © Cambridge University Press 2012.

[1] Eiseman and Haga's estimate in 1999 of "at least 300 million" extant samples and 20 million new samples each year is still the most widely cited reference. The 500 million sample estimate in the text

because they enable researchers to correlate even rare genetic variations in the specimens with documented health effects. Unlike much traditional biomedical research, which involved obtaining individual consent and individual specimens for a single study, biobanks facilitate numerous, future, unspecified research by investigators whose research project and personal identity are unlikely to be known at the time the sample is obtained. Thus, the one study/one consent model does not comport with modern biobank-based research.

Informed consent is the most important and contentious ethical issue in research using biobanks. There is no single rule on whether informed consent is legally required under the Federal Policy for the Protection of Human Subjects (Common Rule) (45 CFR Part 46) or whether authorization is required under the Health Insurance Portability and Accountability Act's Standards for the Protection of Individually Identifiable Information (Privacy Rule) (45 CFR Parts 160, 164). In contemplating the need for informed consent, the following four questions are essential to answer.

First, does the proposed research involve extant or prospectively obtained materials? Some biobanks include tissue samples and pathology slides obtained many decades ago without the knowledge or informed consent of the patient. Other samples were obtained after legal and ethical requirements for informed consent and authorization were established. The age of the samples, the feasibility of obtaining consent (e.g., the likelihood that the patients are deceased), and the feasibility of obtaining alternative samples from other sources are among the considerations an institutional review board (IRB) will use to determine whether to grant a waiver of informed consent. For samples to be obtained in the future, informed consent is presumptively needed.

Second, are the samples identifiable or de-identified? The Common Rule and Privacy Rule apply only to identifiable samples and information. Such a rigid, regulatory distinction is no longer appropriate (Rothstein, 2010a). Moreover, there are inconsistencies between these two sets of rules in defining "de-identified" (Rothstein, 2005a). This issue is further explored below.

Third, if consent was obtained, is it general or limited consent? Under the Common Rule, IRBs generally disapprove of the concept of a general consent to research, but they will often permit general consent for submitting specimens to a biobank. An alternative is to use "tiered consent," in which sample donors select from a menu of possible types of research (e.g., genetics, mental health, cancer, HIV/AIDS) the areas in which they consent to have their samples used. For older samples with only general consent, a frequent issue is whether a specific research protocol comes within the original general consent.

Fourth, does the research involve a sensitive matter? For example, the research might incorporate controversial technologies (e.g., embryonic stem cells), contemplate controversial therapies (e.g., gene therapy), or implicate possible group harms, an issue further discussed below.

There have been a number of proposals to create an additional layer of protection between the individuals who provide the samples and the researchers who use them. One approach, the "tissue trustee" model, permits researchers access only to anonymized information while permitting information to flow in both directions (Knoppers, 2005). With this approach, additional clinical information can be obtained from the sample source, if necessary, and scientific findings can be provided back to the individual or his or her clinician.

was calculated by taking the 300 million figure from 1999 and adding 12 years of at least 20 million samples per year.

Under another approach, the "charitable trust" model, the donor transfers his or her property interest in the specimen to a trust, which has a fiduciary duty to use the specimen only in accordance with the express wishes of the donor (Winickoff and Winickoff, 2003). Under the charitable trust model, the trustee has a more substantive role than merely protecting the privacy of the sample donors, including informing sample donors about all research projects, sharing information, weighing the risks and benefits of participating in certain research, and determining the appropriate mechanisms for obtaining any additional informed consent and authorizations. The main objections to these and similar proposals are their complexity, burden, and expense.

Health records

Researchers often need to correlate genotype with phenotype, and therefore it is essential for them to have the ability to match samples with health records. The conversion from paper records to EHR, established as a national priority by President Bush in 2004 and reaffirmed by Congress and President Obama with enactment of the Health Information Technology for Economic and Clinical Health Act (HITECH Act), Title XIII of the American Recovery and Reinvestment Act of 2009, already has facilitated biobank research at many institutions (Roden et al., 2008). The value of EHR in research will be further enhanced by the development and implementation of the Nationwide Health Information Network (NwHIN), a system of linking EHR that are interoperable (technologically compatible), longitudinal (covering much or all of an individual's lifetime), and comprehensive (containing substantially all health-care encounters).

Three important issues are raised by using health records in research. Two of the issues, de-identification and sequestration, are discussed below. A third issue involves the validity under the Health Insurance Portability and Accountability Act (HIPAA) Privacy Rule of prospective authorizations. The Privacy Rule requires an individual to sign an authorization for the use and disclosure of protected health information in research. For the records to be valuable, they need to be continually updated. Thus, the question arises whether it is possible to have an individual sign a valid authorization that contemplates the future addition of individual health information.

The Privacy Rule does not provide a definitive answer to the question of whether prospective authorization is valid under the Privacy Rule. Even if it is, there would be serious ethical issues raised by such a practice. For example, an individual's health status may change dramatically from the date of an initial authorization, and his or her record might subsequently contain sensitive information, such as information about mental health, substance abuse, domestic violence, or sexually transmitted infections. In such an event, the individual might not want to have this new information automatically added to the research file without additional consent. Individuals also should not be responsible for monitoring their various consents and authorizations and they may not even have the ability to withdraw authorizations for research in progress.

I have previously suggested the following ways to address this issue:

(1) the authorization for future medical records should include a statement that future medical records will be sent to the biobank without notification to the individual

(2) the authorization should expressly mention that it applies to health information relating to the medical conditions specifically listed on the authorization (e.g., lung cancer) as well as other conditions not prohibited from disclosure

(3) additional authorization should be needed for the disclosure of future records containing health information within a research subject-determined list of sensitive conditions, such as psychiatric conditions, HIV/AIDS, sexually transmitted diseases, substance abuse, domestic violence, or sexual or reproductive health

(4) authorizations for future medical records should be limited to 5 years (Rothstein, 2005b: 94).

These recommendations seek to strike a balance between protecting the privacy and confidentiality of the individual and the interests of the researchers in gaining reasonable access to essential health information about research participants.

Interventional research with human subjects

Interventional research involves the examination of, or experimentation on, actual research participants or human subjects (IOM, 2009). Although the ethical principles for interventional research follow the established rules for all research involving human subjects, it is important to recognize that individuals with alcohol dependence or other addictions may be considered "vulnerable" research populations, which may necessitate additional ethical safeguards. The Common Rule provides detailed, special protections for the following categories of vulnerable subjects: pregnant women, fetuses, and neonates (45 CFR 46 Subpart B); prisoners (45 CFR Subpart C); and children (45 CFR Subpart D).

Besides these specific categories, other research subjects may be considered vulnerable because of their impaired decisional capacity or their susceptibility to coercion. The Common Rule provides: "When some or all of the subjects are likely to be vulnerable to coercion or undue influence, such as children, prisoners, pregnant women, mentally disabled persons, or economically or educationally disadvantaged persons, additional safeguards [should] be included in the study to protect the rights and welfare of these subjects" (45 CFR 46.111(b)). Subjects who are vulnerable because of their impaired decisional capacity would include individuals with mental retardation or mental illness. Subjects who are vulnerable because of their susceptibility to coercion or undue influence would include institutionalized mental patients, members of the military, students, nursing-home patients, and workers. These individuals are especially susceptible to coercion when the recruitment is conducted by individuals exercising a degree of control over the individual.

Individuals with alcohol dependence or other addictions could be a part of either category of vulnerable subjects. For example, those with active, major addictions could be decisionally impaired by their addiction to the extent that they lacked the capacity to consider the benefits and risks of participating in the research. In addition, if they were institutionalized or otherwise subject to the control of another person, they might be objectively or subjectively subject to coercion.

Being considered a vulnerable research subject raises the question of what such a designation means in terms of possible additional protections. The federal regulations applicable to research on prisoners are instructive. Because of the history of past abuses involving prisoners as research subjects and the possibility of coercion in enrollment, research on prisoners is generally prohibited except if the research involves studying the causes and effects of incarceration, the institutional structure of prisons, or conditions particularly affecting prisoners as a class (45 CFR § 46.306(a)(2)(A)-(C)). Therefore, it might be appropriate to restrict research on subjects with alcohol dependence or other addictions to research on addiction, including the genetic and environmental factors leading to addiction or of significance in the treatment of addiction. Consequently, individuals with addictions generally should not be used for non-addiction research, thereby limiting the risk of coercion or other impediments to informed consent.

Unique privacy issues in research on alcohol dependence and other addictions

Individual harms

Alcohol dependence and other addictions are extremely stigmatizing. In the case of drug addiction, mere possession of many of the commonly abused substances is illegal; and the abuse of prescription medications through unauthorized diversion and use is also illegal. Although the use of alcohol by adults is lawful, a range of alcohol-related conduct, such as public intoxication and driving while intoxicated, is illegal.

The disclosure of information regarding an individual's alcohol dependence or other addiction can lead to a variety of negative consequences, including loss of employment opportunities and undermining of social relationships. Even though an express provision of the Americans with Disabilities Act (ADA) prohibits discrimination against individuals who are alcoholics or substance abusers who are no longer using drugs (42 USC § 12114(a)), it is often difficult for the individual to prevail in such cases, and merely pursuing them has the effect of further calling public attention to the individual's condition.

Research protocols differ on whether information generated in the research process is shared with the individual's physician for clinical use. On the one hand, sharing such information has the benefit of providing to the treating clinician additional, expert information about the nature of the individual's condition, which could have the effect of aiding in treatment. On the other hand, integrating research data in clinical records could have the effect of increasing the amount of stigmatizing information in the record, where it may be further disclosed within or beyond the health-care setting, without necessarily improving the prospects for treatment.

Family harms

Alcohol dependence and other addictions often have devastating personal, social, and economic consequences for family members and friends of the affected individual. One effect of genetic research on addictions is to expand the ambit of harms to family members from that caused by an affected member with an addiction to other immediate and extended family members who may be at an increased risk of addiction. Thus, in addition to having to deal with their family member's addiction, at-risk family members also are likely to suffer from the social stigma and psychological burden of knowing they or other family members are at a genetically increased risk of addiction.

Individuals vary widely in whether they consider learning predictive genetic information desirable. Thus, it can be assumed that family members of someone with an addiction would vary in whether they wanted to learn predictive information of their genetic risk for addiction. Similarly, at-risk individuals vary widely in their response after learning of their genetic risks. Some of the possible reactions include depression, heightened vigilance, or fatalism. The intra-family dynamics of individuals with varied risk based on a genetic test have been widely observed and described for various conditions, such as Huntington's chorea and breast cancer (Taub et al., 2004). Undoubtedly, similar tensions will arise as predictive genetic testing for predisposition to alcohol dependence and other addictions are developed and offered widely.

Group harms

Because of historical patterns of migration, isolation, endogamy, founder effect, and other principles of population genetics, certain population groups associated with common geographic ancestry often possess similar genotypes or haplotypes (Hartl and Clark, 2007: 519–563). The population groups with similar genetic characteristics may be socially defined by race or ethnicity. When the genetic characteristics involve disease or disfavored social conditions and the population groups affected are minority groups or vulnerable populations in a particular society, there is tremendous potential for group-based harm or "group-mediated harm to individuals" (Hausman, 2007: 354).

The harms caused by associating an increased risk of a stigmatizing condition with a particular group attaches to each member of the group regardless of whether that person participated in the research or any particular person actually has the allele conferring increased risk. The risk of group harms also exists regardless of whether the information has been de-identified. Therefore, researchers need to be concerned about the potential for group-based harms when conducting research on stigmatizing conditions, including addictive behavior, especially when it involves socially disadvantaged individuals and groups.

The principle of group harm is illustrated by a recent incident involving the Havasupai Indian tribe, a 650-member tribe living in a remote part of the Grand Canyon. In 1989, members of the tribe asked researchers at Arizona State University if they would investigate the cause of the tribe's high incidence of diabetes. The tribal council approved the research and individuals signed a general consent for the collection of blood samples and health histories. Allegedly without the consent of members of the tribe, the researchers undertook extensive genetic research and published articles about the tribe members' rate of schizophrenia and inbreeding, as well as the genetic relatedness of the tribe to other native peoples. This latter information was especially hurtful, as it conflicted with the tribe's longstanding creation stories (Drabiak-Syed, 2010). Lawsuits brought by members of the tribe in 2005 were settled in 2010 (Harmon, 2010).

Strategies to protect privacy

De-identification

Although de-identification would seem to minimize the risk of harm from research involving stigmatizing conditions, a closer examination indicates that de-identification is insufficient to protect health privacy in research (Rothstein, 2010a). There are many issues to consider, but first it must be observed that the concept of de-identification is poorly defined (Knoppers, 2005). The literature abounds with confusing and contradictory definitions of anonymization, pseudonymization, linking, and single and double coding (Weir and Olick, 2004; Knoppers, 2005). Most importantly, the definitions under the Common Rule and the

Privacy Rule differ. The Common Rule mentions de-identifiability in very general terms as involving information "recorded by the investigator in such a manner that subjects cannot be identified, directly or through identifiers linked to the subjects" (45 CFR § 46.101(b)(4)).

The Privacy Rule provision on de-identification, notoriously complicated, can be satisfied in either of two ways. First, an expert in statistical and scientific methodologies can determine "that the risk is very small that the information could be used ... to identify an individual who is a subject of the information" (45 CFR § 164.514(b)(1)). Second, the following identifiers must be removed: (1) names; (2) geographical subdivisions smaller than a state except for the first three digits of a ZIP code; (3) all elements of dates (except year) that relate to birth date, admission date, and discharge date; (4) telephone numbers; (5) fax numbers; (6) e-mail addresses; (7) social security numbers; (8) medical record numbers; (9) health plan beneficiary numbers; (10); account numbers; (11) certificate or license numbers; (12) vehicle identifiers, including license-plate numbers; (13) device identifiers and serial numbers; (14) URLs (web locators); (15) Internet protocol (IP) address numbers; (16) biometric identifiers; (17) photographic and comparable images; and (18) any other unique identifying number, characteristic, or code (45 CFR § 164.514(b)(2)(i)).

The Privacy Rule also permits covered entities to use a limited data set for purposes of research, public health, or health-care operations if the recipient of the data set enters into a data use agreement specifying that the recipient will only use the information for limited purposes and the data set may not include "direct identifiers of the individual or of relatives, employers, or household members of the individual" (45 CFR § 164.514(e)(2)). The two categories of identifiers that may be included in a limited data set are dates, including date of birth and dates of service, and "any other unique identifying number, characteristic, or code."

The Privacy Rule and the Common Rule not only differ in degree of detail, but in substance as well. According to the Office of Human Research Protections (OHRP), the agency charged with administering the Common Rule, private information or specimens are "[not] individually identifiable when they cannot be linked to specific individuals by the investigator(s) either directly or through coding systems" (OHRP, 2008). Furthermore, research involving only coded information does not involve human subjects if the investigator cannot "readily ascertain" the identity of the individual. In its guidance, the OHRP recognized that it created a lower standard for de-identification than the Privacy Rule. "Therefore, some coded information, in which the code has been derived from identifying information linked to or related to the individual, would be individually identifiable under the Privacy Rule, but might not be individually identifiable under the [Common Rule]" (OHRP, 2008). Nevertheless, despite the fact that both the Common Rule (OHRP) and Privacy Rule (Office for Civil Rights) are administered by agencies of the Department of Health and Human Services (HHS) and there have been numerous recommendations to end the discrepancy (NCVHS, 2004), there have been insufficient efforts to harmonize the two sets of rules.

Regardless of the definition, de-identified information and specimens are not covered under either the Common Rule or the Privacy Rule. De-identified materials are exempt from the Common Rule pursuant to exemption 4 (45 CFR § 46.101(b)(4)). Similarly, de-identified information is not considered protected health information subject to the Privacy Rule (45 CFR § 164.514(a)). The regulatory dichotomy of all-or-nothing coverage may be criticized, however, as failing to recognize the varying degrees of identifiability of health information and failing to appreciate the privacy risks to individuals and groups caused by research uses of even de-identified health information.

Privacy issues are raised at the beginning of de-identified research, when identifiers are removed. For paper records, the process involves the cumbersome "whiting out" of individual names and other identifiers. For virtually all EHR, because they were not developed for "one-click" de-identification, electronic "white-out" strategies also need to be used for free text and scanned images. The individuals performing these functions may not have any relationship to health care and perform these tasks without the knowledge, consent, or authorization of the patient. During the process of de-identification sensitive health information is easily observable. Nevertheless, the Privacy Rule expressly provides that no consent or authorization is needed before de-identification is undertaken and there is no regulation of the procedures used (45 CFR § 164.502(d)(1)).

Another threat to privacy is the possible re-identification of a large number of de-identified health records using computerized network databases containing voter registration records and other publicly available sources. Most of the US population can be uniquely identified by using only gender, date of birth, and ZIP code (Benitez and Malin, 2010). Although complete compliance with the HIPAA de-identification specification is ordinarily not achieved in practice, even fastidious compliance cannot ensure against the possibility of re-identification. Measures to provide substantial protection against re-identification remain in the theoretical realm (Malin, 2010).

Individuals whose de-identified information is used in research without their consent or authorization often learn of the research through scholarly papers, popular publications, or other means, especially if an institution where the individuals have been treated conducts research into a specific and perhaps uncommon health condition. If the individuals' specimens and health records are used for personally "objectionable purposes," such as stem cell research or germ-line gene therapy, the individuals are likely to believe their rights and interests have been violated. Similarly, if the research leads to commercially viable discoveries, the individuals are likely to feel they were exploited (Rothstein, 2010a).

Although the interest of individuals in the research use of their de-identified specimens and health records is often referred to as a privacy interest, it is more accurate to describe the interest as involving autonomy. Recent survey research overwhelmingly supports the view that most people believe they should have reasonable control over the use of their biological specimens and health records (Westin, 2007; Goldenberg et al., 2009; Kaufman et al., 2009). Significantly, the public does not recognize the regulatory distinction between identifiable and de-identified biological samples and health information (Hull et al., 2008). Most members of the public want to control the use of their samples and information as an element of personal autonomy.

Sequestration of sensitive health information

As mentioned above, the United States is in the process of transitioning from paper-based health records to networks of interoperable, longitudinal, and comprehensive EHR. Today, with unconnected, disaggregated health records, old (and perhaps sensitive) health information is frequently lost or inaccessible, and the health conditions they document can be relegated to the fading recollections of the patient without any appreciable risk they will resurface to cause anxiety or humiliation. By contrast, the newly emerging NwHIN will aggregate an individual's cradle-to-grave health information from substantially all health-care encounters.

Thus, for example, the embarrassing details of a long-ago visit to a college health service will never go away and can be revisited with the click of a mouse by anyone with access to the individual's health records.

There are three situations in which the lawful users of an individual's health record may have access to much more health information than they need. First, physicians in clinical settings often need and only have time to review limited amounts of information. For example, a physician treating a sprained ankle in an emergency department ordinarily does not need to have access to the patient's reproductive health information.[2] Second, non-physician health-care providers, who ordinarily will have access to the same comprehensive EHR, rarely need access to the entire health record. The list of providers with access to a patient's health records includes dentists, chiropractors, optometrists, podiatrists, nutritionists, social workers, audiologists, and physical therapists. Access to complete records, however, is rarely necessary. For example, a podiatrist normally does not need access to an individual's genetic test results. Third, any third party with an interest in the individual's health status, such as an employer or life insurer, can make completion of an authorization for release of the individual's health records a condition of applying for a job or an insurance policy. Each year an estimated 25 million of these "compelled authorizations" are executed in the United States, and most result in the disclosure of the individual's entire health record (Rothstein and Talbott, 2007).

Some old health information, such as surgeries, allergies, and adverse reactions to drugs, has continued medical relevance, but much old information has no current clinical utility. The continued availability of such information raises the following four potential types of harms: (1) tangible harms to the patient, including discrimination, stigmatization, social upheaval, and embarrassment; (2) intangible harms to the patient, including anxiety and lack of trust in the health-care system; (3) individual health harms, including suboptimal care caused by incomplete disclosures to health-care providers by patients engaging in "defensive privacy practices"; and (4) public health harms caused by the reluctance of individuals to seek prompt medical care for stigmatizing conditions (e.g., alcohol dependence, substance abuse, mental illness, sexually transmitted infections) because they fear that the information will become part of their permanent health records.

Protecting the privacy of health information in an era of EHR and other forms of health information technology (HIT) raises numerous challenges, including dealing with the concern of many physicians that they will no longer be able to have access to the information they need to provide safe and effective care (Rothstein, 2010b). The National Committee on Vital and Health Statistics (NCVHS), the statutory public advisory committee to the Secretary of HHS, addressed this issue in its HIT recommendations to the Secretary in 2008: "The design of the NwHIN should permit patients to elect to sequester sensitive health information in one or more predefined categories" (NCVHS, 2008). The NCVHS listed the following as

---

[2] In a study by the California HealthCare Foundation in 2010, even before the widespread adoption of longitudinal, comprehensive EHR, 12% of respondents agreed with the statement that "my doctor has too much information about me on the computer." California HealthCare Foundation, *Consumers and Health Information Technology: A National Survey* (April 2010): 30, available at www.chcf.org/publications/2010/04/consumers-and-health-information-technology-a-national-survey [accessed March 1, 2012].

sample categories of sensitive information: domestic-violence information, genetic information, mental-health information, reproductive-health information, and substance-abuse information.

In 2009, the HITECH Act title of the American Recovery and Reinvestment Act implicitly adopted the NCVHS recommendation to develop the ability of patients to sequester certain sensitive information in their EHR. Section 3002, which established a new HIT Policy Committee in the Department of HHS, charged the committee with certain areas for its consideration. First on the list was technologies that protect the privacy of health information and promote security in a qualified EHR, including for the segmentation and protection from disclosure of specific and sensitive individually identifiable health information with the goal of minimizing the reluctance of patients to seek care (or disclose information about a condition) because of privacy concerns, in accordance with applicable law, and for the use and disclosure of limited data sets of information (ARRA § 3002(b)(2)(i)).

In November 2010, the NCVHS issued detailed recommendations on sensitive health information, following up on recommendations it previously made in 2006 and 2008. The NCVHS recommended that "sensitive information" subject to special sequestration rules should include categories already defined by federal law (genetic information, psychotherapy notes, substance-abuse treatment records, and HITECH Act cash payments), categories defined in many state laws (HIV, sexually transmitted diseases, mental-health information, and health records of children and adolescents), and other categories of potentially sensitive information (mental-health information other than psychotherapy notes or state law definitions, sexuality and reproductive-health information) (NCVHS, 2010).

In December 2010, the President's Council of Advisors on Science and Technology issued a report to the President, *Realizing the Full Potential of Health Information Technology to Improve Healthcare for Americans: The Path Forward* (PCAST, 2010). Among other things, the report recommends the research, development, and use of the "tagged data element approach," which permits patients to restrict the types of health information contained in their EHR. This technical solution would permit the use of sequestration by categories or even more granular control of health information.

Although the concept of patient-directed sequestration of sensitive health information has been added to the national agenda on HIT, thus far there has been glacial movement in both supporting development of the necessary technology and undertaking the substantial policy analysis needed to implement such a fundamental change in health care. All individuals, especially those with stigmatizing conditions such as alcohol dependence and substance abuse, should have the ability to restrict access to certain elements of their health records by the wide range of health-care providers needing access to only a part of the record. The challenge remains to design a system that permits segmentation without burdening either patients or heath-care providers (Rothstein, 2011).

Certificates of Confidentiality

Pursuant to section 301(d) of the Public Health Service Act (42 USC § 241(d)), the Secretary of HHS may authorize persons engaged in biomedical, behavioral, clinical, or other research to protect the privacy of research subjects. The National Institutes of Health (NIH) has been delegated the authority under the law to issue Certificates of Confidentiality, which protect investigators and institutions from being compelled to release information that could be used to identify subjects of research. When issued, a Certificate allows investigators and others with access to research records to refuse to disclose identifying information in any civil, criminal, administrative, legislative or other proceeding, whether at the federal, state, or local level. Without provisions for issuing Certificates of Confidentiality it would be difficult to enroll subjects in many areas of health and behavioral research.

Certificates of Confidentiality can be issued for any "sensitive" research, defined by NIH as research where "disclosure of identifying information could have adverse consequences for subjects or damage their financial standing, employability, insurability, or reputation" (NIH, 2010a). Among the examples of "sensitive research" according to NIH are genetic research and research collecting data on substance abuse or other illegal activities. Clearly, genetic research on alcohol dependence or other addictive behaviors would qualify as sensitive research. In 2002, NIH announced a new policy of encouraging the broader use of Certificates. In particular, NIH recommends as part of its data-sharing policy that Certificates be obtained for genome-wide association studies (NIH, 2010b).

Certificates have been widely promoted, yet their efficacy has not been well established. There have been very few court cases involving Certificates (Beskow et al., 2008), and research subjects are often confused about the provisions and effects of Certificates (Catania et al., 2007). Of importance to research subjects are that Certificates are issued to the institution, not the investigator; research subjects have no right to insist that the Certificate be invoked to prevent disclosure; and there is no private right of action provided by the statute in which research subjects can seek redress for breaches of confidentiality. For genetic research on alcohol dependence and other addictions Certificates are a necessary but not sufficient means of assuring research subjects that their participation in research will be confidential and not lead to social or other harms.

Conclusion

Genetic research on alcohol dependence and other addictions raises familiar themes of modern biomedical research, including the use of biobanks, EHR, high-throughput genome sequencing, and other research methodologies. In addition, it involves behavioral genetic conditions with a high degree of stigma. Therefore, rigorous measures to protect the privacy and related interests of research subjects are essential to enable the enrollment of an adequate number of research subjects as well as to achieve the level of protections they have been promised. Nevertheless, the United States does not have a comprehensive law for the protection of individual privacy, including health privacy.

In the absence of a well-considered legal framework for regulating privacy in genetic research on alcohol dependence and other addictions, the focus must be on the two parties with the greatest ability to protect privacy: investigators and research subjects. As for investigators, they need to understand the privacy implications of their research in such a sensitive field, the range of risks arising from privacy breaches, and the strong autonomy and related interests of research subjects in controlling their specimens and health records. As for research subjects, they need to be informed about the nature of biomedical research, the specific measures that will be used to protect their privacy and the likely success of each measure, and the role of privacy in calculating the risks and benefits of participating in research.

References

Benitez, K. and Malin, B. (2010). Evaluating re-identification risks with respect to the HIPAA Privacy Rule. *Journal of the American Medical Informatics Association*, 17, 169–177.

Beskow, L. M., Dame, L., and Costello, E. J. (2008). Research ethics. Certificates of confidentiality and compelled disclosure of data. *Science*, 322, 1054–1055.

Blum K., Braverman, E. R., Holder, J. M., et al. (2000). Reward deficiency syndrome: A biogenetic model for the diagnosis and treatment of impulsive, addictive, and compulsive behaviors. *Journal of Psychoactive Drugs*, 32 (Supp. 1–4), 1–112.

Caron L., Karkazis, K., Raffin, T.A., Swan, G., and Koenig, B. A. (2005). Nicotine addiction through a neurogenomic prism: Ethics, public health, and smoking. *Nicotine and Tobacco Research*, 7, 181–197.

Catania, J. A., Wolf, L. E., Wertleib, S., Lo, B., and Henne, J. (2007). Research participants' perceptions of the Certificate of Confidentiality's assurances and limitations. *Journal of Empirical Research on Human Research Ethics*, 2, 53–59.

Drabiak-Syed, K. (2010). Lessons from Havasupai Tribe v. Arizona State University Board of Regents: Recognizing group, cultural, and dignitary harms as legitimate risks warranting integration into research practice. *Journal of Health & Biomedical Law*, 6, 175–225.

Eiseman, E. and Haga, S. B. (1999). *Handbook of Human Tissue Sources: A National Resource of Human Tissue Samples*. Rockville, MD: RAND, p. xvii.

Goldenberg, A. J., Hull, S. C., Botkin, J. R., and Wilfond, B. S. (2009). Pediatric biobanks: Approaching informed consent for continuing research after children grow up. *Journal of Pediatrics*, 155, 578–583.

Goldman, D., Oroszi, G., and Ducci, F. (2005). The genetics of addictions: Uncovering the genes. *Nature Reviews Genetics*, 6, 521–535.

Harmon, A. (2010). Tribe wins fight to limit research of its DNA. *New York Times* April 22, 2010, A1.

Hartl, D. L. and Clark, A. G. (2007). *Principles of Population Genetics*, fourth edition. Sunderland, MA: Sinauer Associates.

Hausman, D. M. (2007). Group risks, risks to groups, and group engagement in genetics research. *Kennedy Institute of Ethics Journal*, 17, 351–369.

Hull, S. C., Sharp, R. R., and Botkin, J. R. (2008). Patients' views on identifiability of samples and informed consent for genetic research. *American Journal of Bioethics*, 8, 62–70.

IOM (2009). *Beyond the HIPAA Privacy Rule: Enhancing Privacy, Improving Health Through Research*. Washington, DC: National Academies Press.

Kaufman, D. J., Murphy-Bollinger, J. Scott, J., and Hudson, K. L. (2009). Public opinion about the importance of privacy in biobank research. *American Journal of Human Genetics*, 85, 643–654.

Knoppers, B. M. (2005). Biobanking: International norms. *Journal of Law, Medicine and Ethics*, 33, 7–14.

Malin, B. (2010). Secure construction of k-unlinkable patient records from distributed providers. *Artificial Intelligence in Medicine*, 48, 29–41.

NCVHS (2004). Letter to Secretary of Health and Human Services Secretary Tommy G. Thompson, March 5, 2004. Available online at: www.ncvhs.hhs.gov/040305l2.htm [accessed March 1, 2012].

NCVHS (2008). Letter to Secretary of Health and Human Services Secretary Michael O. Leavitt, February 20, 2008. Available online at: http://ncvhs.hhs.gov/080220lt.pdf [accessed March 1, 2010].

NCVHS (2010). Letter to Secretary of Health and Human Services Secretary Kathleen Sebelius, November 10, 2010. Available online at: http://ncvhs.hhs.gov/101110lt.pdf [accessed March 1, 2012].

NIH, Office of Extramural Research (2010a). Certificates of Confidentiality: Background Information. Available online at: http://grants.nih.gov/grants/policy/coc/background.htm [accessed March 1, 2012].

NIH (2010b). Genome-Wide Association Studies (GWAS), Points to Consider. Available online at: http://grants.nih.gov/grants/gwas/gwas_ptc.pdf [accessed March 1, 2012].

OHRP (2008). Guidance on Research Involving Coded Private Information or Biological Specimens. Available online at: www.hhs.gov/ohrp/policy/cdebiol.html [accessed March 1, 2012].

PCAST (2010). Realizing the Full Potential of Health Information Technology to Improve Healthcare for Americans: The Path Forward. Available online at: www.whitehouse.gov/administration/eop/ostp/pcast [accessed March 1, 2012].

Roden, D. M., Pulley, J. M., Basford, M. A., et al. (2008). Development of a large-scale de-identified DNA biobank to enable personalized medicine. *Clinical Pharmacology and Therapeutics*, 84, 362–369.

Rothstein, M. A. (2005a). Expanding the ethical analysis of biobanks. *Journal of Law, Medicine and Ethics*, 33, 89–101.

Rothstein, M. A. (2005b). Research privacy under HIPAA and the Common Rule. *Journal of Law, Medicine and Ethics*, 33, 154–159.

Rothstein, M. A. (2010a). Is deidentification sufficient to protect health privacy in research? *American Journal of Bioethics*, 10, 3–11.

Rothstein, M. A. (2010b). The Hippocratic bargain and health information technology. *Journal of Law, Medicine and Ethics*, 38, 7–13.

Rothstein, M. A. (2011). Debate Over Patient Privacy Controls in Electronic Health Records. *Bioethics Forum*, February 17, 2011. Available online at: www.thehastingcenter.org/Bioethicsforum/post.aspx?id=5139&blogid=140 [accessed March 1, 2012].

Rothstein, M. A. and Talbott, M. K. (2007). Compelled authorizations for disclosure of health records: Magnitude and implications. *American Journal of Bioethics*, 7, 38–45.

Taub, S., Morin, K., Spillman, M. A., Sade, R. M., Riddick, F. A.; Council on Ethical and Judicial Affairs of the American Medical Association (2004). Managing familial risk in genetic testing. *Genetic Testing*, 8, 356–359.

Weir, R. F. and Olick, R. A. (2004). *The Stored Tissue Issue: Biomedical Research, Ethics, and Law in the Era of Genomic Medicine*. New York: Oxford University Press.

Westin, A. F. (2007). IOM Project Survey Findings on Health Research and Privacy. Available online at: www.iom.edu/~/media/Files/Activity%20Files/Research/HIPAAandResearch/AlanWestinIOMSrvyRept.ashx [accessed March 1, 2012].

Winickoff, D. E. and Winickoff, R. N. (2003). The charitable trust as a model for genomic research. *New England Journal of Medicine*, 349, 1180–1184.

7

Certificates of Confidentiality: Uses and limitations as protection for genetic research on addiction

Zita Lazzarini

Introduction

Certificates of Confidentiality have existed to protect research data for over 40 years, yet they are rarely used (Cooper et al., 2004: 217). Relatively few researchers seek and obtain certificates, even in fields such as genetics where most researchers acknowledge collecting sensitive data. As Professor Mark Rothstein points out in his chapter on protecting privacy in this field of research (Chapter 6 of this volume), "[g]enome researchers often analyze and manipulate vast data sets derived from the 3.2 billion base-pair human genome" and involving the genetic material of thousands of individuals. These very large data sets often include extensive phenotypic data on individuals, including their identities and medical, behavioral, and social histories. In research focusing on alcohol and drug dependence, data collected may include evidence of illegal activities, as well as risky activity, dependence, or addiction. Any such evidence, if disclosed, could have serious negative consequences on participants' employment and education opportunities and on their relationships within families and communities. Such databases could also provide tempting targets for law enforcement under a number of different scenarios (Earley and Strong, 1995: 728), from officials seeking information on possible child abuse or domestic violence (Marshall et al., 2003) to requests to search the database for a match to evidence left at a crime scene or on a victim.

This chapter will focus on Certificates of Confidentiality as one tool to protect the privacy and confidentiality of research data, particularly from the types of third-party requests arising from the legal system (subpoenas and court orders). First, it will review the history of Certificates of Confidentiality. Second, it will consider arguments for their use, particularly in genetic research on addiction. Third, it will review critiques of Certificates of Confidentiality, including whether they are necessary, whether they are effective, and whether they can be relied on to protect subjects' sensitive information.

History

Congress originally created Certificates of Confidentiality through federal legislation in 1970 to protect information collected as part of research involving alcohol or other psychoactive drugs (Comprehensive Drug Abuse Prevention and Control Act, 1970, PL 91–53, 84 Stat. 1236). In 1988, legislation expanded the scope of Certificates of Confidentiality to cover a wide range of health research (Public Health Services Act, 1988, 42 USC § 241(d), Section 301(d)). Today individual institutes of the National Institutes of Health (NIH) are

Genetic Research on Addiction, ed. Audrey R. Chapman. Published by Cambridge University Press.
© Cambridge University Press 2012.

authorized to grant Certificates to any research that: "(1) collects personally identifiable, sensitive information; (2) collects information that, if disclosed, could have adverse consequences for subjects or damage financial standing, employability, insurability, or reputation; and (3) has been approved by an IRB [institutional review board]" (Coffey and Ross, 2004: 209–210; NIH Kiosk, 2009a).

Scope of protection

On its website the NIH describes the purpose of Certificates as follows:

> Certificates of Confidentiality are issued by the National Institutes of Health (NIH) to protect the privacy of research subjects by protecting investigators and institutions from being compelled to release information that could be used to identify subjects with a research project. Certificates of Confidentiality are issued to institutions or universities where the research is conducted. They allow the investigator and others who have access to research records *to refuse to disclose identifying information in any civil, criminal, administrative, legislative, or other proceeding, whether at the federal, state, or local level* [emphasis added].

> Identifying information is broadly defined as any item or combination of items in the research data that could lead directly or indirectly to the identification of a research subject.

> By protecting researchers and institutions from being compelled to disclose information that would identify research participants, Certificates of Confidentiality help achieve the research objectives and promote participation in studies by assuring privacy to subjects (NIH Kiosk, 2003).

Theoretically, researchers who receive a Certificate should be able to use it to protect their research data from almost any third-party requests for data, including subpoenas and court orders. The actual limits, if any, of Certificates of Confidentiality have not been fully tested in court. The few reported court cases are described below.

Arguments in favor of Certificates of Confidentiality

Application to genetic research on addiction

In 1995 Earley and Strong argued that "most investigators should use all available resources to avoid having their data subpoenaed and to prevent having to reveal the identity of participants in research projects..." (Earley and Strong, 1995: 727). Congress first envisioned protecting research on illicit drug use and addiction in the 1970 Act that authorized the creation of Certificates (Comprehensive Drug Abuse Prevention and Control Act, 1970, PL 91–53, 84 Stat. 1236). The NIH currently specifies that Certificates of Confidentiality are appropriate for any research that is sensitive. They define research as sensitive where "disclosure of identifying information could have adverse consequences for subjects or damage their financial standing, employability, insurability, or reputation" (NIH Kiosk, 2003). Studies that collect data including "genetic information... psychological well-being of subjects... [and] ... data on substance abuse or other illegal risk behaviors" are all examples of "research with potential adverse consequences for subjects" that are suitable for a Certificate (NIH Kiosk, 2002b: 6). Given the stigma associated with all forms of addiction in our society, and the acknowledged risks to privacy inherent in genetic research, research on the possible role of genetics in alcohol and drug dependence seems to easily satisfy the NIH criteria. Although the research itself is likely to involve large numbers of people who are not addicted as well as those who are, public perception of anyone participating in such research could be negative and lead to stigma and discrimination.

A study that surveyed three NIH institutes in order to describe the prevalence of Certificates of Confidentiality found that the most common reason investigators gave for obtaining a Certificate was that the research involved genetics (Cooper et al., 2004). Other reasons included that the data, if disclosed, could lead to social stigma and discrimination or that it could damage the subject's financial standing, employability or reputation (both criteria taken directly from the NIH's definition of "sensitive"). A study that looked at authors' documentation of human subjects protections (IRB approval, informed consent, and Certificates of Confidentiality) in articles published in four genetics journals found that documentation rates were similar to earlier studies of the medical literature in general, suggesting that researchers or editors in these journals were no more consistent in their reporting of these human subjects protections than researchers in other, less-sensitive areas (Coffey and Ross, 2004: 211–212). Various guidance materials from the NIH Kiosk also specifically mention both studies involving genetics and those involving substance abuse (NIH Kiosk, 2002b).

Other commentators have tried to operationalize the process of deciding whether research meets the threshold criteria for a Certificate. One commentator has suggested a list of questions that start with the basic NIH criteria, but go beyond them, to help individual researchers decide if they should apply for a Certificate (Lutz et al., 2000). These include: (1) "Is the topic sensitive?"; (2) "Is the target or sample population vulnerable?"; (3) "Are others likely to be interested in participant data for purposes other than the advancement of science?"; (4) "Are traditional methods to protect confidentiality inadequate?"; and (5) "Does the informed consent explicitly detail mandated reporting duties of researchers?" (Lutz et al., 2000: 187, Table 2). Questions (2), (3), (4), and (5) address not just the sensitivity of the information, but also the vulnerability of the subjects. Vulnerability, in this case, means both those who are inherently vulnerable (which can include the poor, marginalized, or disenfranchised, as well as those "at risk for morbidity or premature mortality") and those who have experienced "discrimination, intolerance, subordination, or stigma, or been denied their legal rights" (Lutz et al., 2000: 187, Table 2). Lutz et al. also recommend that researchers evaluate whether third parties are likely to try to obtain the data (for purposes not related to science, such as law enforcement or to establish paternity) and to consider whether other means of protection (pseudonyms or coded identifiers) could be used. Finally, they remind researchers that they must inform participants of any anticipated voluntary disclosures (including for communicable diseases and child or elder abuse reporting) by the researchers. These questions could be adapted to apply to research involving genetics of addiction.

Should IRBs require certificates in some cases?

IRBs also have an obligation to protect the privacy of research subjects and the confidentiality of data that are collected. In practice, some IRBs recommend or even require investigators working in sensitive areas to obtain a Certificate as a condition of approving the protocol (Wolf and Zandecki, 2006). Mandating Certificates, however, places a significant burden on the researcher and may delay the research, as the application process takes from 1–2 weeks to 4–6 months (depending on the NIH institute in question) (Wolf et al., 2004: 16, Table 3).

One commentator has argued that IRBs need a structured framework for determining whether to require a Certificate (Currie, 2005). Such a framework would require a

Certificate where: "(1) the risks of compulsory disclosure are greater than minimal; (2) the research could not otherwise be carried out; and (3) existing legal safeguards do not provide adequate data protection" (Currie, 2005: 7). Thus, IRBs need to conduct a structured risk assessment that includes a "systematic evaluation of: (1) the magnitude of potential harms caused by compulsory disclosure; (2) the probability of compulsory disclosure; and (3) whether the risk of compulsory disclosure is greater than minimal" (Currie, 2005: 9). Although there is little empirical research on any of these three factors, IRBs can do their best to evaluate them in a consistent way relying on any data that does exist. Next, the IRB should determine whether the research could be carried out without a Certificate in place. Some studies will involve such vulnerable populations or seek to elicit such sensitive data, that the researchers will be unable to recruit sufficient subjects in the absence of extensive privacy protections, such as those usually promised by a Certificate (Currie, 2005: 11). Finally, the IRB should determine what other protections for study data exist; these can include the Health Insurance Portability and Accountability Act (HIPAA), federal drug and alcohol treatment rules, and disease-specific and general public health statutes at the state level (Carney et al., 2000). Of course these statutes and regulations do not protect study data from subpoena by law enforcement officials, parties to a civil suit, or court orders. Ultimately, as the author points out, IRBs are responsible for reviewing the whole of the researcher's study design to minimize risks of all kinds to subjects, including risks to confidentiality.

Critiques of Certificates of Confidentiality

Critiques of Certificates fall into three general categories: the Certificates (1) are not really necessary; (2) have only rarely been challenged in court, so their actual function, when needed, remains unknown; and (3) protect against compelled disclosures but not voluntary disclosures.

Do researchers need them to protect their data?

Some of the critics of Certificates of Confidentiality note that there is little empirical evidence to suggest that lawyers (plaintiffs', defendants', or prosecutors) frequently target research data for discovery and even less evidence that subjects have been harmed by this practice (Reilly, 2004). In fact, even in the genetics literature, one commentator explained the relatively low proportion of researchers obtaining a Certificate by hypothesizing that researchers "do not perceive that there is even a minimal risk that they will be forced by a court to disclose genetic data about a research subject" and that "they probably perceive the data as posing little risk to the individual even if it were disclosed..." (Reilly, 2004: 77). This author goes on to conclude that "there is no reason to believe that in the vast majority of genetic research involving human subjects the risk justifies the effort" (Reilly, 2004: 77). However, the majority of the literature considering use of Certificates in genetics assumes they can play a unique role in protecting research data, as they are the only tool that specifically protects data against subpoenas or court orders (Earley and Strong, 1995; Coffey and Ross, 2004; Cooper et al., 2004; Wolf et al., 2004; Wolf and Zandecki, 2006; Beskow et al., 2008; Beskow et al., 2009; Gunn and Joiner, 2009).

Other commentators note that Certificates of Confidentiality are just one of many measures researchers can use to protect subject confidentiality from the range of possible disclosures – others being good study design, training, and oversight of research personnel, implementation of comprehensive security measures, and coding or anonymizing of data (see Chapter 6 in this volume) (Carney et al., 2000; Lutz et al., 2000; Wolf and Zandecki, 2006; Conley et al., 2010).

Will a Certificate withstand a legal challenge?

Because Certificates are a legal mechanism authorized by federal statute, courts can continue to interpret their scope and function. Most sources report one documented case in which a Certificate was tested in court. That case, *People v. Newman* (1973), involved a prosecutor's attempt to subpoena photographs of persons attending a methadone treatment center in New York as part of a homicide investigation. The head of the clinic, Dr. Robert Newman, refused to produce the photographs (or any other data related to clients of the methadone program) based on the original statute's protection for drug treatment program research. He was held in contempt of court by the trial judge and sentenced to 30 days in jail. On appeal, however, the court determined that the Federal Comprehensive Drug Abuse Prevention and Control Act of 1970 did provide protection against subpoena by any court and that the protective clauses of the statute had not been revoked or repealed by the later Drug Abuse Office and Treatment Act 1972 (PL 92–255, 86 Stat. 65) (*People v. Newman*, 1973: 389–390). *Newman* is usually cited as proof that a Certificate will withstand a court challenge from third parties (including law enforcement) seeking research data. However, other commentators find the court's reasoning in *Newman* less reassuring and also note that a single case, from a state court, more than 30 years ago, is not the firmest footing on which to base assumptions about a court's willingness to protect the confidentiality of research data in the twenty-first century.

A second published case, which reached the North Carolina Appeals court (*State v. Bradley*, 2006), presented (and could have resolved) an important issue – whether a Certificate could protect confidential research data when sought by a defendant in a criminal case. *Bradley*, however, was ultimately decided on other grounds, resulting in no precedent one way or the other on this question (Beskow et al., 2009; Gunn and Joiner, 2009). In *Bradley*, when the defendant sought to compel Duke University Health Systems to release research data on a prosecution witness, the trial court judge granted a temporary protective order that prevented the full disclosure of the requested research data, but did require the researchers to hold identifiable information related to the witness in a sealed record pending the appeal (*State v. Bradley*, 2006: 260). On appeal the court ordered the information disclosed to the appellate team and the judge in order to determine whether it was material to the defendant's case (Beskow et al., 2008). The appellate court ultimately determined that the information was not material to the case and the defense attorney's access to the data was revoked. However, by that point, several parties had been able to review the information. This is a critical lesson from *Bradley*, that even where broad disclosure is denied, limited disclosure may be required.

The NIH has maintained that the protections offered by the Certificate supersede federal, state, and local law and will allow a researcher to resist compulsory disclosure in any proceeding. However, the issue that *Bradley* raised, but did not settle, is whether a defendant's constitutional rights to due process would trump the protections of the Certificate (Beskow et al., 2008; Beskow et al., 2009). In cases not involving Certificates, courts have held that constitutional rights, particularly in criminal cases, take precedence over statutes (*Commonwealth v. Craig Neumyer*, 2000).

Relying only on "published" legal cases, although appropriate from the perspective of lawyers seeking to define the contours of settled law, may understate the actual levels of success (or failure) of Certificates of Confidentiality in practice. For example, if in response to a subpoena a researcher notified the attorney that the data were protected by a Certificate and the opposing attorney did not challenge the Certificate, then no easily identifiable court record would result, although the Certificate was effective. Similarly, if a researcher asserted that a Certificate protected the data, but the court disagreed and the researcher did not challenge the resulting court order, the case would be unlikely to be published and there would be no record of it, even though the Certificate would have "failed." In fact, some recent empirical research on Certificates of Confidentiality suggests that they are more widely used to defend data than previously thought, with both successes and failures.

Data collected as part of a qualitative analysis of attitudes and impressions of researchers who have used Certificates suggest that researchers have used Certificates successfully in several instances that have not resulted in reported appellate cases (Wolf and Zandecki, 2006). Wolf and Zandecki (2006) report that 2 out of the 19 researchers they interviewed had used a Certificate in response to a subpoena that could have resulted in disclosure of confidential research data. Because both cases were resolved without the researcher having to defend the Certificate in court, neither resulted in a published legal case. Two other respondents in the same study also reported that researchers they knew had used a Certificate in response to a subpoena. By contrast, one researcher reported knowing a colleague for whom a Certificate had not prevented disclosure of information in response to a subpoena (Wolf and Zandecki, 2006).

Other researchers have noted that *Newman* does not provide a guarantee of complete protection for other reasons (Currie, 2005). Certificates of Confidentiality only protect identifiable data. In at least two reported cases, courts have required researchers to release de-identified data in a court proceeding (*Deitchman v. E.R. Squibb & Sons, Inc.*, 1984; *Farnsworth v. Procter and Gamble Co.*, 1985), although neither involved research protected by a Certificate.

Protection against compelled disclosure but not voluntary disclosure

Many commentators note that a Certificate gives the researcher the power to resist a subpoena or court order, but does not require him or her to do so (Earley and Strong, 1995: 730; Marshall et al., 2003: 57; Tovino, 2007: 458–459). What this means in practice is that a researcher may voluntarily decide to release data in response to legal pressure or to report communicable diseases, child abuse, or other criminal activity. The NIH's instructions to researchers require those who intend to voluntarily comply with state reporting requirements or to voluntarily disclose information for any other reason to clearly inform potential subjects of their intention as part of informed consent (NIH Kiosk, 2009b). Of course, if the researcher has promised not to disclose data and then subsequently chooses to do so, the subject could sue the researcher for breach of contract. However, as one author noted, "being able to sue that researcher for money damages will likely be cold comfort to a subject who ends up in jail, or has her child (or children) removed from her custody based on civil child abuse charges" (Marshall et al., 2003: 58). To partially mitigate this problem Marshall et al. suggest having researchers explicitly promise (in the consent form) that they will not voluntarily disclose any research data.

Do Certificates of Confidentiality provide a false sense of security?

Large genome-wide studies, such as those necessary to advance the field of genetics of addiction and dependence, pose significant risks to privacy and confidentiality, both in terms of the possible sensitivity of the data and the large numbers of individuals who could be affected. Even some proponents of such research agree that it will be impossible to guarantee that participants or their data will never, or could never, be identified (Conley et al., 2010: 349). Because of technological advances, statistical modeling, and the problem of old-fashioned security breaches, even supposedly de-identified or coded data may actually be (or become) identifiable (Greely, 2007: 349–353). Consequently, IRBs and ethicists should ask whether researchers are doing subjects a disservice when they appear to promise (nearly) absolute confidentiality of research data as part of the informed consent form or process. Another way to look at this is to consider whether the entirety of the human subjects protection regulatory system, including IRB review, coding of research data, and even Certificates of Confidentiality, might create a false sense of security for both subjects and researchers.

Of course, researchers can never perfectly protect research subjects from all potential harms – which is why researchers must inform subjects of any foreseeable risks (45 CFR § 46.116(a)(2)) – but researchers must also inform subjects of "the extent, if any, to which confidentiality of records identifying the subject will be maintained" (45 CFR § 46.116(a)(5)). Researchers, however, should be wary about creating the impression of safety, if their assurances go beyond what is realistic. The problem with creating a false sense of security – if that is what happens – is that it might lead subjects to agree to participate or to divulge information beyond what they would do if they appreciated the actual risks.

Fully informing subjects of the known strengths and limitations of Certificates of Confidentiality becomes a critical part of their appropriate use (Beskow et al., 2008; Gunn and Joiner, 2009; Conley et al., 2010: 347–351). Yet some researchers have suggested that describing the Certificate and why the researcher is seeking one may actually dissuade potential subjects from participation (because they had never thought about the potential risks to their privacy from subpoenas or court orders) (Reilly, 2004). Fear of the impact of full disclosure of the risks of a study, however, cannot be used to justify limiting information given to human subjects as part of the consent process (45 CFR § 46.116). Other studies have found a predominantly positive attitude among researchers about the protection offered by a Certificate (Wolf and Zandecki, 2006).

Using Certificates of Confidentiality

Limitations real and potential

In addition to the limitations described above related to possible legal challenges to Certificates of Confidentiality, researchers who work outside the United States cannot rely on Certificates for protection of their data because the protections of the Certificate are based on US federal laws, which have no effect in other countries. This is true even when the research involves sensitive data about subjects that, if disclosed, could expose them to a wide variety of legal and social risks under what may be more punitive foreign laws.

In addition to noting the paucity of case law testing Certificates of Confidentiality, Beskow et al. (2008) note at least four issues that researchers should be aware of that might complicate or compromise their ability to use a Certificate to protect research data: (1) requests for data may come suddenly and unexpectedly, forcing researchers to find legal counsel familiar with Certificates on short notice; (2) the interests of the investigator and the institution may differ and the institution may not be willing to resist a court order to disclose or the threat of being held in contempt of court; (3) even where the institution seeks to enforce a Certificate, some information may be disclosed in the process, including the plain fact of that specific individual's participation in the research; and (4) particularly where research information is being sought by a defendant in a criminal case, "a Certificate may be especially vulnerable" (Beskow et al., 2008: 1055) as courts might find that the protection of the constitutional due process rights of a defendant trump the statute that seeks to protect the rights of research subjects. This was the issue raised in *Bradley*.

Beskow, et al. and others also question whether a Certificate will protect the confidentiality of research records if the government seeks access to information for "national security" reasons. Since the passage of the Patriot Act (USA Patriot Act 2001), government agencies have sought, and often been granted, legal powers to obtain a wide variety of otherwise confidential information (Beskow et al., 2008). Although the durability of Certificates in the context of the Patriot Act has not yet been tested in court, the NIH asserts that a Certificate should protect data from compelled disclosure under any federal law, specifically including the Patriot Act (NIH Kiosk, 2011).

Application process

The NIH provides detailed instructions for obtaining Certificates both for extramural and intramural researchers through its website, the "Certificates of Confidentiality Kiosk" (NIH Kiosk, 2002a, 2009a, 2009b). The site includes step-by-step instructions regarding the documentation required to obtain a Certificate as well as the text of required institutional assurances and examples of informed consent language that must be used (NIH Kiosk, 2009b). Additionally, various authors have published advice and recommendations for researchers considering a Certificate and for those actually in the application process (Carney et al., 2000: 373–374; Lutz et al., 2000; Wolf et al., 2004).

Certificates of Confidentiality only protect data collected after the issuance of the Certificate and before the end of the time specified in the Certificate (although the end date of the research can be extended, if necessary) (NIH Kiosk, 2003). Consequently, to ensure that data are protected, researchers must obtain their Certificate before any data are collected. As it can take anywhere from 1–2 weeks to 4–6 months to obtain a Certificate, depending on the NIH institute involved (Wolf et al., 2004: 16, Table 3), obtaining one imposes a burden on researchers and can cause delays in research (Hermos and Spiro, 2009). Some researchers might be tempted to forgo obtaining one, if a delay will negatively impact their research plan.

Once issued, however, data collected during the dates covered by the Certificate will be protected in perpetuity (NIH Kiosk, 2003). This permanent protection, coupled with the fact that federal funding is not necessary to obtain a Certificate (NIH Kiosk, 2011), makes the protection it offers somewhat unique.

Some delays in issuance of a Certificate, such as those caused by mistakes in the application, are largely avoidable. In one study, seven out of ten NIH institutes surveyed reported that the most common mistake made by applicants was failing to follow the instructions in the application process (Wolf et al., 2004: 16). Eight institutes reported that problems in the consent form also often caused delays (Wolf et al., 2004: 16–17). Mistakes generated by failing to follow the instructions included: failing to obtain the required institutional signature; failing to include basic information; failing to include a letter from the IRB demonstrating IRB approval; use of incorrect wording for required assurances; and lack of background information on personnel (Wolf et al., 2004: 16).

For these reasons, among others, institutions and IRBs should educate researchers to plan ahead, complete documentation carefully, and apply early, in order to avoid delays.

Conclusion

Although there are some ardent critics of Certificates, most commentators agree that they are necessary, but not sufficient, to protect sensitive research data (Wolf and Zandecki, 2004; Conley et al., 2010: 349) (see Chapter 6 of this volume). Particularly in the context of research on genetics of addiction and dependence, the risk of disclosure of research data seems undeniable. Individuals in a study could experience stigma, discrimination, and loss of opportunities, just by being identified as participants. Additionally, those who are identified as carrying specific genes associated with addiction or dependence could experience additional and more concrete harms. Subjects could experience harm regardless of whether the data are disclosed as a result of security breaches, voluntary or compelled disclosure of information, or technical advances that make even anonymized data identifiable when it can be combined with other databases or manipulated by a skilled statistician.

Researchers who gather sensitive data through genetic studies in this field should use all available means to protect the confidentiality and security of their data. Obtaining a Certificate is one step, but one that will require education of researchers and IRBs about their availability, their strengths and limitations, and how to successfully navigate the application process. Additionally, IRBs should carefully review information in informed consent forms about Certificates to ensure both that they fully disclose the strengths and limits of the Certificate and that researchers clearly state their intention regarding voluntary disclosures (if any), or state that they will not voluntarily disclose under any circumstances.

If the institution gives the required institutional assurances as part of the application process, then the institution commits itself to "support and defend the authority of the Certificate against legal challenges" (NIH Kiosk, 2009b). IRBs should also clarify steps a researcher will need to take should any attempt be made to compel disclosure and ensure that the institution is prepared to obtain legal counsel knowledgeable about Certificates.

Finally, IRBs and researchers should not neglect other means to protect subject confidentiality against much more common types of disclosures such as security failures related to data storage or transmission or failures to adequately train and supervise research staff.

Certificates of Confidentiality have allowed researchers to resist subpoenas in several cases. Based on this evidence and the NIH's assertion that Certificates continue to protect researchers against compelled disclosure in "any Federal, State, or local civil, criminal, administrative, legislative or other proceedings" (NIH Kiosk, 2009a), researchers collecting sensitive data, including genetics, substance abuse, psychological and behavioral health, should apply for and obtain a Certificate when their studies fit the published criteria. Although Certificates may not provide absolute protection from subpoena if a future court has to balance a defendant's constitutional right to due process against the rights of privacy and confidentiality of research subjects, this should not deter the vast majority of research projects from taking advantage of this unique source of protection.

References

Beskow, L. M., Dame, L., and Costello, E. J. (2008). Research ethics. Certificates of confidentiality and compelled disclosure of data. *Science*, 322, 1054–1055.

Beskow, L. M., Dame, L. and Costello, E. J. (2009). Research ethics. Certificates of confidentiality and compelled disclosure of data. Author reply. *Science*, 323, 1289–1290.

Carney, P. A., Geller, B. M., Moffett, H., et al. (2000). Current medicolegal and confidentiality issues in large multicenter research programs. *American Journal of Epidemiology*, 152, 371–378.

Coffey, M. J. and Ross, L. (2004). Human subject protections in genetic research. *Genetic Testing*, 8, 209–213.

Commonwealth v. Craig Neumyer (2000). 432 Mass 23 (2000).

Conley, J. M., Doerr, A. K., and Vorhaus, D. B. (2010). Enabling responsible public genomics. *Health Matrix: Journal of Law-Medicine*, 20, 325–385.

Cooper, Z. N., Nelson, R. M., and Ross, L. F. (2004). Certificates of confidentiality in research: Rationale and usage. *Genetic Testing*, 8, 214–220.

Currie, P. M. (2005). Balancing privacy protections with efficient research: Institutional review boards and the use of Certificates of Confidentiality. *IRB: Ethics & Human Research*, 27, 7–13.

Deitchman v. E.R. Squibb & Sons, Inc. (1984). 740 F.2d 556 (7th Cir. 1984).

Earley, C. L. and Strong, L. C. (1995). Certificates of Confidentiality: A valuable tool for protecting genetic data. *American Journal of Human Genetics*, 57, 727–731.

Farnsworth v. Procter and Gamble Co. (1985). 758 F.2d 1545 (11th Cir. 1985).

Greely, H. T. (2007). The uneasy ethical and legal underpinnings of large-scale genomic biobanks. *Annual Review of Genomics and Human Genetics*, 8, 343–364.

Gunn, P. P. and Joiner, S. D. (2009). Certificates should be strengthened. *Science*, 323:1289–90.

Hermos, J. A, and Spiro, A., III (2009). Certificates should be retired. *Science*, 323, 1288–1289.

Lutz, K. F., Shelton, K. C., Robrecht, L. C., Hatton, D. C., and Beckett, A. K. (2000). Use of Certificates of Confidentiality in nursing research. *Journal of Nursing Scholarship*, 32, 185–188.

Marshall, M. F., Meinkoff, J., and Paltrow, L. M. (2003). Perinatal substance abuse and human subjects research: Are privacy protections adequate? *Mental Retardation and Developmental Disabilities Research Reviews*, 9, 54–59.

NIH Kiosk (2002a). Detailed application instructions for Certificates of Confidentiality: Intramural research projects. Available online at: http://grants.nih.gov/grants/policy/coc/appl_intramural.htm [accessed March 9, 2012].

NIH Kiosk (2002b). Slide presentation. Available online at: http://grants.nih.gov/grants/policy/coc/slides_020503/index.htm [accessed March 9, 2012].

NIH Kiosk (2003). Certificates of Confidentiality: Background information. Available online at: http://grants.nih.gov/grants/policy/coc/background.htm [accessed March 9, 2012].

NIH Kiosk (2009a). Certificates of Confidentiality: Homepage. Available online at: http://grants1.nih.gov/grants/policy/coc/?Display=Graphics [accessed March 9, 2012].

NIH Kiosk (2009b). Certificates of Confidentiality: Extramural research projects. Available online at: http://grants.nih.gov/grants/policy/coc/appl_extramural.htm[accessed March 9, 2012].

NIH Kiosk (2011). Certificates of Confidentiality: Frequently asked questions. Available online at: http://grants.nih.gov/grants/policy/coc/faqs.htm [accessed March 9, 2012].

People v. Newman (1973). 32 N.Y.2d. 379, 298 N.E.2d 651 (1973), cert. denied; *New York v. Newman*, 414 U.S. 1163.

Reilly, P. R. (2004). Certificates of Confidentiality. *Genetic Testing*, 8, 77–78.

State of North Carolina v. Bradley (2006). 179 N.C.App. 551.

Tovino, S. A. (2007). Functional neuroimaging information: A case for neuro exceptionalism? *Florida State University Law Review*, 34, 415–489.

USA Patriot Act (2001). *Uniting and Strengthening America by Providing Appropriate Tools Required to Intercept and Obstruct Terrorism Act of 2001*, Public Law 107–56; 115 Stat. 272 (2001).

Wolf, L. E. and Zandecki, J. (2006). Sleeping better at night: Investigators' experiences with Certificates of Confidentiality. *IRB: Ethics & Human Research*, 28, 1–7.

Wolf, L. E., Zandecki, J., and Lo, B. (2004). The Certificate of Confidentiality application: A view from the NIH Institutes. *IRB: Ethics & Human Research*, 26, 14–18.

8

Ethical issues in human genomic databases in addiction research

David B. Resnik

Introduction

Advances in computing, information technology, automated DNA extraction, sequencing, and genotyping have made it possible for researchers to move beyond studying a single gene (or genetic marker) in small populations to studying thousands of genes or even entire genomes in large populations. Genomic databases are playing an increasingly important role in many types of biomedical research involving human participants, ranging from physiological and behavioral studies to epidemiology and clinical trials. To create a genomic database, investigators extract DNA from biological samples such as blood, cheek scrapings, hair, or sputum. The DNA is then sequenced, and the data (e. g., AUGGAGCCU, etc.) is stored in a computer database. Once digitalized, the information can be easily shared with other investigators (Weir and Olick, 2004). The biological samples that serve as the basis for genomic data are usually stored in centralized sites known as biobanks (Weir and Olick, 2004). As biobanks are closely connected to genomic databases, this chapter will also address biobank issues.

Genomic databases may contain information about genes, genetic markers, or common genetic variants or whole genomes (Weir and Olick, 2004). Genomic information can be linked to other types of information pertaining to RNA, proteins, receptors, cellular structures, drugs, and diseases, to study statistical associations. In the last decade, there has been a tremendous increase in the quantity and variety of genomic databases. There are databases for specific populations, nationalities, and diseases, as well general databases. There are public non-profit databases as well as private, for-profit ones. Genomic databases may contain information from a few individuals to hundreds of thousands (Weir and Olick, 2004).

Genomic databases are also playing an increasingly important role in addiction research (Li et al., 2008; Saccone et al., 2009). Investigators can use genomic databases to identify genetic variants related to drug addiction and alcoholism, to study interactions among genes, and to understand the biological basis of addictive behaviors. Although genomic databases are an important tool in addiction research, they raise a number of ethical issues, which will be discussed here. This chapter will describe the issues in general terms, and then highlight important considerations for addiction research.

Informed consent

Informed consent is one of the fundamental ethical and legal requirements for research involving human subjects (Shamoo and Resnik, 2009). For informed consent to be valid, the

Genetic Research on Addiction, ed. Audrey R. Chapman. Published by Cambridge University Press.
© Cambridge University Press 2012.

research subject (or the subject's representative) must freely choose to participate in a study, based on a sound understanding of the relevant information. Informed consent is important for protecting the subject's legal rights and promoting autonomous decision making (Shamoo and Resnik, 2009). The federal research regulations spell out specific types of information that investigators must provide during the consent process, such as information about the nature of the research, study procedures, benefits, risks, alternatives, confidentiality protections, and the right to withdraw (Department of Health and Human Services, 2009).

Consent issues loomed large in one of the world's first large databases to include genomic information, Iceland's health-care database. In 1998, Iceland's parliament passed legislation authorizing the health minister to grant an exclusive license to deCODE genetics, a for-profit US company, to create a database containing the medical records of all Icelanders. As the database can be cross-referenced with information about genetics and genealogy, it allows investigators to study relationships among genotypes, disease, and the environment. The government of Iceland may use the database for health research, planning, and policy, and may license companies to use the data for commercial purposes. To protect confidentiality and privacy, the government included the requirement that no individually identifiable data be disclosed (Annas, 2000; Gulcher and Stefánnson, 2000; Weir and Olick, 2004).

Iceland's health-care database created an ethical controversy because it used a "presumed consent" process: all citizens would be enrolled in the database unless they opted out of it in writing (Gulcher and Stefánnson, 2000). Many argued that community consent and opt-out clauses were no substitute for individual consent. A better approach, according to many, is to use an opt-in procedure (Merz et al., 2004). Additionally, participants who decide to opt out should be able to withdraw their data or samples from the study (Weir and Olick, 2004).

Another important issue is whether a subject's general consent covers the use of their samples and data, as illustrated by the National Health and Nutrition Examination Survey (NHANES), a series of medical and epidemiological studies on adults and children conducted by the Centers for Disease Control and Prevention (CDC) from 1966 to 1984. The original NHANES consent form included detailed language about the study, but because it was judged to be too difficult for laypeople to understand, it was shortened to a six-page document with pictures. The document included only a brief and general statement about how the samples would be used. Some investigators were concerned that the consent form was inadequate, and that the CDC should obtain explicit consent from subjects to cover the use of their samples. Other researchers pointed out that re-consenting the subjects would be expensive and difficult, because of loss of contact information and other logistical problems (Weir and Olick, 2004).

A recent case illustrates the problems of using general consents to cover the use of samples and data. In 1990, investigators from Arizona State University (ASU) collected 200 blood samples from members of the Havasupai American Indian tribe. The consent form stated that the samples and data would be used for research on behavioral and mental illnesses but prior to the initiation of the study investigators told the tribal leaders that it would focus on the genetics of diabetes. Members of the tribe later learned that the investigators had used the samples and data to study diseases other than diabetes and shared the samples with other researchers. They strongly objected to the fact that the samples and data were used to study schizophrenia, inbreeding in the tribe, and the tribe's evolutionary and genetic origins, and they filed a $50 million lawsuit against ASU and the investigators. In the lawsuit, they alleged that the use of the samples and data violated the informed consent provided by the participants. In April 2010, ASU and the tribe agreed to settle the lawsuit out of court.

As part of the agreement, ASU formally apologized to the tribe, returned the samples, and paid $700 000, which was divided among 41 participants. Many members of the tribe vowed never to participate in future research conducted by ASU (Mello and Wolf, 2010).

The Havasupai case demonstrates the importance of clearly describing how samples and data will be used in the consent form and other communications with research participants and community representatives. It also reveals potential flaws with general consents, because research participants may not fully understand the implications of this agreement. They may not understand that samples or data could be used to conduct research that they may have objections to, such as research with potentially embarrassing or disturbing implications for their community or ethnic group (Mello and Wolf, 2010).

There is an ongoing debate among investigators, research organizations, and committees that oversee research with human subjects [such as institutional review boards (IRBs)] about how to approach the issue of general ("blanket" or "generic") consent versus specific consent for the use of samples and data. General consent helps to promote biomedical research by giving investigators a great deal of flexibility, but it may not provide adequate protections for human research participants (Salvaterra et al., 2008). Those who support general consent argue that, as long as participants understand that their samples and data may be used for many different research purposes, general consent does not violate their autonomy (Clayton, 2005). Studies have shown that most research participants are comfortable with giving broad permission for use of their samples and data (Wendler, 2006; Petrini, 2010). Moreover, as it is not possible to anticipate all of the potential uses for data and samples when a study is initiated, specific consent would significantly impede research, because investigators would need to re-consent subjects for new uses of their samples or data not described in the consent form (Clayton, 2005; Wendler, 2006). Opponents of general consent argue that it does not respect the participant's autonomy, even if many people are willing to agree to it, as they may not fully understand its implications. Maximum respect for autonomy requires that subjects consent only for specific uses of their data or samples.

There is no consensus on how to approach the issue of general versus specific consent, and different organizations and groups have adopted different guidelines (Petrini, 2010). Tiered (or "layered") consent strikes a compromise between general and specific content (National Bioethics Advisory Committee, 1999; Salvaterra et al., 2008). Under the tiered approach, subjects are given several options for use of their samples and data, such as no use, uses for research on specific diseases or topics, general uses, and commercial uses. Research participants also decide whether to allow their samples or data to be shared with other researchers. The consent form contains check boxes by which participants can express their choices. Participants that are comfortable with general consent can express this choice on the consent form, while others can choose to limit the use of their samples and data. The tiered approach respects the participant's autonomy but does not impede research. The only major drawback of the tiered approach is that investigators need to keep track of what subjects have consented to, but this problem can be handled with good record-keeping practices (Weir and Olick, 2004).

Another important consent issue is how to deal with biological samples and genomic data provided by children. Ethical and legal rules allow parents or guardians to consent on behalf of their children. Many different research studies involving biobanking and genomic databases include child participants. Some commentators have argued that respect for autonomy requires that when they reach adulthood, child participants should have the opportunity to decide whether to continue participating in a study, as well as the opportunity to withdraw their samples or data (if feasible) (Gurwitz et al., 2009).

Informed consent for genomic studies can present unique challenges for addiction research, because participants may have cognitive or emotional problems that compromise their decision-making abilities. Participants may be suffering from depression, anxiety, drug-withdrawal symptoms, psychosis, dementia, attention deficits, and other medical and psychological problems related to addiction. They may also be socioeconomically disadvantaged, have HIV/AIDS, or a history of physical or sexual abuse or incarceration. As a result, individuals participating in addiction research may be regarded as vulnerable subjects because of difficulties providing consent or protecting their interests (Macklin, 2003), and additional protections may be required to safeguard them from harm or exploitation (Rosenstein and Miller, 2008):

- assessing the individual's decision-making capacity prior to enrollment to determine whether they are capable of providing consent or require assistance
- providing assistance to participants who have difficulties with consent
- making sure that participants who consent to general use of their samples understand what this means
- giving participants the option of consenting to only specific uses of their samples
- obtaining consent from a legally authorized representative, such as a guardian or close family member, if the participant is incapable of consent.

Enrolling minors also presents challenges for addiction researchers. Adolescents with drug addictions or children of addicts may participate in studies involving genomic databases. Parents or guardians can provide consent for these participants. When children reach adulthood, they should be given the opportunity to decide whether they want to remain in the study, and they should be able to withdraw their biological samples. One problem that addiction researchers may encounter is that parents may have compromised decision-making abilities, due to their cognitive or emotional problems (mentioned above). Addiction researchers who enroll children in studies should make sure that the parents are capable of providing consent for their children.

Sharing samples and data

Sharing research materials and data is an essential part of the scientific ethos and facilitates collaboration, peer review, replication of experiments, and other scientific activities (Shamoo and Resnik, 2009). Many different organizations strongly support data sharing in genetics, genomics, and molecular biology. In 1996, leaders of different laboratories working on the Human Genome Project established the Bermuda Rules, which discourage patenting and encourage rapid, unconditional release of DNA sequence data, which should be deposited in a public database (Marshall, 2001). The Bermuda Rules were reaffirmed in 2003. Granting agencies encourage the sharing of genomic data and biological samples, as do many scientific journals (Shamoo and Resnik, 2009).

Although sharing of genomic data and biological samples is crucial to the advancement of biomedical science, it can threaten the confidentiality of research data. Many ethical and legal standards, including the Helsinki Declaration (World Medical Association, 2008) and the US federal research regulations (Department of Health and Human Services, 2009), require investigators to protect the confidentiality of human research subjects. Safeguarding confidentiality helps to protect human research participants from discrimination, bias, embarrassment, and other harms that can result from the disclosure of private information, and also promotes autonomy by allowing human participants to have some control over the disclosure of their private information (Hodge and Gostin, 2008).

Investigators have used different strategies for protecting confidentiality when they share human genomic data. Under the restricted access approach, genomic data are shared only with other researchers who sign a confidentiality agreement that describes how the data will be used, stored, protected, and secured. These agreements usually state that the researchers will not share the data with other investigators without permission and that they will not attempt to identify individual research subjects. Confidentiality agreements may also require that data recipients have IRB approval for the research they are conducting, because the data may include information that could be used to identify individuals (Resnik, 2010). Under the open access approach, investigators share human genomic data freely, without requiring recipients to sign a confidentiality agreement. To do this without violating confidentiality, the investigator removes personal identifiers, such as name, social security number, and address, from the data, which is deemed de-identified. The researchers may maintain a code that links the de-identified data to personal identifiers, but the code is not shared with recipients. Alternatively, they may completely remove personal identifiers so that the data are anonymous. Anonymizing data is only done when investigators have no plans to re-contact participants (see discussion below). Investigators who receive de-identified human genomic data do not need to have an IRB approve their work. It is regarded as "exempt" under federal regulations, as no private information about individuals will be received (Resnik, 2010). In the most open approach, researchers place human genomic data on a public website, so that anyone in the world can access the data freely.

The chief advantage of the open access approach is that it promotes scientific progress by enabling researchers to access data easily without the need to complete paperwork or obtain IRB approval. The restricted access approach could hinder scientific research, because it requires data recipients to comply with more administrative requirements. However, the restricted access approach is the best means for protecting confidentiality.

For more than a decade, investigators believed that de-identifying genomic data was a surefire method of protecting confidentiality, and they shared genomic data freely. However, in the last few years, studies have challenged this assumption (McGuire and Gibbs, 2006). In 2004, scientists demonstrated that individuals could be identified from a de-identified genomic database if one has access to 30–80 statistically independent single nucleotide polymorphisms (SNPs) from that individual (Lin et al., 2004). In 2008, scientists demonstrated that it is possible to identify an individual in a complex DNA mixture of 10 000 to 50 000 SNP, if one already has specific information about that individual's DNA (Homer et al., 2008). Another method for identifying DNA in de-identified genomic databases is to match phenotypes associated with the DNA to identified phenotypes from other databases. For example, if one has access to a criminal or health-care database that identifies individuals, one could use their phenotypes (such as age, gender, disease status, and height/weight) to identify them in a genomic database (Lowrance and Collins, 2007). Although these methods require that one already has access to an identified DNA sample in order to identify an individual in a de-identified genomic database, these studies call into question the reliability of de-identification as a method for protecting confidentiality, as many databases contain identified DNA materials, including databases used for military, scientific, clinical, law enforcement, or commercial purposes. One could also acquire identified DNA by extracting it from a person's blood, sputum, or tissue sample (Resnik, 2010).

One could argue that although scientists have demonstrated that it is theoretically possible to identify individuals in de-identified genomic databases, there is only a remote chance that re-identification will happen, because this requires considerable expertise and resources, such as the use of complex statistical methods to identify individuals (Knoppers, 2010). They also require access to identified samples or data. However, insurance companies, employers, or law-enforcement authorities may have the resources and motivation to identify individuals in de-identified genomic databases. Moreover, as everyone, with the exception of identical twins, has a unique genome, the notion of de-identified genetic information is precarious, as it will become easier to identify individuals in genomic databases as technology advances and more information becomes available (Resnik, 2010).

There are different ways of responding to the possibility of identifying individuals in de-identified genomic databases. One could move away from open access and take a more restrictive approach, which the National Institutes of Health (NIH) recently did. After learning about several papers showing how it is possible to identify individuals in de-identified genomic databases, the NIH decided to remove de-identified genome-wide association study (GWAS) data from its publicly available websites. Access to de-identified GWAS data is granted only to investigators and institutions that submit an application to the data access committee and abide by the terms of the data use agreement (NIH, 2010). In August 2007, the NIH also decided that GWAS data from studies it sponsors must be deposited in the National Cancer Institute's Cancer Genetic Markers of Susceptibility (CGEMS) database or the database of Genotypes and Phenotypes (dbGaP).

Others have taken the opposite approach by asking subjects to consent to open release of their genomic data, with the knowledge that they can or will be identified (Lunshof et al., 2008). The Personal Genome Project (PGP) will sequence the genomes of participants and place their data on a public website. The website will also include phenotypic data, such as height, weight, age, and disease status. The research subjects agree to participate with the understanding that their data will be publicly available, and they forgo traditional confidentiality protections in order to help advance research. The PGP will focus initially on the genotypic and phenotypic data of ten geneticists, including project leader George Church, but it will eventually expand to include 100 000 subjects (Personal Genome Project, 2010). Noted geneticists James Watson and Craig Venter, who are not participants in the PGP, have both agreed to open release of their genomic data (Resnik, 2010).

A third approach is to publicly disclose only the amount of de-identified genomic data necessary for research. Investigators could remove some types of genomic information from the data, such as genetic variants that could more easily be used to identify individuals, thereby reducing the risk of re-identification. Researchers could also use statistical methods to alter the data to reduce the risk of re-identification (Resnik, 2010).

These approaches have their own advantages and disadvantages. The restricted access approach maximizes protection of private information, but impedes research by making it difficult for investigators to obtain genomic data. Some of these difficulties can be overcome by streamlining the application process for access to genomic data. The open access approach promotes research but threatens the confidentiality of the human participants as well as their relatives, as it may be possible to identify the close relatives of someone who is identified in a DNA database. Although it might be acceptable for an individual to sacrifice his or her own confidentiality for the sake of research, one might argue that it is not appropriate to threaten the confidentiality of the subject's close relatives. Investigators have an obligation not only to protect human subjects in research studies, but also to protect third parties who may be placed at risk by those studies (Resnik and Sharp, 2006). The consent form for the PGP warns participants that they may be placing the confidentiality and privacy of their relatives at risk, but one might argue that this warning does not adequately protect third parties (Resnik, 2010). The third approach aims to protect confidentiality while advancing research, but it may fail to do either. In making it impossible to re-identify individuals, investigators may need to remove so much information that the data are useless to other researchers. If investigators release data that are useful to other researchers, they may not adequately protect confidentiality (Resnik, 2010). At present, there is no consensus on the proper way to share genomic information while protecting confidentiality. Different types of research may warrant different approaches, or possibly some combination of all three.

Protecting privacy and confidentiality is especially important in addiction research because of the social stigma related to alcoholism and drug addiction. Someone who is publicly identified as an addict or alcoholic may face embarrassment, guilt, social ostracism, or discrimination in employment or insurance. People who are identified as family members of addicts and alcoholics may also have to deal with social repercussions. Because addiction carries a significant social stigma, investigators must take great care to protect the confidentiality of genomic databases used in addiction research. Restricted access to data may be the preferred approach in addiction research. Investigators should require other researchers to sign a data use agreement in order to have access to genomic databases involving addiction. Public disclosure of de-identified data should be avoided, even if participants are willing to consent to it, in order to protect the privacy and confidentiality of family members of addicts or alcoholics.

Returning individualized research results

Ethical issues also arise when deciding whether to inform participants of individualized results of genomic research (Holtzman, 1999; Renegar et al., 2006; Dressler, 2009). When analyzing genomic data, investigators may discover genetic variants that are associated with increased risks of some types of diseases. These include variants that are investigated as part of the study as well as variants that investigators happen to discover during the course of investigation (i.e., incidental findings) (Wolf et al., 2008). Although information about genetic risks is potentially very useful to human research participants, disclosing test results that have questionable utility, accuracy, or reliability may cause people needless worry, anxiety, and stress. Some people may even make misinformed or ill-advised decisions, such as deciding not to have children or planning to commit suicide before becoming senile, upon learning about genomic research results (Renegar et al., 2006). Investigators should consider the following when deciding whether and how to return individual genomic research results.

First, would the results provide valuable information for medical decision making? The clinical utility of genomic information can vary considerably, depending on the probability of developing a disease, given a particular phenotype, and our ability to treat or prevent the disease. For example, a woman who tests positive for *BRCA1* or *BRCA2* mutations has a 60% lifetime risk of developing breast cancer, compared with a 12% lifetime risk for a woman in the general population, and a 15–40% lifetime risk of developing ovarian cancer, compared with a 1.4% lifetime risk for a woman in the general population (National Cancer Institute, 2010). As there are effective options for preventing breast cancer, women who know that they have *BRCA1* or *BRCA2* mutations can alter their diet, take medications that reduce the risk of breast cancer, opt for more frequent cancer screening exams, or decide to have their breasts or ovaries removed (National Cancer Institute, 2010). Thus, informing women about their *BRCA1/BRCA2* status can benefit them by enhancing their decision making.

However, the clinical utility of many other individualized genomic findings is more uncertain. If the genomic finding pertains to a rare disease (i.e., less than 1/1500 people in the population affected), then the person's absolute risk of developing the disease might still be quite low, even if they have a genetic variant that increases their relative risk of the disease. For example, suppose that an American male is told that he has a genetic variant that increases his risk of penile cancer by 50%. As 1/100 000 males in the United States develops penile cancer, his absolute risk would still only be 1.5/100 000 (American Cancer Society, 2006). Would this information be very helpful to the man, or could it possibly cause him needless worry?

If the genomic finding pertains to a common disease, then it may not add much information that has practical value, because there may be many controllable factors that have more relevance. For example, many of the currently available genetic tests for cardiovascular disease susceptibility yield inconclusive results. Non-genetic risk factors, such as smoking, body mass index, blood pressure, and blood cholesterol levels are often more clinically useful than current genetic tests (Humphries et al., 2004). Genomic information related to cancer, diabetes, Alzheimer's disease, and many other conditions may also add little of diagnostic or therapeutic value (Renegar et al., 2006).

Second, testing methods that are inaccurate or unreliable can yield misleading information (Holtzman, 1999). For instance, a false positive test for a gene that is strongly associated with a serious disease, such as progressive dementia, could cause an individual needless anxiety and worry and lead them to make misinformed medical or reproductive choices. In the United States, the Clinical Laboratory Improvement Amendments (CLIA) require that laboratories that perform clinical testing be certified in order to promote accurate and reliable clinical testing (Holtzman, 1999). Laboratories that perform tests only for research studies are not required to be CLIA certified. If genomic tests are performed by laboratories that lack certification, the results may be questionable (Holtzman, 1999).

Third, does the research protocol include plans for providing counseling, medical referrals, or follow-up for people who receive genomic test results? Receiving tests results without adequate counseling, advice, or follow-up can be distressing and harmful, and subjects who receive genomic information may not understand it or know what to do with it. Investigators have an obligation to help subjects understand the information they receive and to help them obtain an appropriate referral or advice. Investigators may want to collaborate with qualified medical professionals, who can discuss the results with the subjects and help them obtain treatment or a referral. Handouts and other study-related materials may also help subjects understand their test results (Wolf et al., 2008).

Researchers have taken three different approaches on the issue of reporting test results to individuals. The first approach is to report only the results of the entire research study and not to report any individual results. The rationale for this approach is that the purpose of the research is to advance human knowledge, not to provide participants with individualized testing, counseling, or treatment. Additionally, the research results may not be clinically useful, and there may be problems with reliability or accuracy (as discussed above). Researchers who take this approach usually inform participants that they will not receive individual test results. They may also remove any personal identifiers from the samples and data, making it impossible to return individual results (Holtzman, 1999). The shortcoming with this approach is that sometimes researchers will have access to data about individuals that is useful, accurate, and reliable, such as *BRCA1/BRCA2* results. Withholding this information from individuals would seem to violate the investigator's obligations to benefit research subjects and to enhance their decision making (Wolf et al., 2008).

A second approach is to provide all genomic results to individuals. The rationale for this strategy is that providing all of this information can benefit research participants and promote their autonomous decision making (Renegar et al., 2006). Participants can use the information they receive to make medical, lifestyle, or reproduction choices (Shalowitz and Miller, 2005). Additionally, studies have shown the research participants would like to receive all of their individualized test results (Shalowitz and Miller, 2008). Direct-to-consumer genomic testing embodies this tell-all approach. The main drawback of this approach is that the information participants receive may be confusing and not be very useful, and they could be harmed by information that is inaccurate, unreliable, or misleading. Furthermore, some may prefer not to receive any genomic test results. Sharing all test results would seem to be appropriate only if the participants have the requisite knowledge, background, and motivation. For example, the geneticists participating in the PGP would be capable of dealing with uncertain genomic information.

A third approach is a compromise between these two positions, whereby research participants would receive only test results that are useful, reliable, and accurate (Ravitsky and Wilfond, 2006). They would also have the option of not receiving some or all of the results. This approach benefits participants, promotes their autonomy, and protects them from information that may be uncertain or misleading (Renegar et al., 2006). The difficulty with this approach is determining what type of genomic information should be considered useful. While information that has a direct bearing on medical decision making is clearly useful, other information might be viewed as useful if it helps participants make reproductive choices or provides them with peace of mind. One way to handle this issue is to ask participants about the types of information they would consider useful.

Returning individualized research results raises important issues for addiction research. Potentially useful results include genetic variants that increase the risk of the disease being investigated (e.g., addiction), as well incidental findings, such as genomic variants that increase the risk of cancer or heart disease. Investigators should decide when developing the protocol what types of results they will disclose to participants (if any). The informed consent document should also discuss the disclosure of individualized genomic findings. Counseling should be made available to participants to help them understand genomic findings and to provide them with appropriate referrals. The disclosure plan may need to be revised as new discoveries are made that affect the significance of results.

As many of the research participants may have mental or emotional problems that compromise judgment and decision making, an argument can be made that investigators should only disclose clinically significant research results to individuals. Individuals who receive clinically insignificant information concerning genetic variants may not understand how to deal with this information, which may lead to psychic distress or ill-advised decisions. For example, suppose that a recovering drug addict with schizophrenia is informed that he has a genetic variant associated with a 50% increased risk of a rare neuromuscular disease. The variant increases his relative risk of the disease from 1/50 000 to 1.5/50 000. Although his absolute risk of developing the disease is still very low, he might have an unpredictable and potentially dangerous reaction to this information. The information might affirm a paranoid belief that he is doomed to die from a terrible disease. He might decide to stop taking his medication and start using drugs again.

Of course, many people with addictions will suffer no ill effects from receiving genomic information that has little clinical utility. However, because people with addictions may have mental or emotional conditions that interfere with their ability to process and understand information, investigators should be mindful of the risk of disclosure when they decide to share genomic information with individuals.

Another important issue for addiction researchers to consider is whether to share information about addiction risks with non-addicted participants. Many studies on the genomics of addiction also include healthy controls, who are matched to the addicted population in terms of age, race, sex, and other characteristics. Genomic variants found in the cases but not in the controls could be associated with addiction (Levran et al., 2008). Studies of the genomics of addiction also enroll non-addicted family members to study the heritability of addictive behaviors and identify genes (Lachman et al., 2007). It is possible that some of the non-addicted participants might have genomic variants that are found to increase the risk of addiction. Should investigators inform healthy, non-addicted participants that they have an increased risk of drug addiction? While this information could be very valuable to the healthy participants – they could decide to avoid using recreational drugs or alcohol to reduce their risk – this information also might have little value, and could cause them needless worry. Again, clinical significance may prove to be a useful standard for deciding whether to share this information. If information concerning genetic variants possibly linked to addiction is clinically significant (i.e., it is useful in diagnosis, prevention, or treatment) then it should be shared. If not, then sharing the information may be inadvisable.

To get a better understanding of whether it would be appropriate to disclose genomic information to participants in addiction research, it may be useful to survey the relevant population to find out what types of information they would like to receive if they participate in genomic studies. Non-addicted family members of addicted participants might be especially interested in finding out whether they have any genetic variants possibly associated with addiction. As noted above, studies have shown that most participants would like to receive their individualized test results (Shalowitz and Miller, 2008). The preferences of research participants might not be the determining factor in deciding whether to disclose individualized results, but it should be an important consideration.

Commercialization of research

There are also several issues relating to the commercialization of genomic research. The first issue is whether genomic data can be (or should be) patentable (Resnik, 2003). This is both a legal and an ethical issue. A patent is a right granted by the government to exclude others from using, making, or commercializing an invention for a limited period of time (usually 20 years). In the United States and many other countries, patents have been awarded on DNA sequences. The legal basis for this policy is that patents should be awarded for useful, novel, and non-obvious products, processes, or improvements that result from human ingenuity. Naturally occurring products or processes or abstract ideas cannot be patented. Although DNA occurs in nature, patents agencies and courts have held that DNA can be patented for a modified DNA sequence or an isolated and purified sequence, which has a practical use such as DNA sequences used to test for genetic predispositions to develop diseases. While most people agree that modified DNA sequences should be patentable, many have argued that isolated and purified DNA sequences should not be patentable, because they do not qualify as inventions. Since the 1980s, the courts and patent agencies have treated isolated and purified DNA sequences as patentable on the grounds that they are no different from other molecules that occur in nature, such as proteins, hormones, and RNA (Resnik, 2003).

In March 2010, Judge Robert W. Sweet of the United States District Court for the Southern District of New York ruled in *Association for Molecular Pathology et al. v. U.S. Patent and Trademark Office* that isolated and purified DNA is not patentable, because it is not a human invention and that only modified DNA is patentable. The case involved a legal challenge to Myriad Genetics' *BRCA1/BRCA2* gene patents. The plaintiffs argued that the patents were overly broad and that they shouldn't have been awarded in the first place, because naturally occurring DNA sequences should not be patentable (Marshall, 2010). However, the Court of Appeals for the Federal Circuit reversed this decision in part. The court ruled that isolated and purified DNA is patentable because it is markedly different from naturally occurring DNA, but the court also ruled that some of Myriad's methods for analyzing DNA are not patentable because they are too abstract. This case will probably go to the Supreme Court (Pollack, 2011). The ethical and policy arguments for and against DNA patenting are complex and controversial and will not be reviewed here. (For further discussion, see Resnik, 2003.)

Another issue related to commercialization is the ownership of human biological samples from which genomic information is derived. Although patients and research subjects have claimed ownership of the biological samples that they have donated to clinicians or researchers, US courts have not sympathized with this view. In *Moore v. Regents of University of California* (1990), the California Supreme Court ruled that the plaintiff did not have any property interests in a cell line derived from tissue left over from an operation to remove his spleen. The court held that the researchers had property interests in the cell line, as they expended considerable effort to develop it, but that Moore had no property interests in his cells once they were removed from his body. According to the court, granting patients or research participants such interests would greatly impede progress in biomedical research. In Moore's case, his physician, Dr. David Golde, had recommended that Moore have a splenectomy to treat his leukemia. Unbeknown to Moore, Golde saved the tissue left over from the surgery and developed and patented a cell line, which was worth hundreds of millions of dollars because it produced unusually high quantities of immune system hormones. Moore discovered that his cell line had been patented and initiated a lawsuit. Moore sued the university and its researchers for conversion (i.e., unlawful deprivation of property interests), lack of informed consent, and breach of fiduciary duty. Although the court did not recognize Moore's property interests in the cell line, it held that his right to informed consent had been violated, because Golde did not discuss his commercial interests with Moore (Resnik, 2003). Several other courts have followed the reasoning (if not the legal precedent) found in *Moore*.

Even if human participants currently do not have a solid legal basis for claiming ownership of biological samples collected for research studies, the ethical issues remain pertinent. In many cases involving legal disputes about biological samples, there were also ethical questions concerning exploitation and fair sharing of the benefits of research. In the Moore case, the investigators did not tell Moore that they were planning to commercialize tissue left over from his operation, or that his tissue was worth potentially hundreds of millions of dollars. They asked him to return to the medical center to provide additional tissue samples (blood and skin) that they falsely told him were needed for his medical treatment. In truth, the investigators needed the samples for their research, not for Moore's treatment. In discussing his case, Moore said he had been exploited. In the lawsuit, he asked to receive a fair share of the profits from the cell line (Resnik, 2003). Breast cancer advocates have also complained that Myriad Genetics' commercialization of the *BRCA1/BRCA2* tests is exploitative and unfair, and that benefits should be shared fairly (Resnik, 2003).

Various organizations have called for the fair sharing of the benefits of genetic and genomic research (Knoppers, 2000; Schroeder, 2007). Although few would deny the importance of benefit sharing, many conceptual and practical issues need to be addressed for this idea to become a workable policy. First, there needs to be a basic understanding of what constitutes a fair sharing of benefits. Different approaches to social justice would recommend divergent ways of sharing the benefits of research. For example, libertarians would favor a distribution of benefits on the basis of free market principles, whereas egalitarians would favor equal sharing of benefits. Second, many practical questions also need to be addressed, such as "What are the benefits?," "What is a fair distribution of benefits?", "Who shares in the benefits – investigators, participants, populations, sponsors?", and "How will benefit-sharing arrangements be implemented?" (Schroeder, 2007). Investigators who conduct research on human genomic databases should address questions like these when planning their projects. IRBs should also consider these issues when approving research proposals.

Intellectual property is also an important issue in genomic research on addiction, because scientific discoveries might lead to patents on genes related to addiction, such as: genes that code for chemical receptors, neurotransmitters, or therapeutic proteins; genetic tests; or other medical products (Lee et al., 2010). Patenting can play an important role in making products and services available to the public that can help diagnose, treat, or prevent addiction. Although companies that sponsor research and development need to recoup their investments, products and services should be affordable, so that the benefits are shared fairly with the population being studied and the general public. One of the complaints voiced against the Myriad Genetics *BRCA1/BRCA2* test is that it is too expensive. If Myriad had charged reasonable fees, it is possible that the company would not have been sued. Companies that develop products and services related to addiction prevention or treatment should learn from Myriad's mistakes and charge reasonable prices.

Investigators that work for companies should encourage their employers to make their products affordable, and work closely with community representatives in formulating benefit-sharing plans (Schroeder, 2007). Investigators should inform research participants in addiction studies about commercial products that may be developed from research and let them know about any plans to share benefits with participants or the population. Although many consent forms include language informing participants that they will not share in any profits from the commercialization of research, participants should at least be informed of this outcome. Consent documents should also inform participants about their rights pertaining to the ownership of biological samples, including procedures for withdrawing their samples.

Acknowledgments

This research was supported by the National Institute of Environmental Health Sciences (NIEHS), National Institutes of Health (NIH). It does not represent the views of the NIEHS, NIH, or US Government. I am grateful to Bruce Androphy for helpful comments.

References

American Cancer Society (2006). What are the key statistics about penile cancer? Available online at: www.cancer.org/docroot/CRI/content/CRI_2_4_1X_What_are_the_key_statistics_for_penile_cancer_35.asp?sitearea= [accessed March 13, 2012].

Annas, G. (2000). Rules for research on human genetic variation – lessons from Iceland. *New England Journal of Medicine*, 342, 1830–1833.

Clayton, E. (2005). Informed consent and biobanks. *Journal of Law, Medicine & Ethics*, 33, 15–21.

Department of Health and Human Services (2009). Protection of Human Subjects, 45 CFR 46. Available online at: www.hhs.gov/ohrp/humansubjects/index.html [accessed March 13, 2012].

Dressler, L. (2009). Disclosure of research results from cancer genomic studies: State of the science. *Clinical Cancer Research*, 15, 4270–4276.

Gulcher, J. and Stefánnson, K. (2000). The Iceland Healthcare Database and informed consent. *New England Journal of Medicine*, 342, 1827–1830.

Gurwitz, D., Fortier, I., Lunshof, J., et al. (2009). Children and population biobanks. *Science*, 325, 818–819.

Hodge, J. Jr. and Gostin, L. (2008). Confidentiality. In E. Emanuel, C. Grady, and R. Crouch, et al. (eds.), *The Oxford Textbook of Clinical Research Ethics*. New York: Oxford University Press, pp. 673–681.

Holtzman, N. (1999). Promoting safe and effective genetic tests in the United States: Work of the Task Force on Genetic Testing. *Clinical Chemistry*, 45, 732–738.

Homer, N., Szelinger, S., Redman, M., et al. (2008). Resolving individuals contributing trace amounts of DNA to highly complex mixtures using high-density SNP genotyping microarrays. *PLoS Genetics*, 4, 8: e1000167.

Humphries, S., Ridker, P., and Talmud, P. (2004). Genetic testing for cardiovascular disease susceptibility: A useful clinical management tool or possible misinformation? *Arteriosclerosis, Thrombosis, and Vascular Biology*, 24, 628–630.

Knoppers, B. (2000). Population genetics and benefit sharing. *Community Genetics*, 3, 212–214.

Knoppers, B. (2010). Consent to "personal" genomics and privacy. *Embo Reports*, 11, 416–419.

Lachman, H., Fann, C., Bartzis, M., et al. (2007). Genomewide suggestive linkage of opioid dependence to chromosome 14q. *Human Molecular Genetics*, 16, 1327–1334.

Lee, J., Jung, M., and Lee, J. (2010). 5-HT2C receptor modulators: a patent survey. *Expert Opinion in Therapeutic Patents*, 20, 1429–1455.

Levran, O., Londono, D., O'Hara, K., et al. (2008). Genetic susceptibility to heroin addiction: A candidate gene association study. *Genes, Brain, and Behavior*, 7, 720–729.

Li, C. Y., Mao, X., and Wei, L. (2008). Genes and (common) pathways underlying drug addiction. *PLoS Computational Biology*, 4, 1, e2.

Lin, Z., Owen, A., and Altman, R. (2004). Genomic research and human subject privacy. *Science*, 305, 183.

Lowrance, W. and Collins, F. (2007). Identifiability in genomic research. *Science*, 317, 600–602.

Lunshof, J., Chadwick, R., Vorhaus, D., et al. (2008). From genetic privacy to open consent. *Nature Reviews Genetics*, 9, 406–411.

Macklin, R. (2003). Bioethics, vulnerability, and protection. *Bioethics*, 17, 472–486.

Marshall, E. (2001). Bermuda rules: Community spirit, with teeth. *Science*, 291, 1192.

Marshall, E. (2010). Cancer gene patents ruled invalid. *Science*, 328, 153.

McGuire, A. and Gibbs, R. (2006). No longer de-identified. *Science*, 312, 370–371.

Mello, M. and Wolf, L. (2010). The Havasupai Indian tribe case – lessons for research involving stored biologic samples. *New England Journal of Medicine*, 363, 204–207.

Merz, J., McGee, G., and Sankar, P. (2004). "Iceland Inc.?" On the ethics of commercial population genetics. *Social Science and Medicine*, 58, 1201–1209.

National Bioethics Advisory Commitee (1999). *Research Involving Human Biological Materials: Ethical Issues and Policy Guidance*, Volume 1. Rockville, MD: National Bioethics Advisory Committee.

National Cancer Institute (2010). BRCA1 and BRCA2: Cancer risk and genetic testing. Available online at: www.cancer.gov/cancertopics/factsheet/Risk/BRCA. [accessed March 13, 2012].

NIH (2010). Policy for sharing of data obtained in NIH supported or conducted genome-wide association studies (GWAS). Available online at: http://grants.nih.gov/grants/guide/notice-files/NOT-OD-07-088.html [accessed March 14, 2012].

Personal Genome Project (2010). Available online at: www.personalgenomes.org/ [accessed March 13, 2012].

Petrini, C. (2010). "Broad" consent, exceptions to consent and the question of using biological samples for research purposes different from the initial collection purpose. *Social Science and Medicine*, 70, 217–220.

Pollack, A. (2011). Ruling upholds gene patent in cancer test. *New York Times*, July 29, A1.

Ravitsky, V. and Wilfond, B. (2006). Disclosing individual results to research participants. *American Journal of Bioethics*, 6, 8–17.

Renegar, G., Webster, C., Stuerzebecher, S., et al. (2006). Returning genetic research results to individuals: Points-to-consider, *Bioethics*, 20, 24–36.

Resnik, D. (2003). *Owning the Genome*. Albany, NY: State University of New York Press.

Resnik, D. (2010). Genomic research data: Open vs. restricted access. *IRB*, 32, 1–6.

Resnik, D. and Sharp, R. (2006). Protecting third parties in human subjects research. *IRB*, 28, 1–7.

Rosenstein, D. and Miller, F. (2008). Research involving those at risk for impaired decision-making capacity. In E. Emanuel, C. Grady, R. Crouch, et al. (eds.), *The Oxford Textbook of Clinical Research Ethics.* New York: Oxford University Press, pp. 437–445.

Saccone, S., Bierut, L. and Chesler, E., et al. (2009). Supplementing high-density SNP microarrays for additional coverage of disease-related genes: addiction as a paradigm. *PLoS ONE*, 4, e5225.

Salvaterra, E., Lecchi, L., and Giovanelli, S., et al. (2008). Banking together. A unified model of informed consent for biobanking. *EMBO Reports*, 9, 307–313.

Schroeder, D. (2007). Benefit sharing: It's time for a definition. *Journal of Medical Ethics*, 33, 205–209.

Shalowitz, D. and Miller, F. (2005). Disclosing individual results of clinical research: Implications of respect for participants. *Journal of the American Medical Association*, 294, 737–740.

Shalowitz, D. and Miller, F. (2008). Communicating the results of clinical research to participants: Attitudes, practices, and future directions. *PLoS Medicine*, 5, e91.

Shamoo, A. and Resnik, D. (2009). *Responsible Conduct of Research*, second edition. New York: Oxford University Press.

Weir, R. and Olick, R. (2004). *The Stored Tissue Issue*. New York: Oxford University Press.

Wendler, D. (2006). One-time general consent for research on biological samples. *British Medical Journal*, 332, 544–547.

Wolf, S., Lawrenz, F., Nelson, C., et al. (2008). Managing incidental findings in human subjects research: Analysis and recommendations. *Journal of Law, Medicine and Ethics*, 36, 219–248.

World Medical Association (2008). Declaration of Helsinki: Ethical principles for medical research involving human subjects. Available online at: www.wma.net/en/20activities/10ethics/10helsinki [accessed March 13, 2012].

Chapter

Should addiction researchers accept funding derived from the profits of addictive consumptions?

Peter J. Adams

It is surprising just how easy it is for one's mind to find justifications for what one wants to do. Similar to the way a knee reflex responds to a strike from a doctor's rubber mallet, justifications seem to emerge smoothly and automatically; they swing into action to counter even the slightest prod of conscience: I eat meat because where else will I get sufficient protein; I drive a car to work because the city's public transport system is so lousy; I avoid giving to that charity because that organization is corrupt.

But, of course, one's mind does not pull these justifications out of thin air.

This was brought home to me some time back while in the throes of preparing a grant application on behalf of our department. Our university had established a new fund for staff to invite international experts into departments to promote teaching and research endeavors. It was a generous allowance with enough money to host an overseas visitor for 1 to 3 months. Since such opportunities were rare, we quickly arranged a meeting of interested staff and began brainstorming a proposal. We settled on the idea of inviting a leading academic in community development from overseas who could help boost our fledgling development projects. That person could present in seminars, guide our current projects, input into student research, and help us devise and compile a funding application for a large new project. We were excited. The visit would raise our efforts to a new level.

I took the ideas from the meeting and sat down at my computer to fill in the application form. The first boxes asked for the usual information about the location, the people involved, their roles ... this was easy enough to complete. The boxes then asked for the aims of the visit and the activities we had in mind ... this took a little longer to formulate ... then my eyes scanned a box at the bottom of the page. Inside the box was a familiar brand logo and next to it a statement: "Proudly supported by the Lion Foundation." I instantly recognized the logo as belonging to the nation's largest brewery. I also knew that the Lion Foundation was the largest of the six main organizations involved in distributing community benefit grants from the profits of slot machines.

This complicated matters considerably. I could see the association was very inconvenient. The money we were seeking had come directly from people playing slot machines in bars and, as I knew very well, it was these machines that contributed to the majority of gambling-related harm in our country (Wheeler et al., 2006; Livingstone and Adams, 2011). An unwelcome query was prodding at me from the back of my mind: Is this acceptable? Is it okay to proceed?

Genetic Research on Addiction, ed. Audrey R. Chapman. Published by Cambridge University Press. © Cambridge University Press 2012.

My first response – I am ashamed to admit – was to pretend I had not seen the logo. Well, we had already put so much work into the ideas for the project and our hopes were ablaze. The initiative now had momentum and the financial support would be an ideal stimulus for what our department was seeking to achieve. Maybe I could pretend I hadn't seen it? That's it, I didn't really see it. Perhaps later, if people were to point it out, I could claim I didn't know and by then it would be too late to stop. Maybe my colleagues would follow my example and choose to ignore it as well. It would be so simple to turn the page and continue filling in the boxes without thinking about the logo any further. But, alas, I had seen it and I was already worrying about it. The idea of deceiving myself was beginning to lose its appeal. I was going to have to find another approach.

My second response was more measured. Okay, I can't pretend I didn't see it, but perhaps it's not really such a bad thing to receive money from this source. After all, gambling has its positive side: most people gamble purely for enjoyment and gambling venues help create rich opportunities for family and friends to gather together and to have some fun. Only a churlish spoilsport would stand in the way of people having fun. Besides, it is really only a very small minority of those who gamble who experience serious problems, and they would probably have formed an addiction to that or another product anyway. No harm would be done in making good use of this money.

Such justifications might work in an ordinary university department but, unfortunately, in this arena our department is not so ordinary. It contains three active groups devoted to research on harm from tobacco, alcohol, and gambling. How would it look to others if we were seen to fund our activities from the very sources that generate these harms? On a daily basis our work reminds us of the widespread harm and misery inflicted on individuals, communities, and populations by these consumptions. In addition to the conflict we would experience in our own minds, we would find it difficult to stand up and, with any credibility, criticize the activities of these industries. We could not with any seriousness get away with pretending the impacts of addictive consumptions are minimal. Besides, we had known for a long time that locating the origins of these harms with certain individual "addictive personalities" was in reality a convenient fiction, a fiction that only industry spokespeople appear committed to promoting (Davies, 1992; Kerr, 1996).

My third response drew on a complex mix of justifications. Its spontaneous logic flowed somewhat as follows: the money is sitting there already; our views regarding how it was collected won't make any difference; it is still going to be distributed, so someone has to make use of it, and if we don't access it then somebody else will. Similar to the way gambling profits are distributed to sports clubs to fund overseas travel or new uniforms, if we don't access these funds then it is likely to end up supporting activities far less deserving than our own. It could end up funding obscure research projects in fields such as sports science or literary criticism or plant morphology or archeology – areas of research with little relevance to the problems associated with these consumptions (Stone and Siegel, 2004). Surely it is better that these profits are channeled back into addressing the source of these harms? And our work on strengthening communities will in the long run provide a very important platform for relevant initiatives. We almost have, therefore, a duty to apply. We mightn't succeed, but, after all, you need to be in to win. Besides, it would be very irksome to watch researchers in these unrelated fields scoring without us having at least had a shot at obtaining some of it for our more worthy endeavors.

Now, this is indeed a complex cluster of rationalizations. How do I sort out what these thoughts all mean? Behind it I recognized my primary motive was a raw desire to take the money. But can I trust these thoughts when my desire is so strong?

I sat back and reflected on some of what I was telling myself: gambling is okay, you need to be in to win, we deserve to succeed, our cause is more worthwhile … I could see how these messages resonated with the many very familiar messages we use to justify engagement in addictive consumptions: drinking is fun, it's worth having a flutter, I deserve a smoke … I realized that, while my justifications appeared to bubble up from within, they were in fact connected to the many messages that circulate in advertisements, in films, and in everyday conversations about the permissibility of such consumptions. I concluded that instead of me coming up with these justifications, they were coming from outside; they were already a resource out there, standing ready to service decisions that enable me to attain what I desire. The link between the justification and my desire for the money was too strong and I could not trust it. What I really needed was some way of weighing up and sifting out what is important in this decision; some sort of guide that would assist in methodical deliberation on the issues.

No ordinary consumption

Corporations that trade in legalized addictive consumptions seek to position themselves as legitimate businesses alongside other legitimate businesses trading in commodities in much the same way as other producers. However, as argued by Thomas Babor and his coauthors in their book *Alcohol: No Ordinary Commodity* (Babor et al., 2010a), addictive consumptions are not like other consumptions; they differ in both their capacity to generate harm and their capacity to generate profits. With addictive consumptions, the dynamics of supply and demand are shaped in different ways compared with ordinary consumer products, such as soap, cereals, and vegetables. For example, those addicted to alcohol will devote escalating amounts of time and energy to acquiring and consuming the product and will pursue this commitment way beyond normal constraints of safety and good sense (Adams, 2008a). Acting collectively, their devotion to the product stimulates an almost unquenchable demand that guarantees to producers sustainable and highly profitable markets.

Although trade in illicit drugs – such as those from Mexico, Colombia, and Afghanistan – highlights the profit-generating capacity of addictive consumptions, it is with legalized addictive consumptions that the value add-on of addicted consumers ensures the largest and most enduring profits. As the trade in tobacco, alcohol, and gambling integrates into an economy, more and more people find themselves benefiting from the profits. The network of beneficiaries expands to not only include the producers and retailers but also governments, associated businesses, community agencies, helping organizations, and research groups. This network ensures that the demand for these profits becomes embedded into social and financial structures, and this in turn provides the impetus for further increases in demand for profits.

What beneficiaries may not fully appreciate is the extent to which the profits they receive are derived specifically from addiction. Although addicted consumers comprise a small part of any one population, the money they spend contributes disproportionally to the profits. In other words, the few heavy consumers spend far more money than the many light consumers. In countries with developed economies (such as those in Europe, North America, Australasia, and East Asia) although 15–30% of an entire population are typically physically dependent on nicotine, these people account for 90–98% of expenditure (Mackay and Eriksen, 2002). For alcohol, although 3–6% of a population are drinking addictively and a further 10–18% drinking hazardously, these people account for 50–70% of expenditure (Greenfield and Rogers, 1999; Foster et al., 2006; Kerr and Greenfield, 2007). Similarly, for gambling, although 1–3% are problem gamblers, they account for 30–50% of expenditure (Australian Productivity Commission, 1999; Caraniche Pty Ltd, 2005). Unfortunately for the recipients of the profits from each of these consumptions, it is impossible to work out which portion comes directly from addicted consumers and which part is derived from normal consumption; the profits from both are mixed up together. It follows, therefore, that when a beneficiary accepts funding from these sources, they are drawn in unavoidably to supporting the practices that exploit the vulnerabilities of people struggling with addiction.

Moral jeopardy

Moral jeopardy is generated when researchers or research organizations committed to public good opt to receive profits from addictive consumptions in ways that generate real or perceived conflicts of interest, which in turn jeopardize their purpose, autonomy, and academic integrity (Adams and Rossen, 2006; Adams, 2007; Adams, 2008a; Stenius and Babor, 2010). For example, a health research institute that accepts funds directly from a brewery risks a level of dependency on these profits that could compromise or be seen to compromise their academic independence. As discussed above, a common response to inconvenient questions of morality is to call on easily available justifications to silence any nagging doubts. However, brushing the concerns aside could entail ignoring some areas of risk that may have serious consequences at a later stage. A better approach involves engaging in some form of deliberation before making a decision. The following describes six types of risk that research groups could consider when deliberating on the moral jeopardy associated with receiving industry funds. Each description also specifies indicators that can help in assessing these risks.

Ethical risks

Simply put, an ethical risk emerges when a person or an organization accepts money in order to achieve good from a source that does harm. For example, a charity that is striving to alleviate poverty might consider accepting money from a liquor retailer whose sales are clearly associated with street violence in that community. In accepting the money, it is in a position to reduce some of the misery in that community, but by doing so it also tacitly endorses an activity that contributes to another form of misery. Indeed, a broad range of harms are attributable to addictive consumptions. According to the World Health Organization (2002), of the ten leading risk factors contributing to the burden of disease in developed countries, tobacco is estimated to be the first leading factor, with alcohol as the third. Alcohol, although causing fewer deaths, contributes to a wide range of impacts, which include reductions in the physical, mental, and social well-being of a population (Anderson et al., 1993; Edwards et al., 1994; Babor et al., 2010a). High-intensity gambling has only recently emerged in modern democracies, but already researchers are finding consistent links with poverty, mental health issues, family disruption, crime, and other determinants of health and well-being (Livingstone and Woolley, 2007; Australian Productivity Commission, 2010). This suggests that at some fundamental level it is ethically inconsistent for those trying to achieve good in a community to do so with profits that cause undeniable harm in that same community.

For people attempting to work out the extent of ethical risk associated with accepting such money, two key indicators can help with their deliberations: namely, *purpose* and *harmfulness*. The first indicator, *purpose*, focuses on the extent to which the primary purpose of the research activity clashes with the primary purpose of the activities of the donor corporation. For example, if the primary purpose of a research program is to assist in reducing levels of youth illicit drug use, then this purpose would clash significantly if the donor corporation is involved in selling ready-to-drink 'alcopops' to young people for the purpose of increasing their engagement in alcohol consumption (Miller and Kypri, 2009). Although this example is fairly clear cut, deliberations on purpose are not always as straightforward. Some effort may be required to uncover more clearly the intent of the funding. For example, what might appear on the surface as a generous offer by a tobacco company to fund research on the genetics of nicotine dependence may, on further inspection, turn out to be part of a strategy by the tobacco industry to deflect legal responsibility by attributing the drivers for this addiction to the individual and not industry marketing practices (Hong and Bero, 2006; Gundle et al., 2010).

The second key indicator is the level of *harmfulness* associated with that particular product. The extent of harm generated by different forms of consumption will vary. For example, lower potency products such as smokeless cigarettes, low-alcohol beer, and lottery products are less likely to cause harm than more potent products such as unfiltered roll-your-own cigarettes, easily available spirits, and electronic gambling (slot) machines (Berdahl and Azmier, 1999; Jackson et al., 2000; Shahab et al., 2009). Furthermore, environments and the way a product is presented can add to the extent of harm. For instance, venues that encourage binge drinking are more likely to lead to harm than venues with an accent on socializing and moderate consumption. In this way, forming a judgment on the relative *harmfulness* of how people are encouraged to engage with the product can assist further in understanding purposes.

Contributory risks

Contributory risk occurs when the act of accepting funds either directly or indirectly contributes to sales of the product. Indirect contributions might occur when the funding relationship is used by corporations to reduce negative perceptions and to boost their positive public profile. For example, donations from a tobacco company to disaster relief will not only contribute positively to its public image but could also elevate its standing in policy-making circles (MacKenzie and Collin, 2008). In both these ways, a stronger positive image could help in reducing obstacles to increases in consumption. Direct contributions occur when the consumer's awareness of the funding relationship actually leads to increases in consumption. For example, at the point of sale a person may be more likely to feel inclined to purchase a lottery ticket when they believe some of the profits are going toward worthy causes such as cancer or addiction research (Morgan, 2000).

Two key indicators that can help in assessing contributory risk are the extent to which *purposes* clash (as already discussed) and the *visibility* of the relationship. *Visibility* is understood here as the extent to which the funding relationship can be observed by outsiders. For example, in Hong Kong two large and highly visible identifiers stretch the full length of a long building: the top sign declares "The University of Hong Kong Li Ka Shing Faculty of Medicine," and, with the same size lettering, the sign stretching across the middle of the building declares, "The Hong Kong Jockey Club Clinical Research Centre." This, of course, is a case of extreme visibility. In most situations the extent of visible association takes on more subdued forms such as logos on conference programs, discreet plaques in departmental corridors, or cursory mention of the funding relationship buried in acknowledgments at the end of an article or a report.

Despite the efforts by researchers to contain the visibility of the funding relationship, the donor is unlikely to feel similarly constrained. Corporations involved in addictive consumptions are unlikely to contribute anonymously because, for them, one of the main goals of their contribution is to highlight the visible association with public good activities for the purposes of positive branding (Brammer and Millington, 2005; Tesler and Malone, 2008). The researcher may have hoped to confine the association to discreet acknowledgment, but the corporations will be inclined to exploit the association by profiling it in their promotional and advertising materials, particularly when they involve exposure to policymakers and the general public.

Reputational risks

A researcher who accepts industry funding risks damage to his or her reputation from the negative perceptions of surrounding stakeholders. For example, colleagues researching in the same field might take a dim view of the morality of receiving these funds. They might see the association as undermining the perceived integrity of that particular type of research or perhaps the integrity of the field as a whole (Turcotte, 2003; Munro, 2004). Moreover, these negative reputational associations have a nasty way of sticking around over time. It might be the case that a research group has only once ever received such funds, but in the eyes of their research community, each member of that group risks being perceived as willing, and therefore possibly willing again, to link up with similarly unethical sources. Such perceptions can be particularly bruising for trainee researchers who may, for example, have naively accepted an industry-funded doctoral scholarship only to encounter negative judgments later in their career. These negative judgments may continue to tar those involved well after the completion of the research in question and, in addition, can spread to negative perceptions by other stakeholders. For example, a government funding agency might choose to reduce their own reputational risk by only funding research groups devoid of industry associations. Similarly, community agencies and service consumers might shy away from involvement. For example, a service client with an alcohol-dependent family member might seek to actively avoid involvement with any researcher that they have heard receives alcohol-industry support. The impact of these perceptions on the research group will vary according to the importance of the stakeholder, but as they accumulate over time they can have a lasting impact on its credibility. For example, in 2000 a gambling-industry funding agency, the National Center for Responsible Gaming, promised Harvard Medical School's Division on Addictions US$2.4 million for 2 years' work and in 2002 a further US$1.2 million. This led to widespread condemnation in the media and among other researchers in the field (Mishra, 2004).

Key indicators that are helpful in ascertaining reputational risk are *purpose* and *visibility* (both already discussed) and a third indicator, *reliance*. The extent to which a research group *relies* on such funds can be assessed in much the same way as client alcohol consumption is assessed: that is, by reviewing the quantity, frequency, and heavy use episodes in receiving these funds (Cohen et al., 1999; Cohen, 2001; Rampton and Stauber, 2002). One addiction research group might choose to accept small amounts of industry funding on a regular basis, another group might accept the occasional large amount, and another group might confine acceptance to only one occasion, but the amount involved might entail a multi-million dollar contribution. When tracked over time, each of these groups could end up receiving roughly similar amounts of industry funding. So, in order to accommodate different patterns of acceptance, the extent of *reliance* can be estimated by working out what proportion of their income is derived from that source over the course of a year. A group that derives

30% of its annual income from industry sources is more likely to develop reliance on these sources than a group that receives 10%.

Governance risks

Governance, or the capacity for independence and self-determination, is placed at risk when outsiders have a greater say in the direction of a group than its owners. For example, as an alcohol research group receives an increasing proportion of its funding from one external source, the funder is able to exert increasing influence on the nature and direction of its research. When this proportion of funding reaches high levels (say, over 50%) the funder is likely to be in a position to influence and perhaps dictate the research agenda. For example, a gambling research institute that is 80% funded by a casino would have little alternative but to respond to the interests of casino management.

The governance of most research groups is complex. Ownership of a research unit in a university tracks up officially to the university's overarching board of governance (or council). Unofficially such units are in effect governed through a complex set of relationships that include departmental affiliations, faculty management structures, and the ambitions of the researchers themselves. Similarly complex governance arrangements occur for research groups based in hospitals and other health services. In more independent research agencies and institutes, governance boards are likely to exert more direct control, but they are also typically subject to several layers of internal influence. In these ways, the majority of research groups can be viewed as having complexly layered governance with input from a wide range of people operating at different levels.

Two key indicators that are helpful in identifying risks to independent governance are *reliance* and *directness*. Although *reliance* was discussed in the previous section, in the context of governance, calculating the proportion of industry funding comprises only part of the picture. Another important consideration is the extent to which people at varying levels *perceive* the survival of the research group as relying on these funds. Such perceptions create a dynamic all of their own. For example, the manager of a research unit who is intimately acquainted with the precariousness of the unit's finances may perceive a small fund from a brewery as making all the difference between the unit continuing or collapsing. Accordingly, he or she is likely to attempt to impress on staff the need to avoid any activity that may potentially ruffle the feathers of this funder and thereby disturb ongoing positive relationships. Staff in the unit are urged to avoid making statements or pursuing research activities that might encourage the funder to reconsider its investment. In time, even when a governance board on balance opposes this source on ethical grounds, on pragmatic grounds it may have little choice but to continue with the funding: the members cannot imagine their unit continuing to operate without it. This perceived reliance may result in a growing reluctance to jeopardize funding through any activity that might be seen as unacceptable or upsetting to the donor (Cohen et al., 1999; Doughney, 2002).

The second indicator of risk to governance, *directness*, focuses on the way in which funding is obtained. Funding could be received directly from the industry donor or it could come indirectly via a variety of mediated arrangements or through contractual protections. Research agencies that receive significant funding directly from corporations risk jeopardizing their independence. The exchange of money builds relationships, it forges ongoing connections, and it establishes expectations and obligations. These obligations are further reinforced through multiple exchanges, and the links can gradually build into a lasting interdependence. In an effort to protect the independence of research establishments, governments have set up a variety of intermediary agencies to handle the distribution of such funds. As long as there are no major conflicts of interest for the intermediary agency, the separation reduces the likelihood that recipients would feel obligated – or perhaps coerced – into complying with the interests of the donor. For example, many governments (such as those in Ontario, Queensland, Victoria, and the UK) have set up tripartite funding mechanisms to distribute funds from gambling profits to research groups. These funding committees are typically composed of industry, government, and "community" representatives. However, as has been observed elsewhere (Adams et al., 2010), in reality these arrangements are dominated by the interests of the two main parties, the industry and the government sectors, both of whom have clear interests in protecting the profits they access from gambling consumption.

Relationship risks

An area of concern that is not often taken into account is the various ways in which a decision to accept industry funding can negatively affect relationships both inside and outside an organization. This can occur internally on a person-by-person basis or between different sections of larger organizations. For example, individual researchers may find themselves excluded from research teams according to whether they are willing or are not willing to be associated with those who receive industry funds. Alternatively, tensions may arise in a university between one research group that accepts such funds and another group that refuses them. Our small group of gambling researchers recently faced such tension when our university decided to accept NZ$5 (US$3.7) million from a slot machine source to fund a professorial chair in emergency medicine. In a better-known example, Richard Smith, who was at the time the chief editor of the *British Medical Journal* and who had published several editorials challenging the willingness of scientists to receive tobacco funding (Smith, 1998), had the rug pulled out from under him when his own institution, the University of Nottingham, accepted US$7 million from British American Tobacco to fund an international centre for the study of corporate responsibility. Besides the degree of internal conflict that ensued, the University also lost out when Richard Smith himself decided to resign, taking with him his research activity and his credibility. Broadening the focus to relationships outside the research institution, the prospect for intergroup collaborations are often hampered by having to negotiate around sensitivities associated with differing positions on industry funds. This is particularly challenging in gambling research, where many of the main players currently opt to accept gambling industry funds (Adams et al., 2009).

Two key indicators that can help in ascertaining relationship risks are *purpose* (already discussed) and the likelihood of *dissent*. A research group that embraces addictive consumption funding also embraces the potential for conflict and disagreement within the research team. For example, in circumstances where those in charge of a research unit have decided to accept alcohol-industry funding, a number of staff members are likely to feel dissatisfied with that decision on ethical grounds, but how they each respond will vary. More diplomatic dissenters will, for the sake of retaining their employment, opt to remain silent. The less diplomatically inclined might speak out but may soon find themselves marginalized within the team. The objections are troublesome and threaten organizational coherence. Consequently those in charge might seek ways to reduce levels of open dissent through strategies such as transfers and performance management. This, in turn, reinforces the silence of the diplomatic dissenters who, over time, begin to experience their silence as increasingly burdensome and isolating and may begin seeking out other employment opportunities. Unfortunately, these dissenters (of both the open and the silent variety) are also likely to be those individuals with the greatest passion and ideological commitment to the overall goals of the research program and, accordingly, a longer-term casualty of accepting such funds is likely to be a gradual erosion of the quality and vitality of the work of the group. A similar pattern of deterioration can occur with relationships outside the group. One set of colleagues in associated and partnering organizations (other research groups, relevant services, professional associations) may openly criticize the decision; relationships with these people are likely to gradually wane. Another set of colleagues, those with a stronger interest in maintaining links, might choose not to comment but, over time, they too are likely to lose enthusiasm for the relationship.

Democratic risks

The risks to democratic systems are more subtle and emerge over a longer period of time, but they are just as important to consider when deciding whether to receive industry funding (Adams, 2008b; Orford, 2011). Researchers play a special role in the long-term evolution of a democracy. Their activities generate the knowledge base that informs all layers of society of the impacts and opportunities associated with harm from addictive consumptions. For example, the quality of a magazine article on the physical effects of heavy drinking can only be as informative as the availability and quality of the research that underpins its main points. Knowledge can only exist when knowledge generators are willing to focus their efforts on answering relevant questions, but, as enquiry can proceed in many different directions, the very nature of that knowledge base can be shaped by influences that determine which questions are addressed and which are shelved for later generations.

The disruptive potential of well-conducted research cannot afford to be underestimated. Inconvenient health research has the capacity to disrupt well-established and profitable businesses. Consider, for example, the impact on relevant corporations of the research on harms from hormone replacement therapy, the research on fat content in fast foods, and the research on environmental tobacco smoke. Well-funded and high-quality research provides a critical information source upon which health lobbyists can influence the policy agenda, which in turn will build their descriptions through the media (Jahiel and Babor, 2007). Hence, those with a strong stake in the profits from addictive consumptions – which includes corporations, governments, and community agencies – are unlikely to support research activities that could threaten these profits. For example, internal industry documents recovered from Philip Morris reveal a 40-year commitment to grooming a leading tobacco researcher, Ernst Wynder, in assisting with opposing and stalling progress with tobacco policy (Drope and Chapman, 2001; Fields and Chapman, 2003). Similarly, alcohol-industry-funded "social aspects/public relationships organizations" such as the International Center for Alcohol Policy (Foxcroft, 2005) and Drinkwise in Australia (Miller and Kypri, 2009) have supported activities aimed at diverting research activity away from consumption drivers. Moreover, in several Australian states, where tax revenue from gambling profits have been trending up as high as 15% of their total revenue (Banks, 2003), there is little appetite for research focused on effective modifications to slot machines (Livingstone and Adams, 2011).

The two key indicators that are useful in assessing democratic harm are the current levels of *dissent* (discussed above) and the potential of participating in *diversion* of the research agenda. A pattern of differential investment in research calls into question the processes that determine research funding and prompts an interest in those people who are in positions to influence how funding is allocated. Such a pattern can be detected by monitoring shifts of investment from high-inconvenience to low-inconvenience research; in other words, shifts away from the determinants of harmful consumption to research that either focuses neutrally on trends in consumption or focuses on dislocated aspects of individual consumers. Common examples of low-inconvenience research include large population telephone surveys of consumption, surveys of attitudes and beliefs about addictive products, biomedical and genetic research on addiction (Midanik, 2006; Gundle et al., 2010; Kalant, 2010), clinical research into treatment interventions (Munro, 2004), and evaluations of public education packages (McCambridge, 2007; Petrosino, 2003). These more routinely funded areas of research contrast with the less often funded and highly inconvenient research topics such as social and economic impact studies, behavioral research on product modifications, studies on product promotion and investigations into industry–government relationships (Chapman and Shatenstein, 2001; Adams, 2008b; Babor et al., 2010b).

A continuum of risk

As already implied, a person deliberating on the moral jeopardy of industry funding is not faced with an all-or-nothing decision. Overall estimates of risk can be seen as graded on a continuum from low to high moral jeopardy. This variability increases the importance of conversation and deliberation before deciding whether to accept such funds.

Binary ways of looking at the world involve slotting key aspects of one's reality into category pairs; the weather is either fine or wet, people are either good or bad, patients are either compliant or disruptive. Thinking in binary categories is tempting and powerful. Their use helps organize a complex picture and facilitates decisive action, such as when needing to know who to trust in a crisis situation. However, despite these benefits, their use also runs the risk of oversimplifying and stereotyping the subject material (Derrida, 1982; Marmot, 1998). For example, a common binary related to alcohol is the division of drinkers into those who drink "socially" and those who drink "dependently." The distinction is useful in helping to identify people who require some form of assistance, but it also oversimplifies the diversity of possible relationships to alcohol and runs the risk of stigmatizing dependent drinkers as weak and qualitatively different from those who drink in other ways. The consequent negative stigma discourages people from discussing pertinent issues, thereby making it less likely that they reflect on their own vulnerability. A continuum interpretation involves looking at the world less in terms of fixed categories, and more in terms of gradations of intensity across a particular dimension (Rose, 1992; Ioannou, 2005; Buetow and Adams, 2006). As with other moral binaries – such as fat/normal weight, alcoholic/social drinker, mad/sane, and weak/resilient – the shift from thinking in terms of binaries toward positioning oneself more along a continuum of risk legitimizes the activities of self-reflection and discussion. Thinking on a continuum reduces the impact of negative categorizations and promotes deliberation as a normal and legitimate activity (Ockene et al., 1997; Fleming, 2004).

The key disadvantage of a binary interpretation of morality risks over-categorizing people into either willing or not willing to accept profits from addictive consumptions: either they are morally sound or they are not; either they are good or they are corrupt. This oversimplified perspective can play a strategic role in putting pressure on organizations to consider rejecting such funding, but in the longer term it runs many of the risks of binary categorization outlined above. It discourages both deliberation and discussion, because raising the topic is tantamount to accusing someone of ethical cowardice. For example, a government funder who questions a research group regarding whether they receive industry contributions is likely to encounter a wall of justifications or hostile denials, either of which would discourage further conversation.

The concept of a continuum of moral jeopardy avoids these pitfalls. Instead of distancing those who are ambivalent, it recognizes that the extent to which someone engages with dangerous consumption industries can vary and that it is less a matter of whether or not to accept such funding and more a question of at what point someone views the relationship as too risky. Another reason for moving away from a binary perspective concerns the extent to which this form of funding is now available in communities. As the profits from addictive consumptions circulate more into an economy, it becomes increasingly difficult for public good organizations to avoid such connections. For example, in nations such as Canada and New Zealand alcohol and gambling industry sources provide large portions of the charitable funding available to academic, health, and community organizations and refusing all such funds may threaten organizational viability. Viewing this in terms of a continuum recognizes that these relationships are possible, but unlike a binary perspective, it normalizes the process of ongoing discussion and deliberation.

Where on the continuum do I wish to be positioned?

When faced with the immediate and tangible prospect of industry funding, the first impulse is to suppress doubts, then to reach out and accept the money, and then perhaps to abandon regrets to a later time. A more cautious approach involves research groups clarifying their position well in advance of it becoming a reality. Members of research teams and their management could make use of the moral jeopardy framework outlined above as a basis for conversations that clarify whether or not and/or under which circumstances accepting such funds would be acceptable. The following takes three case circumstances of funding opportunities and examines the overall estimates of moral jeopardy according to the six types of risk and their key indicators. Estimates according to type are graded at four levels: low risk, moderate risk, high risk, and extremely high risk. These estimates are then combined into an overall estimate of moral jeopardy.

Case 1: Public health research on youth alcohol consumption

A research team in a commercially run independent research institute has an opportunity to access funds offered by an agency distributing funds provided by the state alcohol companies. The institute specializes in public health research, and this funding would enable them to further develop their reputation in work on youth at risk.

Risks	Context	Key indicators	Probable outcome
Ethical	Youth drinking contributes to a wide range of harms in this community	Strong clash of *purpose* with alcohol corporations who target increases in youth consumption and high *harmfulness* in that drinking is clearly linked to youth problems	Extremely high risk
Contributory	The funder specifies the need to acknowledge the source of the funding	Strong clash of *purpose* and moderate *visibility* in having to identify the source, although this could be moderated by only providing discreet acknowledgments	Varying high to moderate risk

Risks	Context	Key indicators	Probable outcome
Reputational	High levels of public concern about youth drunkenness	Strong clash of *purpose*, moderate *visibility*, and high *reliance* in that the team may end up isolated and forced to rely more heavily on funding from the same source	High risk
Governance	This source could become critical in ensuring commercial viability	High risk of *reliance* and high *directness* in that the agency distributing the funding is wholly controlled by the alcohol corporations contributing to the fund	High risk
Relationship	Strongly opposed by several research staff and outside agencies	Strong clash of *purpose* and high levels of *dissent* by people both inside and outside the research team	Extremely high risk
Democratic	The companies would strongly oppose any study of advertising or sponsorship	High levels of *dissent* and the strong pressure for diversion of research energy from more influential factors (e.g., promotion and access) to less influential factors (e.g., drug education)	High risk

In this circumstance, the research team's deliberations indicate an overall position of high to extremely high risk on the moral jeopardy continuum.

Case 2: University chair in gambling studies

A casino negotiates with management of a local university to fund a professorial chair in gambling studies. The casino indicates they would like to fund it directly and that their contribution is acknowledged in the naming of the chair.

Risks	Context	Key indicators	Probable outcome
Ethical	The majority of funds are derived from gambling by problem gamblers	A very strong clash of *purpose* in that this casino focuses strongly on marketing to vulnerable populations and high *harmfulness* in that casino gambling is most potent and most harmful	Extremely high risk
Contributory	The casino will reference the position in its promotional materials	Clash of *purpose* and high *visibility* where the casino is likely to encourage consumers to see their expenditure as going to a worthy cause	High risk
Reputational	Likely strong condemnation by gambling public health lobbyists	Clash of *purpose*, high *visibility*, and very high *reliance* in that the professorial chair will provide a focal point in terms of both reputation and research leadership	Extremely high risk
Governance	The chair is likely to form the indispensible hub for the research activity	Very high *reliance* and the relationship has high *directness* without an intermediary body to soften or cushion the influence of the funders	Extremely high risk

Risks	Context	Key indicators	Probable outcome
Relationship	Strong opposition from some in the research team and from other parts of the university	Strong incompatibility of *purpose*, which will encourage high levels of *dissent* in the team, across the university, and from outside agencies with a commitment to public health	Extremely high risk
Democratic	The casino discourages research into strategies that might affect consumption	High levels of *dissent* and as a reference point the position will help with *diversion* of research activity away from effective interventions in moderating harm from gambling	Extremely high long-term risk

In this circumstance, the deliberations by university management indicate an overall position of extremely high risk on the moral jeopardy continuum.

Case 3: Product design research funded by the tobacco industry

A university-based addiction research unit is considering whether to apply to a government-brokered fund provided by the tobacco industry for the purpose of developing cigarettes that deliver less toxic tobacco smoke.

Risks	Context	Key indicators	Probable outcome
Ethical	Nearly all the profits from tobacco sales comes from people addicted to nicotine	Strong clash of *purpose* with the nicotine industry aiming to promote sales and high *harmfulness* with high numbers of deaths directly attributable to smoking	Extremely high risk
Contributory	The claim of designing less-harmful cigarettes will be used to engage more smokers	Strong clash of *purpose* and high *visibility* in that the donors will be wanting to profile the participation of the research unit in improvements to the product	High risk
Reputational	Linkage with tobacco industry funding is now generally seen as unacceptable	Strong clash of *purpose*, high *visibility*, and high likelihood of *reliance* because the funding is substantial and is planned to fund a series of studies	Extremely high risk
Governance	Involved government officials express enthusiasm for the partnership	High *reliance* and moderate *directness* with government as intermediary, but their enthusiasm could expose the unit to undue influence	High risk
Relationship	Other units and departments express strong objections	Strong clash of **purpose** and very high **dissent** both internally and externally, with a likelihood of affecting other funding sources	Extremely high risk
Democratic	This research generates expectations of smoking as less harmful	High **dissent** and likelihood of some **diversion** of interest and energy for public health and smoking-cessation initiatives	High risk

In this circumstance, the research team's deliberations indicate an overall position of extremely high risk on the moral jeopardy continuum.

Conclusion

Should addiction researchers accept funding derived from the profits of addictive consumptions? On the basis of criteria and indicators presented above, I find myself unable to provide any other response but a decisive "NO"! Indeed it is difficult to conceive of circumstances in which *addiction researchers* might avoid high levels of moral jeopardy. Had the focus been on whether *sports organizations* or *community charities* should accept such funds, I can imagine many circumstances where the risk would be considerably lower. For example, a sports club receiving lottery funding or an arts group receiving wine-industry funding is, arguably, unlikely to involve high levels of contributory, reputational, or relationship risk. But addiction researchers, whose efforts focus primarily on reducing the misery associated with addictions, will surely compromise their efforts at so many levels when they rely on profits from the same place that generates this suffering.

Returning to my situation as I sat with the application form displayed on my computer monitor, part of me felt irresistibly drawn to embrace this opportunity: the money would have enabled us to do such good, it would have contributed to both my career and the careers of my colleagues, it was important work and it would have enabled us to further our worthy initiatives within the community. I felt sorely tempted to brush any moral deliberations aside, but, as my mind scanned through the layers of risk, the likely downstream costs became glaringly obvious. The conclusion was unpalatable, inconvenient, and unwelcome, but the time I put aside for deliberation overcame all the automatic and surface justifications that would normally make accepting such funds permissible.

References

Adams, P. J. (2007). Assessing whether to receive funding support from tobacco, alcohol, gambling and other dangerous consumption industries. *Addiction*, 102, 1027–1033.

Adams, P. J. (2008a). *Fragmented Intimacy: Addiction in a Social World*. New York: Springer.

Adams, P. J. (2008b). *Gambling, Freedom and Democracy* (Volume 53 in Routledge Studies in Social and Political Thought). New York: Routledge, pp. 101–123.

Adams, P. J. and Rossen, F. (2006). Reducing the moral jeopardy associated with receiving funds from the proceeds of gambling. *Journal of Gambling Issues*, 17, 1–21.

Adams, P. J., Raeburn, J., and Silva, K. D. (2009). A question of balance: Prioritizing public health responses to harm from gambling. *Addiction*, 104, 688–691.

Adams, P. J., Buetow, S., and Rossen, F. (2010). Poisonous partnerships: Health sector buy-in to arrangements with government and addictive consumption industries. *Addiction*, 105, 585–590.

Anderson, P., Cremona, A., Paton, A., Turner, C., and Wallace, P. (1993). The risk of alcohol. *Addiction*, 88, 1493–1508.

Australian Productivity Commission (1999). *Australia's Gambling Industries: Final Report*. Canberra: Productivity Commission.

Australian Productivity Commission (2010). *Gambling: APC Report no. 50*. Canberra: Productivity Commission.

Babor, T. F., Caetano, R., Casswell, S., et al. (2010a). *Alcohol: No Ordinary Commodity-Research and Public Policy*, second edition. Oxford: Oxford University Press.

Babor, T. F., Miller, P., and Edwards, G. (2010b). Vested interests, addiction research and public policy. *Addiction*, 105, 4–5.

Banks, G. (2003). The Productivity Commission's gambling inquiry: 3 years on. *Gambling Research*, 15, 7–27.

Berdahl, L. Y. and Azmier, J. (1999). *Summary report: The impact of gaming upon Canadian non-profits: A 1999 survey of gaming grant recipients*. Calgary: Canada West Foundation.

Brammer, S. and Millington, A. (2005). Corporate reputation and philanthropy: An empirical analysis. *Journal of Business Ethics*, 61, 29–44.

Buetow, S. and Adams, P. J. (2006). Is there any ideal of "high quality care" opposing "low quality care"? A deconstructionist reading. *Health Care Analysis*, 14, 123–132.

Caraniche Pty Ltd (2005). *Evaluation of electronic gaming machine harm minimization measures in Victoria*. Melbourne: Victoria Department of Justice.

Chapman, S. and Shatenstein, S. (2001). The ethics of the cash register: Taking tobacco research dollars. *Tobacco Control*, 10, 1–2.

Cohen, J. E. (2001). Editorial: Universities and tobacco money. *British Medical Journal*, 232, 1–2.

Cohen, J. E., Ashley, M. J., Ferrence, R., and Brewster, J. M. (1999). Institutional addiction to tobacco. *Tobacco Control*, 8, 70–74.

Davies, J. B. (1992). *The Myth of Addiction: An Application of the Psychological Theory of Attribution to Illicit Drug Use*. Chur, Switzerland: Harwood Academic.

Derrida, J. (1982). *Dissemination*. Chicago: University of Chicago Press.

Doughney, J. R. (2002). *The Poker Machine State: Dilemmas in Ethics, Economics and Governance*. Melbourne: Common Ground.

Drope, J. and Chapman, S. (2001). Tobacco industry efforts at discrediting scientific knowledge of environmental tobacco smoke: A review of internal industry documents. *Journal of Epidemiological Community Health*, 55, 588–594.

Edwards, G., Anderson, P., Babor, T. F., et al. (1994). *Alcohol Policy and the Public Good*. Oxford: Oxford University Press.

Fields, N. and Chapman, S. (2003). Chasing Ernst L Wynder: 40 years of Philip Morris' efforts to influence a leading scientist. *Journal of Epidemiological Community Health*, 57, 571–578.

Fleming, M. F. (2004). Screening and brief intervention in primary care settings. *Alcohol Research and Health*, 28, 57–62.

Foster, S. E., Vaughan, R. D., Foster, W. H., and Califano, J. A. (2006). Estimate of the commercial value of underage drinking and adult abusive and dependent drinking to the alcohol industry. *Archives of Pediatric Adolescent Medicine*, 160, 473–478.

Foxcroft, D. (2005). International Center for Alcohol Policies (ICAP)'s latest report on alcohol education: A flawed peer review process. *Addiction*, 100, 1066–1068.

Greenfield, T. K. and Rogers, J. D. (1999). Who drinks most of the alcohol in the US? The policy implications. *Journal of Studies on Alcohol*, 60, 78–89.

Gundle, K. R., Dingel, M. J., and Koenig, B. A. (2010). "To prove this is the industry's best hope": Big tobacco's support of research on the genetics of nicotine addiction. *Addiction*, 105, 974–983.

Hong, M.-K. and Bero, L. A. (2006). Tobacco industry sponsorship of a book and conflict of interest. *Addiction*, 101, 1202–1211.

Ioannou, S. (2005). Health logic and health-related behaviours. *Critical Public Health*, 15, 263–273.

Jackson, M. C., Hastings, G., Wheeler, C., Eadie, D., and MacKintosh, A. M. (2000). Marketing alcohol to young people: Implications for industry regulation and research policy. *Addiction*, 95, 597–608.

Jahiel, R. and Babor, T. F. (2007). Industrial epidemics, public health advocacy and the alcohol industry: Lessons from other fields. *Addiction*, 102, 1335–1339.

Kalant, H. (2010). What neurobiology cannot tell us about addiction. *Addiction*, 105, 780–789.

Kerr, J. S. (1996). Two myths of addiction: The addictive personality and the issue of free choice. *Human Psychopharmacology*, 11, S9–SI3.

Kerr, W. C. and Greenfield, T. K. (2007). Distribution of alcohol consumption and expenditures and the impact of improved measurement on coverage of alcohol sales in the 2000 national alcohol survey. *Alcoholism: Clinical and Experimental Research*, 31, 1714–1722.

Livingstone, C. and Adams, P. J. (2011). Harm promotion: Observations on the symbiosis between government and private industries in Australasia for the development of highly accessible gambling markets. *Addiction*, 106, 3–8.

Livingstone, C. and Woolley, R. (2007). Risky business: a few provocations on the regulation of electronic gaming machines. *International Gambling Studies*, 7, 361–376.

Mackay, J. and Eriksen, M. P. (2002). *The Tobacco Atlas*. Geneva: World Health Organization.

MacKenzie, R. and Collin, J. (2008). Philanthropy, politics and promotion: Philip Morris' "charitable contributions" in Thailand. *Tobacco Control*, 17, 284–285.

Marmot, M. (1998). Improvement of social environment to improve health. *Lancet*, 351, 57–60.

McCambridge, J. (2007). A case study of publication bias in an influential series of reviews of drug education. *Drug and Alcohol Review*, 26, 463–468.

Midanik, L. T. (2006). *Biomedicalization of Alcohol Studies: Ideological Shifts and Institutional Challenges*. New Brunswick, NJ: Transaction Publishers.

Miller, P. and Kypri, K. (2009). Why we will not accept funding from Drinkwise. *Addiction*, 28, 324–326.

Mishra, R. (2004). Gambling industry link to Harvard draws questions. *The Boston Globe*, November 6, p. A1.

Morgan, J. (2000). Financing public goods by means of lotteries. *Review of Economic Studies*, 67, 761–784.

Munro, G. (2004). An addiction agency's collaboration with the drinks industry: Moo Joose as a case study. *Addiction*, 99, 1370–1374.

Ockene, J. K., Wheeler, E.V., and Adams, A. (1997). Provider training for patient-centered alcohol counseling in a primary care setting. *Archives of Internal Medicine*, 57, 2334–2341.

Orford, J. (2011). *An Unsafe Bet: The Dangerous Rise of Gambling and the Debate We Should Be Having*. Chichester, UK: Wiley-Blackwell.

Petrosino, A. (2003). Standards for evidence and evidence for standards: The case of school-based drug prevention. *The Annals of the American Academy of Political and Social Science*, 587, 180–207.

Rampton, S. and Stauber, J. (2002). Research funding, conflicts of interest, and the "meta-methodology" of public relations. *Public Health Reports*, 117, 331–339.

Rose, G. (1992). *The Strategy of Preventive Medicine*. Oxford: Oxford University Press.

Shahab, L., West, R. and McNeill, A. (2009). A comparison of exposure to carcinogens among roll-your-own and factory-made cigarette smokers. *Addiction Biology*, 14, 315–320.

Smith, R. (1998). Beyond conflict of interest: Transparency is the key. *British Medical Journal*, 317, 219–212.

Stenius, K. and Babor, T. F. (2010). The alcohol industry and public interest science. *Addiction*, 105, 191–198.

Stone, M. and Siegel, M. B. (2004). Tobacco industry sponsorship of community-based public health initiatives: Why AIDS and domestic violence organizations accept or refuse funds. *Journal of Public Health Management and Practice*, 10, 511–517.

Tesler, L. E. and Malone, R. E. (2008). Corporate philanthropy, lobbying, and public health policy. *American Journal of Public Health*, 98, 2123–2133.

Turcotte, F. (2003). Editorial: Why universities should stay away from the tobacco industry. *Drug & Alcohol Review*, 22, 107–108.

Wheeler, B. W., Rigby, J. E., and Huriwai, T. (2006). Pokies and poverty: Problem gambling risk factor geography in New Zealand. *Health & Place*, 12, 86–96.

World Health Organization (2002). *The World Health Report 2002: Reducing Risks to Health, Promoting Healthy Life*. Geneva: World Health Organization.

Chapter

10

Ethical issues related to receiving research funding from the alcohol industry and other commercial interests

Thomas F. Babor and Katherine Robaina

Introduction

Using terms of justification such as "corporate social responsibility" and "partnerships with the public health community," the alcohol, tobacco, and gambling industries (mainly large producers, trade associations, interest groups, and social aspects organizations[1]) fund a variety of scientific activities that involve addiction scientists or overlap with their work. In addition, the pharmaceutical industry funds clinical trials and supports other activities related to scientific research, such as the preparation of manuscripts and the sponsorship of lectures by speakers who investigate their products. The aim of this chapter is to evaluate the ethical challenges that have emerged from industry involvement in addiction science, particularly in relation to genetic research.

At the center of the ethical challenges are issues of trust, credibility, and conflict of interest. Trust in the addiction research world can be affected when commercial interests are perceived to outweigh health considerations. The credibility of scientific findings may be affected when evidence emerges that industry-sponsored research is flawed, biased, or methodologically weak. Conflict of interest is a situation in which the researcher has a personal or financial interest that may be put above the integrity of the research being conducted. After reviewing the extent of industry involvement in addiction research, we discuss the moral hazards of research funding from commercial interests, and offer ways in which individual investigators as well as professional organizations can work to minimize these risks.

Background

Types of funding

The alcohol, tobacco, gambling, and pharmaceutical industries are involved directly or indirectly in the conduct of scientific research by setting up funding mechanisms that specify the kinds of research they will support and the amounts they will pay for it (Miller et al., 2008;

Genetic Research on Addiction, ed. Audrey R. Chapman. Published by Cambridge University Press. © Cambridge University Press 2012.

[1] Social aspect organizations (SAOs) are non-profit organizations funded in whole or in part by the alcohol beverage industry and other producers of commercial products, such as tobacco, that cause damage to health. Their main purpose is to manage issues that may be detrimental to industry

Gundle et al., 2010). There are a number of ways that money from industry sources becomes available for research and research dissemination.

Direct (apparent and unapparent)

In a direct funding situation the link between funder and researcher is apparent and often clearly visible through a contract or other formal declaration. A few examples of apparent direct funding include the Ernest Gallo Clinic and Research Center, established by the E. & J. Gallo Winery, and research on the genetics of tobacco smoking funded by the R.J. Reynolds Tobacco Company to support studies at the University of Colorado on the genetics and neurobiology of nicotine response (Gundle et al., 2010).

Direct funding also includes consulting fees, paid travel expenses, or other monetary rewards for addiction scientists. For example, the International Center for Alcohol Policies (ICAP), a social aspect organization funded by a consortium of alcohol producers, pays alcohol scientists as much as $13 000 for a chapter-sized contribution to the books it publishes on alcohol policy (Jernigan, 2012). ICAP also pays travel expenses for academics to make presentations at conferences organized by the alcohol producers interested in expanding into developing countries (Bakke and Endal, 2010).

When research is directly funded by the industry but the link is not so clear, or when the relationship is not declared, or when the recipient of the funding is unaware of the funding source, it is termed "unapparent." For example, Bitton et al. (2005) found that researchers and journal editors with ties to several tobacco companies participated in the dissemination of research that cast doubt on the link between smoking and the *p53* tumor suppressor gene mutations[2] without clear disclosure of their tobacco industry links. The researchers, funded by British American Tobacco (BAT), Lorillard, and Philip Morris, published critical reviews of the evidence. These reviews instead offered histological tumor type, gender, age, and ethnic origin as explanations for mutations in *p53*. Journal editors of *Oncogene* and *Mutagenesis*, who had undisclosed ties to the tobacco industry, both published widely on the subject, undermining information that might have led to increased restriction of tobacco use.

Conflicts of interest may also be difficult to detect in situations when the funding source is declared, but the connection to the industry is not clear or not specified in the article. An analysis comparing a disclosure statement in a peer-reviewed journal with information on the authors' financial ties obtained from an independent source and internal tobacco industry documents (Bero et al., 2005) found that the lead author had numerous financial ties with the industry that were not disclosed. The coauthor also had an ongoing relationship with the industry that had not been divulged. Moreover, the analysis showed that even an extensive financial disclosure statement can fail to provide key information, such as who was actually involved in the design, conduct, and publication of the study.

---

interests. They also engage in information dissemination and other activities designed to minimize harm to individuals and society.

[2] Mutations in the *p53* tumor suppressor gene are found in 60% of lung cancers and 50% of all human tumors. Research, first published by Mikhail Denissenko et al. in 1996, provides evidence that benzo[a]pyrene, a carcinogen present in tobacco smoke, caused mutagenic effects on *p53* (Bitton et al., 2005).

Indirect (third-party organizations)

The tobacco, alcohol, and gambling industries also support research activities indirectly through third-party organizations that give the appearance of being independent of industry influence. These organizations include the Center for Indoor Air Research (CIAR), formed by Philip Morris, R.J. Reynolds Tobacco Company, and Lorillard Corporation in 1988; the National Center for Responsible Gaming (NCRG), the European Research Advisory Board (ERAB); the Alcoholic Beverage Medical Research Foundation (ABMRF); the Institut de Recherches Scientifiques sur les Boissons (IREB) and a number of trade organizations and social aspect organizations. ICAP, for example, attempts to influence alcohol control policies by recruiting scientists, disseminating research findings, hosting conferences, and promoting publications. Tied to industry interests, their viewpoints include the idea that moderate consumption of alcohol is beneficial, that only irresponsible drinking makes alcohol dangerous, and that marketing should be regulated by the industry rather than by government (Jernigan, 2012). Similar themes have been identified in the genetic studies funded by the tobacco industry's Council for Tobacco Research (CTR), which provided university-based scientists with grants to establish the genetic influence on nicotine dependence in order to exonerate the industry from responsibility for the health effects of tobacco products and specifically litigation from individuals and government authorities (Wallace, 2009; Gundle et al., 2010).

Many of these industry-supported research organizations have organizational features that separate their funding decisions from the direct influence of industry executives. ERAB, for example, funds biomedical and psychosocial research on beer and alcohol (ERAB, 2011a). It is managed through a board of directors, which consists of people drawn from business (including the beer industry), public relations, the legal profession, banking, and the medical sciences (ERAB, 2011b). The board of directors oversees an advisory board, which is responsible for soliciting grant applications, arranging grant reviews, and awarding grants. This group currently consists of academics with expertise in epidemiology, liver disease, genetics, heart disease, social science, and clinical treatment of alcohol problems (ERAB, 2011c). According to their website (www.erab.org), applications are "independently externally peer reviewed," with a funding limit of 100 000 euros for a 2-year grant. Currently funded projects include research on genetics, chronic disease, and protective effects of alcohol (ERAB, 2011d).

The ABMRF, now renamed the Foundation for Alcohol Research, describes itself as "a nonprofit independent research organization that provides support for scientific studies on the use and prevention of misuse of alcohol." Established in 1982, it is supported by the brewing industries of the United States and Canada (ABMRF, 2011a), as a partnership that grew out of the industry's concern over the perceived lack of information about the health benefits of alcohol for the majority of consumers who drink in moderation (ABMRF, 2011b). The Foundation funds biomedical and psychosocial research on alcohol through small grants that initially focused on the benefits of moderate drinking but have since expanded to include other topics (ABMRF, 2011c, 2011d). Industry members hold minority seats on the ABMRF Board of Trustees but do not participate in the grant selection process, which is done by senior alcohol researchers recruited from a broad spectrum of disciplines and universities (ABMRF, 2011e). Advisory Council members receive consulting fees and are encouraged to fraternize with senior industry executives at the Foundation's International Medical Advisory Group conferences. The Foundation's activities provide an example of how the alcohol industry promotes goodwill and takes credit for supporting science while at the same time controlling the research agenda (Babor, 2009; Miller et al., 2011).

Industry involvement in genetic research

There is growing evidence that the tobacco, alcohol, and gambling industries have a strong vested interest in the outcomes of genetic research related to addiction and to the health effects associated with the use of their products (Wallace, 2009; Gundle et al., 2010; Miller et al., 2011; Carter and Hall, 2012). In an effort to expand the market for health-care products to large numbers of healthy people, pharmaceutical companies also fund research targeting drugs at individual differences in disease susceptibility suggested by research on the human genome. In the case studies that follow, we describe examples of organized efforts by industry sources to promote genetic research for reasons that may be more connected with public relations than with public health.

Case study 1: Tobacco

In many respects the tobacco industry can be considered a prototype for other dangerous consumption industries in terms of its strategic approach to genetic research (Caron et al., 2005). Internal industry documents made public through US federal and state court cases reveal that the tobacco industry began to endorse genetic research and the notion that a minority of smokers are "genetically predisposed" to lung cancer in the 1950s. From 1954 to 1999, the CTR, the main tobacco-industry-funded research body, ran a $20 million a year research program in which genetics played a central role (Gundle et al., 2010). According to Wallace (2009), it was Clarence Cook Little, eugenicist and first director of the CTR, who promoted the idea that a gene both leads people to smoke and predisposes them to cancer. By the mid-1990s, the CTR was among the largest sponsors of medical research in the United States and had given close to $225 million to around 1000 researchers. The research was directed at identifying familial cancers, the role of genetic factors in cancer formation, and the identification of oncogenes responsible for causing lung cancer in cigarette smokers.

In addition to the CTR, more than half of funding allocated by BAT's Scientific Research Group (SRC) from 1990 to 1995 went to genetic research, primarily related to cancer (Wallace, 2009). According to the environmental campaign group GeneWatch, internal memos obtained from BAT reveal that research into "bad genes" was the largest area of university funding by BAT during these years (Doward, 2004). The largest of these projects involved a pharmacogenetic research unit whose main endeavor was to identify a minority of smokers who were allegedly "genetically susceptible" to lung cancer. Research on genetic predisposition to disease continued at SRC until at least 2000 (Wallace, 2009).

Case study 2: Alcohol

In 1980, the Ernest Gallo Clinic and Research Center (2011a) was established at the University of California to study basic neuroscience and the effects of alcohol and drugs on the brain. The Center, initially funded through a reported $6.5 million endowment from major wine producer Ernest Gallo, now has a staff of over 150 employees funded from multiple sources. The board of directors is made up of: John De Luca, President and CEO of the Wine Institute for 28 years and Senior Advisor on the Gallo Winery Board;

Joseph Gallo, President and Chief Executive Officer of E. & J. Gallo Winery; and Mary Gallo, widow and member of the Gallo Winery Advisory Board (Ernest Gallo Clinic and Research Center, 2011b). Much of their research is designed to identify the genetic components of susceptibility to alcohol abuse and alcoholism (Ernest Gallo Clinic and Research Center, 2011a).

ABMRF is devoted to the support of research on the effects of alcohol on health and the prevention of alcohol-related problems. Despite the priority given to prevention, an analysis of its funding portfolio (2008–2010) indicated that more than half of all grants (58%) were given for biomedical research, including genetics, and no funds went to environmental and public health research (Miller et al., 2011). Similar trends have been identified for other industry-supported research funding organizations, supporting the conclusion that industry funding of research is guided by an agenda favoring biological over environmental causes of alcohol-related problems (Miller et al., 2011).

Case study 3: Gambling

The NCRG was set up by the American Gaming Association (AGA) in 1996 with the purpose of funding research related to gambling disorders. In turn, the NCRG awarded a multimillion-dollar contract to Harvard Medical School to create the Institute for Research on Pathological Gambling and Related Disorders at the Division on Addictions in 2000. From 2000 to 2009, the Institute was supported by a multimillion-dollar grant from the NCRG. In total, the Division received more than $7 million from the NCRG from 1996 to 2009 (NCRG, 2011). The Institute's research has in part supported the idea that an addictive personality, rooted in genetics, puts a small number of people at risk of developing gambling-related problems (Mishra, 2004). A thematic analysis of 45 projects listed on the NCRG's website found that neuroscience received 32% of its funding, behavioral sciences 51%, and mental illness 17%, with all research focused on the pathological gambler (Miller et al., 2011). None of the research addressed the environmental contributions to gambling problems, such as easy access to casinos, gambling machine design, or advertising promotions.

Other commercial interests

Pharmaceutical companies also have a vested interest in genetic predisposition or susceptibility, as it is a means to identify subgroups that might respond to specific pharmacotherapies (GeneWatch UK, 2004). The industry has invested billions of dollars into the development of gene-related cures and treatments, and medication is increasingly prescribed to reduce the risk of future illness. Genetic testing could significantly expand the market for "preventive" medication to healthy people identified as "genetically susceptible." Roche, a multinational pharmaceutical company, is one of the world's leading providers of diagnostic tests. The company is developing genetic tests for "predisposition" to common diseases, which will be marketed along with lifestyle advice or medication (Hoffmann-La Roche Inc., undated).

In a more general sense, this is part of a trend within biomedical science toward the "geneticization" of explanations for complex behaviors such as addiction, which may "inadvertently grant priority to certain theories of causation, e.g., privileging either a molecular or an environmental cause for complex disorders and behaviours" (Caron et al., 2005). This trend has been reinforced by government funding of neuroscience research, which has invested substantially in the pharmacological treatment of addictive disorders without any major breakthroughs (Miller et al., 2011).

Industry objectives and strategies

Regardless of the validity of genetic explanations for addiction and disease, such an interpretation is consistent with policies that remove responsibility from industry products and marketing strategies, and is likely to have implications for profits and sales if it results in weaker regulations and controls on availability and marketing (Gundle et al., 2010; Hall et al., 2010). Also, by spending significant amounts of money on scientific research, industries can portray themselves as "good corporate citizens" (Bond et al., 2010).

The tobacco industry documents, made available as part of the US Master Settlement Agreement, revealed that the industry devoted significant amounts of money to promote genetic research findings, even launching a campaign about "junk science" to generate confusion about the health effects of smoking (Bero, 2005). The documents also disclosed corporate motives. One analysis of the Legacy Tobacco Documents (Gundle et al., 2010) showed how the search for a genetic basis for smoking was used by the industry as a strategy to shift blame from tobacco onto individuals' genetic dispositions. By suggesting that a necessary component of nicotine addiction is genetic, and that most people are "addiction-free" smokers, with the exception of a small number who are genetically susceptible to addiction, the industry was free to argue that cigarettes are a product used by those making an informed choice. As mentioned previously, the industry also carried out another line of genetic research, which supported the idea that some individuals have a "genetic predisposition" to lung cancer (Wallace, 2009).

In a confidential memorandum, industry lawyers wrote that several of these projects "…were primarily a means of attracting researchers to areas of scientific inquiry not being addressed and, in particular, were focused on satisfying the needs of lawyers involved in defending the tobacco industry in litigation" (quoted in Gundle et al., 2010: 5). This indicates that the industry had much to gain from funding research bolstering a genetic basis of tobacco dependence and related disease. Research on the genetics of smoking not only serves to absolve nicotine as the cause of dependence and smoking as the cause of disease, but also allows the industry to advocate that smoking-cessation measures can more effectively be targeted at a small number of people rather than the general population (Wallace, 2009). It has also been hypothesized that the industry may have an interest in using genetic screening for disease vulnerability to persuade smokers that they do not need to quit (Hall et al., 2002).

A report by ICAP (2001) states that the vulnerability of some individuals (or "special populations") to the adverse effects of alcohol consumption is "generally not psychological or due to social or economic conditions," but is "instead, a biological predisposition [which] makes them especially susceptible." The report argues that the genetic makeup of individuals is largely responsible for an increased risk for alcohol abuse and dependence, as well as low tolerance to alcohol. ICAP believes this has important policy implications – that genetic research may help identify markers for individuals at risk for alcohol dependence and offer options for early diagnosis and treatment, producing new approaches to both screening and education measures.

Critics of the Institute for Research on Pathological Gambling and Related Disorders at the Harvard Division on Addictions say that the Institute's research is used by the gambling industry to invalidate claims that gambling is commonly addictive and that this argument has been used in testimony before state legislatures and in lawsuits. Critics also show that their focus on gambling addiction is being used by the industry to influence the public's opinions about gambling – that it is harmless fun and has few, if any, negative consequences – with the exception of a small percentage of people who have "pathological" addictions. Two well-known treatment experts resigned from the NCRG board because of such concerns (Mishra, 2004; Strickland, 2008).

As no internal documents from the alcohol and gambling industries have been made available, their research funding objectives remain less clear. However, both the alcohol and gambling industries assert that prevention strategies can be developed to discourage alcohol use and gambling in the minority of the population who are genetically susceptible to addiction and disease (Hall et al., 2010). The alcohol industry, in particular, has undertaken an active role in research and in the area of policy, challenging effective environmental strategies such as those increasing price and limiting availability (Jernigan, 2012). Instead, the alcohol industry generally supports strategies that focus on the individual drinker, such as education, which has been shown to be relatively ineffective (Babor et al., 2010). The industry's policy objectives ignore epidemiological research (Rossow and Romelsjö, 2006; Babor et al., 2010) that shows that the majority of alcohol-related harm is attributable to the large group of hazardous and harmful drinkers, rather than a relatively small number of individuals with severe alcohol-related problems or alcohol dependence.

The alcohol industry has even taken their research agenda one step further by sponsoring research and disseminating information promoting the positive effects of alcohol on health. The International Scientific Forum on Alcohol Research (ISFAR) is a joint undertaking of Boston University's Institute on Lifestyle and Health and Alcohol in Moderation (AIM) – both of which are industry-funded. The purpose of ISFAR is to provide "open website timely critiques and comments by Forum members on emerging scientific publications and policy statements related to alcohol and health" (Boston University School of Medicine Institute on Lifestyle and Health, 2011a). The site consists of critiques which praise research articles that speak of the benefits of alcohol and critique those that provide evidence of the burden of alcohol on health, including several studies suggesting that alcohol is the cause of an increase in breast cancer risk among drinkers (Boston University School of Medicine Institute on Lifestyle and Health, 2011b). Often, more than one member will write a critique of the same article. The Forum and the critiques have received a good deal of positive attention from wine journalists and trade associations (see, for example: http://vinigator. finewinepress.com; http://winedoctors.com; www.indianwineacademy.com; www.newyork-wines.org).

By emphasizing individual voluntary (rather than legislative) solutions, the dangerous consumption industries are able to minimize regulatory controls, avoid being held accountable, and maintain and enlarge their consumer base. This strategy diverts attention and policymaking efforts away from the chief environmental determinants of addiction and their adverse health and social outcomes in the general population, most of whom are not "addicts" (Hall, 2006). Most research, however, highlights the effectiveness of population-based strategies (Babor et al., 2010; Gundle et al., 2010).

Further, the sponsorship of research can be used as a public relations strategy, demonstrating that industry philanthropy toward science is a responsible way to deal with societal problems. Contributions may also be perceived as counteracting the harms caused by industry products and practices (Tesler and Malone, 2008). Several industry players have made large investments in public relations through their promotion of "corporate social responsibility" and social aspect organizations in order to improve their reputation and portray an image of itself as an ethically responsible company (Babor, 2009). Corporate social responsibility, although touted as having a positive societal impact, is clearly focused toward commercial interests. At one meeting with business executives, the chief executive of Diageo, one of the largest alcohol multinational companies, was quoted as saying that his company's generous funding of university research on binge drinking was designed in part to discourage governments from placing higher taxes on its products and thus eating into revenues (Babor, 2006). Although many corporations use corporate social responsibility activities as a public relations strategy, there is evidence that the tobacco and alcohol industries have used these activities to influence public policies that may affect sales and profits (Tessler and Malone, 2008; Jernigan, 2012).

Implications

As discussed above, research funded wholly or in part by the tobacco, alcohol, and gambling industries has the potential to increase a company's profit margin and improve public perceptions of an industry as a "good corporate citizen." Industry-funded research also has several ethical implications for the integrity of science, including biased research, the potential to undermine public trust, and its negative effect collegiality within the scientific community.

Research bias in industry-funded research

Industry involvement in research funding can be controversial for both institutions and researchers and can pose a direct conflict of interest. A growing number of studies have found troubling correlations between financial relationships with industry and problems with research, including a tendency for funding sources to influence study design and hypothesis formulation. There is also a greater likelihood that researchers will use poor study designs, produce pro-industry results, publish biased interpretations of trial results, and even suppress the publication of negative findings (Bero and Rennie, 1996; Davidson, 1986; Friedberg et al., 1999; Djulbegovic et al., 2000; Yaphe et al., 2001; Kjaergard and Als-Nielsen, 2002; Als-Nielsen et al., 2003; Bekelman et al., 2003; Lexchin et al., 2003; Melander et al., 2003; Bhandari et al., 2004; Friedman and Richter, 2004; Montgomery et al., 2004; Perlis et al., 2005; Bero et al., 2007; Etter et al., 2007; Nieto et al., 2007; Tungaraza and Poole, 2007; Yank et al., 2007; DeAngelis and Fontanarosa, 2008; Sismondo, 2008a, 2008b; Jagsi et al., 2009). Wallace (2009) reported that interpretative bias played a role in the research funded by the tobacco industry claiming a genetic predisposition to lung cancer, and that studies tended to overestimate genetic risk. Barnes and Bero (1998) found that review articles funded by the tobacco industry were 88 times more likely than non-industry-funded studies to conclude that passive smoke is not harmful to health.

Research bias are often unintentional, but are nevertheless common when a conflict of interest (or competing interest) exists. A conflict of interest is a situation in which professional judgment or objectivity concerning a primary interest (such as the validity of research findings) has the potential to be influenced by a secondary interest (such as financial gain or personal rivalry). Conflicts of interests can be: financial, professional, or personal; hidden or declared; actual or perceived (Public Library of Science in the United States, 2009). Any of these can be problematic if they are related to the product under study or the sponsor of the research.

Although conflict of interest motivations are difficult to investigate, there is a substantial literature on the psychological mechanisms that influence behavior when a competing interest exists. At an individual level, conflicting interests and biased behavior may be produced by financial considerations, academic–professional ambitions, or personal relationships and experiences (Bion, 2009). Self-interest has been described as an automatic response and "viscerally compelling," unlike giving consideration to one's ethical and professional obligations to others, which requires a more thoughtful process (Moore and Loewenstein, 2004). Conflicts of interest can further influence behavior by imposing a "sense of indebtedness," and thereby the obligation to reciprocate (Katz et al., 2003).

The findings from social science and neuroscience tell us that the impact of financial contributions and gifts is often unconscious, shaping behavior without a person's awareness (Gold and Appelbaum, 2011), and that even when individuals try to be objective, their judgments are "subject to an unconscious and unintentional self-serving bias" (Dana and Loewenstein, 2003). Therefore, surrendering to a conflict of interest may often be a result of unintentional bias rather than intentional dishonesty (Cain and Detsky, 2008).

Mechanisms of influence at the institutional level include the need for organizational funding and responsiveness to stakeholders (Bion, 2009). The boundaries between funding organizations, social aspect organizations, and their parent corporations or private funders can become unclear. Often, directors of the boards of foundations also sit on the boards of private corporations, adopting multiple roles, presenting potential conflicts of interests. University-based scientists are under increasing pressure to support their research through extramural funding, and are even encouraged to develop partnerships with industries that can rapidly translate their research into products or other applications.

Loss of creditability and trust

The tobacco, alcohol, and gambling industries have vested interests in promoting the idea of "genetic susceptibility" to addiction and its effects on health, such as cancer. Promotion of this idea by those with commercial interests can distort the health research agenda and divert resources from more effective public health approaches. Another risk is the loss of public trust in research. When assertions of conflict of interest are raised toward scientists, academics, and other professionals who have received industry funding or who are employed by the industry, it tends to diminish the credibility of the individual, the institution, or a study.

Over a span of 15 years, University of California, Los Angeles (UCLA) epidemiologist James Enstrom received more than $1.4 million in undeclared consulting fees from the tobacco industry, producing research that backed industry views. In 2007, a federal judge cited Enstrom's research in a racketeering case as evidence of the tobacco industry's manipulation of science. Later, a public meeting of the University of California Board of Regents called the ethics of his research into question (Paddock, 2007). Similarly, a public health researcher from the University of Geneva faced legal proceedings for scientific fraud in three different courts when it was discovered that he had been secretly paid as a consultant for the tobacco company Philip Morris for several decades. The federal court and the University concluded that he could not be considered to be independent from the tobacco industry, that his research was part of a deliberate strategy by the tobacco industry to raise controversy about the health risks of passive smoking, and that the interests of the industry were inconsistent with those of public health and medical science. He was also removed from a

European Commission's advisory committee (Diethelm et al., 2005). Instances such as these raise doubts about the results of scientific research and can challenge the integrity of the researcher, the institution, or even an entire profession.

Effects on collegiality among scientists

In addiction research, the increasing competition for research positions and financial resources can foster the temptation to neglect ethical rules as well as the ethos of science. Career considerations can orient one's research to what is popular or fundable, rather than toward what is interesting or important. The growth in private research funding may lead to secrecy instead of the open exchange of new ideas and research results, and to new priorities that favor business interests rather than the public good (Babor, 2009). There is also growing concern about the climate of accusation, recrimination, and guilt by association that sometimes accompanies the imposition of conflict of interest declaration procedures in scientific publishing and grant applications. For example, some scientists have objected to "blacklisting" of reputable academics just because they accept small amounts of industry funding (Kuhar, 2009). Others have accused those who support more rigorous conflict of interest policies as being guilty of "McCarthyite" tactics (Gmel, 2010; Peele, 2010). As these examples suggest, industry funding of research and research scientists can lead not only to controversy over ethics, but also acrimonious debates and complaints about false accusations, either actual or implied. The net effect is often the destruction of collegiality within a field of science.

How to minimize effects of conflict of interest

As evidence and concern grows about the consequences of conflicts of interest, ethicists, journal editors, and scientists have proposed several procedures to handle conflict of interest.

Three approaches have been proposed to deal with conflict of interest in the addiction field: regulatory guidelines, awareness training using ethical analysis techniques, and total bans on acceptance of industry funding for research (Stenius and Babor, 2010).

Regulatory guidelines

Several organizations and self-appointed groups have developed consensus statements and voluntary guidelines to serve as a guide for research scientists and professional organizations. The Federation of American Societies for Experimental Biology (FASEB, 2007) has developed a "toolkit" that can be used by institutions, journal editors, and scientific and professional societies to construct conflict of interest policies relevant to their own particular needs (see also Stenius and Babor, 2010). Another approach is described in the professional and ethical codes for socioeconomic research in the information society, better known as the RESPECT Code of Practice (Dench et al., 2004). This is a voluntary model code designed to protect researchers from unprofessional or unethical demands. Researchers are required to ensure factual accuracy, avoid misrepresentation or misinterpretation of data, and declare any conflict of interest that may arise in their research.

To promote uniform conflict of interest guidelines for scientific journals that publish alcohol research, the International Society of Addiction Journal Editors (ISAJE) issued a consensus statement stating that all sources of funding and possible conflicts of interest should be declared when a scientific manuscript is submitted for editorial review (Farmington

Consensus, 1997). In a related development, Goozner et al. (2009) drafted a common standard for conflict of interest disclosure. These guidelines call for the disclosure of *all* potential conflicts of interest, including financial and nonfinancial interests and relationships. They also suggest that journals require that senior editorial staff avoid financial relationships that might constitute a conflict of interest. This model policy also provides guidelines for enforcement.

Ethical analysis

Ethical analysis is the second approach that the addiction field has used to deal with conflict of interest issues. This approach recommends the use of moral reasoning skills to resolve ethical conflicts. For example, Peter Adams (2007) posits three kinds of risk in relation to the acceptance of industry research funding: (1) reputational risks, or damage to an individual's reputation; (2) governance risks, where industry funding affects an organization's capacity to make choices about their future; and (3) relationship risk, which is the potential damage done to an individual's or organization's working relationships over disagreements about industry funding. Adams recommends that individuals and organizations engage in a consciousness-raising exercise to consider all information relevant to an understanding of the degree of moral jeopardy involved in a particular choice. This can be done by answering five kinds of questions: (1) To what extent do the *purposes* of the industry (e.g., return on investment, increased alcohol sales) differ from those of the scientist (e.g., to find out how best to prevent alcohol-related problems)? (2) Is the *extent* or amount of research support offered sufficient to compromise the independence of an individual scientist or an academic institution? (3) Is there *relevant* harm associated with continued marketing of the industry's products (for example, beer and alcopops are the beverages of choice for adolescent binge drinkers)? The greater the relevant harm, the greater the investigator's risk of being compromised by collaboration. (4) Will the recipient of the funds be *identified* with the funder and will the industry-related organization derive a public relations benefit from its support of scientists? Could the scientists or their institutions eventually be exposed to reputational risk? (5) Finally, is the nature of the *link* between recipient and donor direct or indirect? If it is indirect, in some cases it may not involve a major conflict of interest (Stenius and Babor, 2010). Adams' analysis is similar to one proposed by ISAJE to allow members of the scientific community to evaluate the extent of "moral jeopardy" associated with a particular decision to accept funding from a particular funding source (McGovern et al., 2008).

Total bans

As bias resulting from a conflict of interest is often unintentional (Dana and Loewenstein, 2003; Cain and Detsky, 2008), disclosing a conflict of interest may be an inadequate solution to the problem. A number of prominent hospitals, medical schools, and schools of public health have therefore established policies prohibiting tobacco-industry research funding, citing the health effects of smoking, the industry's denials of the science linking cigarettes to disease and death, and the massive public-relations campaign mounted by the companies to create a scientific controversy. Experts also argue that the aims of institutions committed to public health and those of the tobacco and alcohol industries are intrinsically incompatible (Clarion Declaration, 2008; Brant, 2010).

In May 2008, an international group of alcohol policy researchers, public health professionals and nongovernmental organization experts met in Dublin to discuss the role of the alcohol industry in the positioning of science, knowledge, and policy. Considerable concern was expressed about the involvement of the alcoholic beverage industry in research activities, and their involvement in activities which impede research. It was agreed that alcohol research is no different from other areas of science, where a significant number of studies have shown that conflicts of interests are associated with biased research findings that favor commercial interests at the expense of public health. The meeting concluded by adopting the Clarion Declaration, which states that no funding relationships with the alcohol industry should be entered into in the field of alcohol research in order to protect the integrity and legitimacy of alcohol research, and the reputation of academic institutions (Clarion Declaration, 2008).

Conclusion

This chapter has considered the ethical challenges associated with various funding sources for addiction research, and the responsibilities of addiction scientists, academic institutions, and professional organizations in protecting the integrity of science from funding sources that have a commercial and corporate interest in the outcomes of research. At present there is no consensus in the field about whether or not a scientist should accept funding from these kinds of vested interests. Nevertheless, the growth of concern about conflict of interest issues has resulted in a set of policies, procedures, and precedents that individual investigators can use to make an informed decision about how to proceed. What is clear from the literature reviewed in this chapter is that commercial interests seem to be complicating, if not impairing, the evolution of genetic research in the addiction field, and that some corporate entities (e.g., the tobacco industry) have violated the public trust to such an extent that collaboration is considered damaging to the scientist, the field, and the public. To protect the scientific integrity of the field from further influence from commercial interests, the best advice is that under most circumstances collaboration with the alcohol and gambling industries is neither warranted nor advisable, and that research funded by the pharmaceutical industry needs to be conducted in ways that protect, if not advance, the public interest.

References

ABMRF (2011a). About us. Available online at: www.abmrf.org/about_us.asp [accessed March 13, 2012].

ABMRF (2011b). Unique partnership. Available online at: www.abmrf.org/unique_partnership.asp [accessed March 13, 2012].

ABMRF (2011c). Grants and alcohol funding. Available online at: www.abmrf.org/grants2.asp [accessed March 13, 2012].

ABMRF (2011d). Medical Advisory Council. Available online at: www.abmrf.org/medical_advisory_council.asp [accessed March 13, 2012].

ABMRF (2011e). Board of Trustees. Available online at: www.abmrf.org/board_of_trustees.asp [accessed March 13, 2012].

Adams, P. J. (2007). Assessing whether to receive funding support from tobacco, alcohol, gambling and other dangerous consumption industries. *Addiction*, 102, 1027–1033.

Als-Nielsen, B., Chen, W., Gluud, C., and Kjaergard, L. L. (2003). Association of funding and conclusions in randomized drug trials: A reflection of treatment effect or adverse events? *JAMA: The Journal of the American Medical Association*, 290, 921–928.

Babor, T. F. (2006). Diageo, University College Dublin and the integrity of alcohol science: It's time to draw the line between public health and public relations. *Addiction*, 101, 1375–1377.

Babor, T. F. (2009). Alcohol research and the alcoholic beverage industry: Issues, concerns and conflicts of interest. *Addiction*, 104, 34–47.

Babor, T., Miller, P., and Edwards, G. (2010). Vested interests, addiction research and public policy. *Addiction*, 105, 4–5.

Bakke, Ø. and Endal, D. (2010). Alcohol policies out of context: Drinks industry supplanting government role in alcohol policies in Sub-Saharan Africa. *Addiction*, 105, 22–28.

Barnes, D. E. and Bero, L. A. (1998). Why review articles on the effects of passive smoking reach different conclusions. *JAMA: The Journal of the American Medical Association*, 279, 1566–1570.

Bekelman, J. E., Li, Y., and Gross, C. P. (2003). Scope and impact of financial conflicts of interest in biomedical research: A systematic review. *JAMA: The Journal of the American Medical Association*, 289, 454–465.

Bero, L. A. (2005). Tobacco industry manipulation of research. *Public Health Reports*, 120, 200–208.

Bero, L. A. and Rennie, D. (1996). Influences on the quality of published drug studies. *International Journal of Technology Assessment in Health Care*, 12, 209–237.

Bero, L. A., Glantz, S., and Hong, M. K. (2005). The limits of competing interest disclosures. *Tobacco Control*, 14, 118–126.

Bero, L. A., Oostvogel, F., Bacchetti, P., and Lee, K. (2007). Factors associated with findings of published trials of drug-drug comparisons: Why some statins appear more efficacious than others. *PLoS Medicine*, 4, 184.

Bhandari, M., Busse, J., Jackowski, D., et al. (2004). Association between industry funding and statistically significant pro-industry findings in medical and surgical randomized trials. *CMAJ: Canadian Medical Association Journal*, 170, 477–480.

Bion, J. (2009). Financial and intellectual conflicts of interest: Confusion and clarity. *Current Opinion in Critical Care*, 15, 583–590.

Bitton, A., Neuman, M., Barnoya, J., and Glantz, S. (2005). The p53 tumour suppressor gene and the tobacco industry: research, debate, and conflict of interest. *Lancet*, 365, 531–540.

Bond, L., Daube, M., and Chikritzhs, T. (2010). Selling addictions: Similarities in approaches between Big Tobacco and Big Booze. *Australasian Medical Journal*, 3, 325–332.

Boston University School of Medicine Institute on Lifestyle and Health (2011a). International Scientific Forum on Alcohol Research. Available online at: www.bu.edu/alcohol-forum [accessed March 13, 2012].

Boston University School of Medicine Institute on Lifestyle and Health (2011b). Archives: Summaries of critiques: April 2010–April 2011. Available online at: www.bu.edu/alcohol-forum/archives-april-2010-april-2011 [accessed March 13, 2011].

Brant, A. (2010). A not-so-slippery slope. *Academe*, 96, 25–27.

Cain, D. and Detsky, A. (2008). Everyone's a little bit biased (even physicians). *JAMA: The Journal of the American Medical Association*, 299, 2893–2895.

Caron, L., Karkariz, K., Raffin, T. A., Swan, G., and Koenig, B. A. (2005). Nicotine addiction through a neurogenomic prism: Ethics, public health, and smoking. *Nicotine and Tobacco Research*, 7, 181–197.

Carter, A. and Hall, W. (2012). *Addiction Neuroethics: The Promises and Perils of Neuroscience Research on Addiction*. New York: Cambridge University Press.

Clarion Declaration. (2008). *Nordic Studies on Alcohol and Drugs*, 25, 316.

Dana, J. and Loewenstein, G. (2003). A social science perspective on gifts to physicians from industry. *JAMA: The Journal of the American Medical Association*, 290, 252–255.

Davidson, R. A. (1986). Source of funding and outcome of clinical trials. *Journal of General Internal Medicine*, 1, 155–158.

DeAngelis, C. and Fontanarosa, P. (2008). Impugning the integrity of medical science: The adverse effects of industry influence. *JAMA: The Journal of the American Medical Association*, 299, 1833–1835.

Dench, S., Iphofen, R., and Huws, U. (2004). *An EU Code of Ethics for Socio-Economic*

Research (Brighton, UK: Institute for Employment Studies). Available online at: www.respectproject.org/ethics/412ethics.pdf [accessed March 13, 2012].

Diethelm, P., Rielle, J. C., and McKee, M. (2005). Links with the tobacco industry. *Lancet*, 365, 211–212.

Djulbegovic, B., Lacevic, M., Cantor, A., et al. (2000). The uncertainty principle and industry-sponsored research. *Lancet*, 356, 635–638.

Doward, J. (2004). Tobacco giant funds "bad gene" hunt. *The Observer*, May 30, 2004.

Ernest Gallo Clinic and Research Center (2011a). About the Gallo Center. Available online at: www.galloresearch.org/about.htm [accessed March 13, 2012].

Ernest Gallo Clinic and Research Center (2011b). Board of Directors. Available online at: www.galloresearch.org/board.htm [accessed March 13, 2012].

ERAB (2011a). About ERAB. Available online at: www.erab.org/asp2/about_erab/index.asp?doc_id=428 [accessed March 13, 2012].

ERAB (2011b). Board of Directors. Available online at: www.erab.org/asp2/about_erab/board_of_directors.asp [accessed March 13, 2012].

ERAB (2011c). Advisory Board. Available online at: www.erab.org/asp2/about_erab/advisory_board.asp [accessed March 13, 2012].

ERAB (2011d). Details of ERAB grants funded in 2010/11. Available online at: www.erab.org/documents/research_grants/Research_funded_03_-_10.pdf [accessed March 13, 2012].

Etter, J. F., Burri, M., and Stapleton, J. (2007). The impact of pharmaceutical company funding on results of randomized trials of nicotine replacement therapy for smoking cessation: A meta-analysis. *Addiction*, 102, 815–822.

Farmington Consensus (1997). The Farmington Consensus. *Addiction*, 92, 1617–1618.

FASEB (2007). Association of American Medical Colleges – Office of Research Integrity Responsible Conduct of Research Program for Academic Societies. Toolkit. Available online at: http://opa.faseb.org/pages/Advocacy/coi/Toolkit.htm [accessed March 13, 2012].

Friedberg, M., Saffran, B., Stinson, T. J., Nelson, W., and Bennett, C. L. (1999). Evaluation of conflict of interest in economic analyses of new drugs used in oncology. *JAMA: The Journal of the American Medical Association*, 282, 1453–1457.

Friedman, L. S. and Richter, E. D. (2004). Relationship between conflicts of interest and research results. *Journal of General Internal Medicine*, 19, 51–56.

GeneWatch UK (2004). GeneWatch UK submission to the Health Committee Inquiry: "The influence of the pharmaceutical industry." Available online at: www.genewatch.org/pub-507666. [accessed March 13, 2012].

Gmel, G. (2010). The good, the bad and the ugly. *Addiction*, 105, 203–205.

Gold, A. and Appelbaum, P. S. (2011). Unconscious conflict of interest: A Jewish perspective. *Journal of Medical Ethics*, 37, 402–405.

Goozner, M., Caplan, A., Moreno, J., et al. (2009). A common standard for conflict of interest disclosure in addiction journals. *Addiction*, 104, 1779–1784.

Gundle, K., Dingel, M., and Koenig, B. (2010). To prove this is the industry's best hope: Big tobacco's support of research on the genetics of nicotine addiction. *Addiction*, 105, 974–983.

Hall, W. (2006). Avoiding potential misuses of addiction brain science. *Addiction*, 101, 1529–1532.

Hall, W., Madden, P., and Lynskey, M. (2002). The genetics of tobacco use: Methods, findings and policy implications. *Tobacco Control*, 11, 119–124.

Hall, W., Mathews, R., and Morley, K. I. (2010). Being more realistic about the public health impact of genomic medicine. *PLoS Medicine*, 7, pii: e1000347.

Hoffmann-La Roche, Inc. (n.d.) Genetic testing in research & healthcare. Available online at: www.roche.com/sci-genetictesting.pdf [accessed March 13, 2012].

ICAP (2001). Alcohol and "special populations": biological vulnerability. *ICAP Reports 10*. Available online at: www.icap.org/LinkClick.aspx?fileticket=jMev%2FS7JOa4%3D&tabid=75 [accessed March 13, 2012].

Jagsi, R., Sheets, N., Jankovic, A., et al. (2009). Frequency, nature, effects, and correlates of conflicts of interest in published clinical cancer research. *Cancer*, 115, 2783–2791.

Jernigan, D. H. (2012). Global alcohol producers, science, and policy: The case of the International Center for Alcohol Policies. *American Journal of Public Health*, 102, 80–89.

Katz, D., Caplan, A. L., and Merz, J. F. (2003). All gifts large and small: Toward an understanding of the ethics of pharmaceutical industry gift-giving. *American Journal of Bioethics*, 3, 39–46.

Kjaergard, L. L. and Als-Nielsen, B. (2002). Association between competing interests and authors' conclusions: Epidemiological study of randomised clinical trials published in the BMJ. *British Medical Journal (Clinical Research Ed.)*, 325, 249.

Kuhar, M. J. (2009). Blacklisting among scientists. *Synapse*, 63, 539–540.

Lexchin, J., Bero, L. A., Djulbegovic, B., and Clark, O. (2003). Pharmaceutical industry sponsorship and research outcome and quality: Systematic review. *British Medical Journal (Clinical Research Ed.)*, 326, 1167–1170.

McGovern, T., Babor, T. F., and Stenius, K. (2008). The road to paradise: Moral reasoning in addiction publishing. In T. F. Babor, K. Stenius, S. Savva, and J. O'Reilly (eds.), *Publishing Addiction Science: A Guide for the Perplexed*. London, UK: Multi-Science Publishing Company, pp. 172–189.

Melander, H., Ahlqvist-Rastad, J., Meijer, G., and Beermann, B. (2003). Evidence b(i)ased medicine – selective reporting from studies sponsored by pharmaceutical industry: review of studies in new drug applications. *British Medical Journal (Clinical Research Ed.)*, 326, 1171–1173.

Miller, P., Carter, A., and De Groot, F. (2011). Investment and vested interests in neuroscience research of addiction: Ethical research requires more than informed consent. In A. Carter, W. Hall, and J. Illes (eds.), *Addiction Neuroethics: The Ethics of Addiction Neuroscience Research and Treatment*. Chennai, India: Academic Press, pp. 278–296.

Miller, P., Babor, T. F., McGovern, T., and Büringher, G. (2008). Ethical issues related to academic relationships with the alcoholic beverage industry, pharmaceutical companies and other funding agencies: Holy Grail or poisoned chalice? In T. F. Babor, K. Stenius, S. Savva, J. O'Reilly (eds.), *Publishing Addiction Science: A Guide for the Perplexed*, second edition. London, UK: Multi-Science Publishing Company, pp. 190–212.

Mishra, R. (2004). Gambling industry link to Harvard draws questions. *The Boston Globe*, November 6. Available online at: www.boston.com/news/local/articles/2004/11/06/gambling_industry_link_to_harvard_draws_questions/ [accessed March 13, 2012].

Montgomery, J., Byerly, M., Carmody, T., et al. (2004). An analysis of the effect of funding source in randomized clinical trials of second generation antipsychotics for the treatment of schizophrenia. *Controlled Clinical Trials*, 25, 598–612.

Moore, D. and Loewenstein, G. (2004). Self-interest, automaticity, and the psychology of conflict of interest. *Social Justice Research*, 17, 189–202.

NCRG (2011). About NCRG. Available online at: www.ncrg.org/about-ncrg [accessed March 13, 2012].

Nieto, A., Mazon, A., Pamies, R., et al. (2007). Adverse effects of inhaled corticosteroids in funded and nonfunded studies. *Archives of Internal Medicine*, 167, 2047–2053.

Paddock, R. C. (2007). Tobacco funding of research reviewed. *Los Angeles Times*, March 28.

Peele, S. (2010). Civil war in alcohol policy: Northern versus southern Europe. *Addiction Research and Theory*, 18, 389–391.

Perlis, R. H., Perlis, C. S., Wu, Y., et al. (2005). Industry sponsorship and financial conflict of interest in the reporting of clinical trials in psychiatry. *American Journal of Psychiatry*, 162, 1957–1960.

Public Library of Science in the United States (2009). PLoS policy on declaration and evaluation of competing interests. Available online at: www.plosmedicine.org/static/competing.action [accessed March 13, 2012].

Rossow, I. and Romelsjö, A. (2006). The extent of the "prevention paradox" in alcohol problems as a function of population drinking patterns. *Addiction*, 101, 84–90.

Sismondo, S. (2008a). How pharmaceutical industry funding affects trial outcomes: causal structures and responses. *Social Science and Medicine*, 66, 1909–1914.

Sismondo, S. (2008b). Pharmaceutical company funding and its consequences: a qualitative systematic review. *Contemporary Clinical Trials*, 29, 109–113.

Stenius, K. and Babor, T. F. (2010). The alcohol industry and public interest science. *Addiction*, 105, 191–198.

Strickland, E. (2008). Gambling with science. *Salon News*, June 16.

Tesler, L. E. and Malone, R. E. (2008). Corporate philanthropy, lobbying, and public health policy. *American Journal of Public Health*, 98, 2123–2133.

Tungaraza, T. and Poole, R. (2007). Influence of drug company authorship and sponsorship on drug trial outcomes. *British Journal of Psychiatry*, 191, 82–83.

Yank, V., Rennie, D., and Bero, L. A. (2007). Financial ties and concordance between results and conclusions in meta-analyses: retrospective cohort study. *British Medical Journal (Clinical Research Ed.)*, 335, 1202–1205.

Yaphe, J., Edman, R., Knishkowy, B., and Herman, J. (2001). The association between funding by commercial interests and study outcome in randomized controlled drug trials. *Family Practice*, 18, 565–568.

Wallace, H. (2009). Big tobacco and the human genome: Driving the scientific bandwagon? *Genomics, Society and Policy*, 5, 1–54.

11

The public health implications of genetic research on addiction

Rebecca Mathews, Wayne Hall, and Adrian Carter

Introduction

Genetic research has identified a number of genetic variants that are believed to increase the risk of developing addictive disorders or predict responses to treatments for these disorders (see Chapter 2 of this volume for a review of the genetic research on alcohol dependence). This research has the potential to enhance public health through improved prevention and treatment of addiction. Predictive genetic screening might be used to identify persons at a greater risk of developing addiction and prevent them from doing so. Pharmacogenetic research may enable clinicians to better match persons with addictive disorders to more effective treatments, thereby minimizing side effects and relapse.

As well as having the potential to improve public health, research identifying genes predictive of addiction liability and treatment response may also be misused or misinterpreted in ways that harm individual and population health. It may negatively influence community attitudes to persons with a genetic predisposition to addiction, resulting in stigmatization of such individuals (Berghmans et al., 2009). Individuals may interpret genetic risk information in a deterministic way and believe they are powerless to change their behavior or their risk of addiction. Genetic risk information about addiction liability may also be used in a discriminatory way by employers or insurance companies (Taylor et al., 2008). Alcohol and tobacco industries may misuse this research to discourage population-level interventions aimed at reducing hazardous alcohol consumption and increasing smoking cessation (Gundle et al., 2010; Miller et al., 2012).

Genetic risk information on addiction may also be exploited by companies seeking to commercialize it. Commercial companies are already selling putative genetic tests for addiction liability and addiction treatment response (e.g., response to naltrexone treatment of alcohol dependence) direct to the consumer, even though these tests have not been approved by the US Food and Drug Administration for use in clinical practice (e.g., Janssens et al., 2006).

This chapter discusses these concerns and other possible public health issues raised by genetic research on addiction. We focus on research on alcohol and nicotine dependence, two of the leading preventable causes of disease burden globally. First, we briefly discuss the potential benefits of this research – namely, improved prevention and treatment of addiction – the likelihood of these applications being realized, and the factors that may affect their uptake. We then turn to the potential misunderstandings and misuses of this research by individuals, the media, industry, and commercial companies. We highlight the potential

Genetic Research on Addiction, ed. Audrey R. Chapman. Published by Cambridge University Press.
© Cambridge University Press 2012.

implications of such misuse by alcohol and tobacco companies for individual and population health. Finally, we discuss the potential consequences of an overemphasis on genetic research on addiction for responses to this disorder by the public and in the research, prevention, and treatment arenas.

The potential public health benefits of genetic research on addiction

Better prevention of addiction?

As outlined in Chapter 2, the potential for genetic research on alcohol and nicotine dependence to be useful in preventing these disorders at present seems doubtful. The future feasibility of population-level predictive genetic screening for alcohol and nicotine dependence remains uncertain because: (1) the candidate alleles identified so far have small effect sizes and have not always been replicated; (2) there may be complicated multiple gene–gene and gene–environment interactions that predict disease liability in ways that are difficult to identify in genome-wide association studies (GWAS); and (3) disease liability may also be affected by epigenetic modifications (that is, environmentally induced changes in which the nuclear DNA is expressed). Even if more than 200 susceptibility alleles for these disorders were found, modeling suggests simultaneous testing of this many alleles will provide little useful information, as most consumers will find themselves in the middle of log-normal distributions with an "average" genetic risk (Janssens et al., 2006; Wray et al., 2007, 2010; Clayton, 2009).

Population screening for nicotine and alcohol dependence would also be prohibitively expensive, owing to the small effect sizes for susceptibility alleles; extremely high numbers of people would need to be screened to detect one "high-risk" case. Triaging screening on the basis of family history of disorder, and thus restricting to those with a higher likelihood of the genetic and or environmental factors that predispose a disorder, would be a less expensive proposition. However, the costs of screening even this more select group could only be justified if the addition of genetic information improved upon predictions based on family history. For smoking, the evidence suggests it does not (Gartner et al., 2009); it is unclear as yet if this is also true for alcohol dependence.

Better treatment of addiction?

Pharmacogenetic research on addiction seems more promising and more likely to benefit public health in the near future. Pharmacogenetic testing has the capacity to help clinicians to select the treatment and determine the dose of treatment that will yield the best outcomes in an individual, minimizing side effects and relapse. Pharmacogenetic studies of treatment for alcohol dependence have examined a number of polymorphisms, including the *Asp40* allele of *OPRM1* (mu opioid type 1 receptor) for naltrexone response (e.g., Anton et al., 2006); the LL genotype of the *5-HTT* (serotonin transporter) gene for ondansetron response (Johnson et al., 2011); variants in *GABRA2/GABRA6* for response to acamprosate (Ooteman et al., 2009); and a single nucleotide polymorphism (SNP) in intron 9 of the glutamate receptor 5 (GluR5) gene (*GRIK1*) for topiramate response (Ray et al., 2009). Pharmacogenetic studies of smoking cessation have also examined a variety of polymorphisms, such as *DRD2* (e.g., Berlin et al., 2005; Lerman et al., 2006), *OPRM1* (Munafò et al., 2007), *SLC6A3* (Lerman et al., 2003), *SLC6A4* (Munafò et al., 2006; David et al., 2007), *DBH* (Johnstone et al., 2004), *FREQ* (Dahl et al., 2006), and *COMT* genes (Berrettini et al., 2007).

For a pharmacogenetic test to be clinically useful, the genes tested need to be highly prevalent and predictive of differential treatment response. The candidate genes examined in pharmacogenetic studies of smoking cessation struggle to meet these criteria. Some trials have reported a differential response to treatment (typically to nicotine replacement therapy or bupropion compared to placebo), but the differences have been small, have often weakened over time, and most findings have not been replicated (e.g., Lerman et al., 2004; Munafò et al., 2006; David et al., 2007; Munafò et al., 2007). The positive results are also of uncertain utility because the polymorphisms that have been tested are not SNPs (Lee and Tyndale, 2006), but copy number variants (i.e., variations in the number of copies of nucleotides that have been inserted or deleted from the usual DNA sequences). The latter genetic variations are not as straightforward to genotype as SNPs, which can be sequenced more rapidly, efficiently, and cheaply.

With respect to treatment for alcohol dependence, the *Asp40* allele of the *OPRM1* gene for response to naltrexone treatment best meets the aforementioned criteria, at least in Asian and Caucasian Americans. *Asp40* is found in 48% of Americans of Asian descent, and 15 to 18% of Caucasian Americans, but less than 5% of African Americans (Kuehn, 2009). Those possessing the allele are three times more likely to respond to naltrexone therapy for alcohol dependence than those homozygous for the *Asn40* allele (Oslin et al., 2003; Anton et al., 2006; Ray and Hutchison, 2007). Cost-effectiveness analyses are needed to determine whether using this test provides a sufficient gain in treatment outcome to justify the costs of its use in the whole population, as there is a lower prevalence of this variant in Caucasian and African Americans than in those of Asian descent. If the test does prove to be cost-effective and acceptable to both clinicians and patients, it will provide a good model of how a pharmacogenetic test may be used in the addiction field.

Factors affecting uptake of pharmacogenetic testing for addiction

For the public health benefits of such testing to be realized, clinicians must understand and be willing to use these tests; so must patients. Evidence suggests that clinicians may be concerned about inadvertently misusing, misinterpreting or mis-communicating genetic test results, and this may be a barrier to the use of such tests in clinical contexts (Shields and Lerman, 2008; Shields et al., 2008). One study suggested that clinicians may be reluctant to use genetic tests for fear of the liability consequences if they incorrectly or inaccurately interpret or communicate genetic test results to patients (Shields and Lerman, 2008). These concerns may be a result of their lack of training and expertise in interpreting genetic tests, which may be a particular problem among older cohorts of physicians who have received little formal education in molecular genetics and who may not be familiar with the breadth of human genome variation or with clinical applications of this knowledge (Gurwitz and Manolopoulos, 2007). For some clinicians, keeping abreast of the abundant new pharmacogenetic research may be seen as an additional burden and a complicating factor in therapeutic decision making, rather than as an enabler of optimal therapeutic decision making (Kirchheiner et al., 2005). These difficulties are seen elsewhere in medicine, and should not prevent the use of pharmacogenetic tests. Efforts to provide concise clinical guidance to clinicians on pharmacogenetic tests, including about their evidence base, suitable populations for use, and other implementation issues should be encouraged.

There is clearly a need for more comprehensive education about genetic testing and its interpretation both in medical training and for registered physicians as part of ongoing professional development. The provision of genetic counseling both before and after ordering a genetic test may also be one way to mitigate these personal liability concerns, although this would be expensive to implement in all clinical consultations. Guidelines on this matter exist to assist clinicians in determining when genetic counseling is and is not warranted. Such guidelines could be adapted for specific application to addiction medicine.

Bodies such as the US Center for Disease Control and Prevention's Evaluation of Genomic Applications in Practice and Prevention (EGAPP) Working Group may play an important role in providing reputable independent advice on which pharmacogenetic tests have sufficient evidence to justify their clinical use. For instance, EGAPP has published statements about the validity and strength of the evidence around pharmacogenetic testing for response to serotonin-specific reuptake inhibitors for depression and genotyping for response to a particular form of chemotherapy (EGAPP, 2009). At present, they have not issued any statements about the evidence for a pharmacogenetic test for using naltrexone to treat alcohol dependence.

Physicians may also be reluctant to order genetic tests if the genotype is more prevalent in certain racial groups, for fear that the information will be used to further marginalize such groups, or that they will be perceived as racist (Shields et al., 2008). This concern is likely to be salient in pharmacogenetic testing for responses to treatment for alcohol dependence, given that the allele that confers a better response to naltrexone is most prevalent in persons of Asian descent and rare in African Americans (Kuehn, 2009). The same variant has also been examined for predicting responses to smoking-cessation treatment (Munafò et al., 2007), so the same concerns may also apply for pharmacogenetic testing for smoking cessation.

Concerns about managing the ancillary risk information generated from genetic tests may also be a barrier to their use by clinicians. Many of the genes that confer increased susceptibility to addiction are also associated with susceptibility to other diseases – a phenomenon known as pleiotropy. A study of primary care physicians showed they were less likely to order a pharmacogenetic test designed to tailor smoking-cessation treatment if the genotypes being tested had pleiotropic associations with other conditions (including other addictions and mental health disorders) (Shields et al., 2008). This is likely to be an issue for genetic tests for alcohol dependence, for which many of the genes likely to be tested also confer increased risks for other types of addictions and medical conditions (e.g., cancers). For example, ALDH2*2 has been associated with an increased risk of oral, pharyngeal, laryngeal, and esophageal cancer (Boffetta and Hashibe, 2006), whereas variants in ADH1B*1 and ADH7 have been shown to be protective against aerodigestive cancers (Hashibe et al., 2008). A variant in the CHRNA5 gene that encodes the neuronal acetylcholine receptor subunit alpha-5 is associated with an increased risk of alcohol dependence (Wang et al., 2009) but protects against cocaine dependence (Grucza et al., 2008). As more genetic research is undertaken, no doubt further examples of pleiotropy will emerge.

Public understanding of pharmacogenetic testing for addiction will affect the public health gains yielded by this technology. A pharmacogenetic test may provide a useful marker of a more *likely positive* treatment response to a drug in an individual, but other nongenetic factors, such as co-occurring diseases or other medications that the individual is taking, may mean that the drug is contraindicated (Shah, 2006). This is an important message for clinicians to give to prospective users of pharmacogenetic tests so that unnecessary drug use and adverse responses to drugs can be minimized, along with overinflated expectations.

The availability and funding sources for these tests may also influence their uptake. Policymakers need to decide from where such tests will be accessed (i.e., from a clinician, over the counter, or on the Internet?) and who will pay for them. Will the patient pay for the costs of the genetic test, or will they be subsidized, either in part or in full, by health insurance? Consideration would also need to be given as to whether a patient is entitled to be subsidized to use a medication if they do not want to take the predictive genetic test.

Possible misuses and misunderstandings of genetic research on addiction

The way genetic risk information about addiction is communicated by researchers, the media, clinicians, and individuals will be important factors in the impact of genetic research on public health. Misunderstanding of such research, even if unintentional, could adversely affect community attitudes to addicted persons and their relatives. It could also undermine addicted persons' beliefs about their capacity to cut down or abstain from smoking and alcohol consumption.

The misuse of genetic research or risk information about addiction, whether inadvertent or deliberate, has the potential to cause harm not only to genetically predisposed individuals, but to the greater population. Third parties such as employers and insurance companies may misuse this information in a discriminatory way to exclude individuals from eligibility for insurance or to justify employment decisions. Tobacco, alcohol, and gambling industries may also use genetic research on addiction to discourage attempts to reduce population-level consumption of the products that they represent (and seek to promote). We discuss these issues next.

Effects of genetic information on public attitudes and behavior

One common misunderstanding of genetic research is that having a genetic predisposition to a disorder means one either has, or is very likely to develop, the disorder. When applied to genetic research on addiction, such misunderstandings could lead to unnecessary stigmatization and discrimination of genetically vulnerable individuals. They could also create unnecessary anxiety in genetically vulnerable individuals and in their relatives.

Public misunderstandings of genetic information may in part be a by-product of a lack of health literacy (including genetic literacy) among the general public. The US Department of Health and Human Services estimates that 50% of Americans lack what they define as functional health literacy, that is: "the degree to which individuals have the capacity to obtain, process, and understand basic health information and services needed to make appropriate health decisions" (US Department of Health and Human Services, 2000).

Rates of population-level genetic literacy are less well established. However, the results of recent surveys on public understanding of basic genetics suggest that genetic literacy is likely to be even more limited than health literacy. For instance, a recent survey of 1200 Americans found that 75% incorrectly believed that a single gene could control specific human behaviors (Christensen et al., 2010). Similarly, an Australian survey of a representative sample of 1009 persons found that only a minority correctly understood the meaning of increased genetic risk (Molster et al., 2009). None of this is too surprising, perhaps, given the lack of concerted attempts to improve public understanding of the genetics of common disorders.

The way genetic research is reported and portrayed in the media may also influence public attitudes to those suffering from an addiction. The media often portrays the role of genetics in disease susceptibility in a deterministic way. For instance, in reporting on genetic research on addiction, media articles detailing discoveries of "the gene for addiction" (BBC News, 2004; Doyle, 2004) are not uncommon. Media reporting of the NicoTest, for example, described it as a test for "the smoker's gene" or the "addiction gene" (BBC News, 2004; Doyle, 2004). Such reports can reinforce common misunderstandings by suggesting that people with "the gene" are very likely to develop a particular disorder, and that those who do not have it are at low risk of doing so (Khoury et al., 2000). These views may reflect the media's focus on Mendelian disorders, such as Huntington's chorea and cystic fibrosis (Khoury et al., 2000), for which such portrayals are more appropriate. However, for polygenic disorders such as addiction, in which multiple gene–gene and gene–environment interactions predict disease outcome, these interpretations are not warranted.

A major challenge for genetics researchers and for policymakers is to ensure that the reporting of research on common, non-Mendelian disorders effectively communicates the complex interactions that occur between environmental, social, and cultural factors and genes in influencing behavior (Wensley and King, 2008). This is particularly true for research on disorders such as addiction that tend to attract stigma. Failure to do so may result in discrimination against populations in which susceptibility genes are more prevalent. An example of this was the reporting on the discovery of a "warrior gene" in the Maori population of New Zealanders (Lea and Chambers, 2007). This research linked a mutation in the *MAOA* (monoamine oxidase) gene that was highly prevalent in the Maori population with a range of antisocial behaviors, which included alcoholism, violence, criminality, and gambling. It sparked much media controversy, and the researchers were accused of using the research to justify discriminatory attitudes toward Maori individuals.

The challenge for public education on genetic research will be to better explain the personal and public health implications of polygenic disorders in which individual alleles weakly predict risk, and interact with each other and with the person's environment (McBride et al., 2010). Researchers have a role to play in public education through the responsible dissemination of aggregate research results in the community, and their responsible disclosure of individual genetic test results to research participants. When researchers disclose results to research subjects, they have a responsibility to communicate clearly what the information does and does not mean. If successful, such public education could help to allay some anxieties about third-party misunderstanding of genetic information about addiction risk because people would better understand that this information is not sufficiently predictive of disease risk to be able to be misused in discriminatory ways.

Public education will also need to avoid any unintended message that high-risk genomic medicine strategies can replace, rather than supplement, public health strategies (Willett, 2002; Merikangas and Risch, 2003; Carlsten and Burke, 2006). Measures such as applying a volumetric tax to alcoholic beverages, increasing the tax on cigarettes, reducing the availability of alcohol, and requiring plain packaging for cigarettes will remain more cost-effective policies than attempting to identify those at higher genetic risk of becoming alcohol or nicotine dependent (Hall et al., 2002; Khoury et al., 2004; Doran et al., 2010).

Impacts of genetic information on smoking and alcohol use

A key consideration in the public health policy implications of genetic research on addiction is whether and how genetic information on disease risk influences an individual's behavior. It is often assumed that giving genetic risk information will prompt individuals to change their behavior in desired directions (Haga et al., 2003; Hunter et al., 2008). It is not clear that this will always be the case (Peto, 2001; Khoury, 2003). Inappropriate communication of genetic risk information may undermine individuals' beliefs about their ability to change their behavior (Senior et al., 2000; Wright et al., 2003). It may also raise unnecessary anxiety about disease risk in persons who are in fact at low risk of developing the disorder (Marteau and Croyle, 1998).

For example, the assumption that telling persons they are genetically predisposed to tobacco-related diseases will prompt them to quit smoking is not supported by the research to date. In two randomized trials, smokers who were advised they had a positive test for genetic susceptibility to lung cancer (*CYP2D6* status) were no more likely to attempt to quit or to succeed in quitting than smokers who were not advised of their genetic risk (Audrain et al., 1997; Lerman et al., 1997).

The few studies that have suggested personalized feedback about genetic susceptibility to tobacco-related diseases may encourage smoking-cessation attempts found that these changes were not sustained in the long term. For example, one study showed that testing positively for a genetic predisposition to lung cancer increased smoking-cessation attempts (McBride et al., 2002) and another showed it reduced the number of cigarettes smoked (Sanderson et al., 2008), but neither of these changes was sustained for more than 6 months.

There is also the possibility that if persons are told they are at lower genetic risk of tobacco-related diseases, they may be less motivated to quit smoking. There is little evidence on this issue. The few studies that do exist suggest a lower motivation to quit among smokers given hypothetical genetic feedback indicating a "low risk" of disease (Hoff et al., 2005). One randomized trial found that smokers who were told that they were at low risk of tobacco-related diseases had lower smoking-cessation rates than those not given any genetic risk information (Ito et al., 2006). A more recent randomized controlled trial found some evidence of a beneficial effect of pharmacogenetic feedback about responsiveness to a particular nicotine replacement therapy (NRT) medication in adherence to that medication; there was no evidence that genetic feedback reduced the future quit preparedness of those at high genetic risk who failed to quit on the occasion studied (Marteau et al., 2010).

Similarly, there is the possibility that persons who are told that they have a genetic variant that confers high protection against alcohol dependence could believe they could drink as much as they liked with no adverse consequences (Spooner et al., 2001). They would need to be told that they were still at risk of experiencing the multiple adverse social consequences associated with heavy drinking, such as road traffic and other accidents, violence, and abuse.

To date, no studies have examined the impact of genetic feedback about the high risk of alcohol dependence on consumption, but two have examined the impact of hypothetical genetic feedback about protection against alcohol dependence on alcohol consumption. Both randomized trials examined the impact on alcohol consumption of being told that one had the variant in *ALDH2*2* that is protective against alcohol dependence and increases the risk of alcohol-related cancers. The first randomized trial (Komiya et al., 2006) found slightly higher alcohol consumption in those who had been notified of their genetic risk, compared with those who had not, although the differences were not statistically significant.

The second trial, which used web-based personalized genetic feedback, showed that participants who were told they tested positive for the *ALDH2*2* allele had significant reductions in 30-day drinking frequency and quantity compared with controls (Hendershot et al., 2010). Given its links with cancer susceptibility (Boffetta and Hashibe, 2006), knowledge of possession of the *ALDH2*2* allele should provide a strong impetus to reduce alcohol consumption. It is unclear whether similar changes would be seen in persons who tested positive for an allele that predicted a lower risk of alcohol dependence but had no implications for susceptibility to alcohol-related cancers.

A more speculative possibility is that persons who know that they have a higher genetic risk of developing an addiction may be less inclined to seek treatment because they believe that their disorder is incurable. In the case of smokers, one study suggests that genetic factors did not reduce smokers' beliefs in their ability to quit (Hughes, 2009). However, it is unclear whether this was a result of participants' lack of knowledge of the genetic determinants of smoking, as this was not assessed in the study. It is also not clear whether these results would translate to alcohol dependence.

Genetic risk information may also incline addicted individuals to believe that they require a pharmacological intervention to quit (Marteau and Weinman, 2006). Two studies suggest smokers who were told that they had a genetic predisposition to nicotine dependence were more likely to believe that they needed to use a drug to quit smoking (Wright et al., 2003; Cappella et al., 2005). This may not be desirable, because many smokers in the population quit without such medical aids (Chapman and Mackenzie, 2010). However, a recent study found that individuals were equally willing to try a nicotine vaccine for smoking cessation regardless of whether they were told nicotine dependence was genetically or environmentally determined (Leader et al., 2010). It is unclear how a genetic predisposition to alcohol dependence would affect addicted persons' beliefs about the interventions that they required to stop drinking. Research is needed to examine this.

Misuse of genetic information by industry stakeholders

Public health professionals are concerned that industries with an interest in promoting high levels of consumption of their product will misuse genetic research to achieve this end (Gundle et al., 2010). In the case of alcohol dependence, for example, genetic research has been misused by the alcohol industry to argue that alcohol-related problems occur only in a minority of genetically susceptible individuals (Hall, 2005). The alcohol industry has a vested interest in advocating high-risk policies as alternatives to population-level policies. The policy implication favored by the industry is that alcohol problems are better addressed by identifying and intervening with problem drinkers rather than adopting effective strategies for reducing population-level alcohol consumption, such as increased taxation and reduced availability of alcohol (Babor et al., 2010). It could, for example, advocate population-wide genetic screening to identify the minority at increased risk for alcohol dependence (Hall et al., 2008).

The tobacco industry has also promoted genetic explanations of smoking and of tobacco-related diseases in this way (Hall et al., 2008). In the 1970s and 1980s, it funded behavioral and genetic research on smoking and tobacco-related disease as a strategic decision that located the risks of smoking in the genome of the individual smokers and implicitly exonerated tobacco smoking as a cause of disease (Hall et al., 2008; Gundle et al., 2010). The potential for industry to misuse research also raises important ethical questions around researchers' engagement with industry-funded research. We do not discuss these issues here: a comprehensive analysis is provided elsewhere in this volume (see Section 2).

Premature commercialization of direct-to-consumer genetic tests

Genetic research may also be misused by companies who are seeking to prematurely commercialize it. As the pace of genetic research increases, biomarkers are rapidly moving from discovery to commercial application [in the form of direct-to-consumer (DTC) tests] with little oversight, regulation, or respect for scientific rigor (Hogarth, 2010). There is no longer an intervening period in which test results are replicated and gradually adopted by the medical profession before their commercial application.

Genetic tests for alcohol and nicotine dependence are no exception. Even though these tests are not yet available in clinical practice, a number of commercial companies are selling putative genetic tests for alcohol dependence liability, nicotine dependence liability, and response to naltrexone treatment for alcohol dependence direct to consumers. In 2011, five companies offered genetic testing for nicotine dependence (23andMe, deCODE genetics, GenePlanet, Lumigenix, and BioMarker Pharmaceuticals), four for alcohol flush response (23andMe, deCODE genetics, GenePlanet, and Lumigenix) and three for alcohol dependence (23andMe, BioMarker Pharmaceuticals, and Lumigenix). One company, 23andMe, also offered pharmacogenetic testing for individual's response to naltrexone treatment for alcohol dependence. These tests are accessible over the Internet. Consumers send the company a swab of cells from the inside wall of their cheeks, which are subsequently sent to the company's laboratories for genetic testing, in some cases for as little as $200 (e.g., 23andMe). Table 11.1 summarizes the DTC genetic tests available for phenotypes related to alcohol and nicotine dependence as at January 2011. Some companies publish the genetic variants they test for on the Internet, in some cases including links to empirical literature about the variants and their association with disease risk. We have included this information where available.

The predictive power, reliability, validity, and clinical utility of the genes tested for alcohol and nicotine dependence via these DTC tests is extremely limited. With the exception of the variant for alcohol flush reaction, the genes tested are only weakly predictive of addiction risk. None of the other DTC genetic tests for alcohol or nicotine dependence liability provides the consumer with actionable information: most will be told that they are at average, or slightly above or below average, risk of disease. Also, the prevalence of some of the genetic variants being tested (e.g., *Asp40* of *OPRM1* and *ALDH2*2*) is extremely rare or absent in certain cultural groups (see Chapter 2 of this volume). None of these factors is transparently communicated to the consumer to inform their decision about whether to take the test. Furthermore, in the United States, the laboratories in which DTC genetic tests are conducted are not always subject to the same rigorous Clinical Laboratory Improvement Amendments standards as clinical laboratories are. Consequently, the quality and analytical validity of their tests results is also questionable.

Furthermore, there are wide variations between companies in the estimates of the genetic risk for the same diseases (Ng et al., 2009). An in-depth discussion of all the public health concerns raised by the use of DTC genetic tests for addiction is beyond the scope of this chapter: interested readers should see Janssens et al. (2006). Most of these concerns are largely due to the absence of any regulation of DTC genetic testing.

Regulation of DTC genetic testing has been a hotly debated issue. Advocates of DTC testing believe regulation of these tests is unnecessary and may risk undermining an individual's right to "know their DNA" and make "empowered" decisions about their health (Bender et al., 2010). Caulfield (2011) questioned the need for regulation, citing an analysis of Internet hits of DTC genetic testing company websites which suggested that DTC testing has not had a high uptake to date (Wright and Gregory-Jones, 2010), and the lack of evidence that genetic risk information causes anxiety in consumers or influences their health behaviors.

We argue that there is a case for regulation to protect the public health of consumers. Even though it is unclear what the actual uptake of DTC genetic tests currently is, it seems

Table 11.1. Genetic tests offered direct to the consumer for addiction-related disorders/phenotypes by company

	23andMe	deCODE	GenePlanet	BioMarker Pharmaceuticals	My Gene Profile	Lumigenix
Alcohol dependence	Taq1 A SNP of DRD2			Yes*		Yes*
Alcohol flush response	ALDH2*2	ALDH2*2	ALDH2*2			Yes*
Alcohol metabolism					Yes*	
Alcohol intoxication	OPRM1 (Asp40)				Yes*	
Naltrexone response for alcohol dependence treatment	OPRM1 (Asp40)					
Nicotine dependence	CHRNA3, CHRNA5, and CHRNB4	CHRNA3, CHRNA5, and CHRNB4	Yes*	Yes*		Yes*
Heroin addiction	OPRM1 (Asp40)					

* But not gene specified

Source: Table adapted from (Genetics & Public Policy Center, 2010).

likely that use of these tests will increase, especially as the costs of DTC tests continue to fall. Furthermore, we believe the fact that the market of DTC test users is small is not sufficient grounds not to regulate their use. There are many other examples in which regulation is enforced to protect the public health of a small minority of people who may be at risk of harm. Similarly, in the interests of protecting the public health of DTC genetic test consumers, governments have a responsibility to oversee these tests and ensure that they provide valid genetic risk information to avoid causing unnecessary anxiety or harmful behaviors or interventions.

The US Food and Drug Administration (FDA) has proposed that DTC genetic testing be regulated in the United States largely because of concerns about the questionable validity and clinical utility of the alleles tested (United States Government Accountability Office, 2010). If regulation does proceed, an immediate priority should be to set minimum standards for the clinical validity and utility of tests. These standards would need to be met before a test could be made available for purchase by consumers.

The pharmacogenetic test for naltrexone response, unlike the tests for alcohol-dependence liability, does have the potential to provide actionable information, assuming the consumer can correctly interpret the test result. This raises another important issue for regulation of DTC genetic tests: the need for genetic counseling. At present, many DTC genetic testing companies provide genetic information in the absence of genetic counseling before and after testing (McGuire and Burke, 2008). Navigenics is one exception, although it does not offer testing for addiction-related genotypes.

Developing standards to protect the privacy of consumers' genetic information should also be a priority for regulation. DTC tests raise greater privacy concerns than laboratory-based tests, given that they are purchased over the Internet, and genetic information can be shared with others. For example, 23andMe has a social networking component on its website that is similar to a Facebook group for people with common genetic vulnerabilities. The potential for surreptitious testing via these companies (i.e., family members of individuals collecting a sample of DNA without their permission) is an emerging privacy concern, although it is not clear how common this may be (Udesky, 2010). It is vital to develop measures to safeguard the privacy of genetic information derived through DTC genetic testing, including preventing surreptitious testing (e.g., of minors in the case of disputed paternity).

Possible social impacts of the medicalization of addiction

Many of the important public health policy implications of genetic research on alcohol dependence emanate from concerns that it will *medicalize* the disorder (Midanik, 2006; Berghmans et al., 2009). Medicalization involves focusing on the individual-level neurobiological and genetic factors involved in disease with little regard to the social and cultural determinants. A medicalized view of addiction has implications both for how those that suffer from it are viewed in society, and how society responds to addiction as a public health issue.

Impacts on stigma and discrimination

Proponents of a medicalized view of addiction believe it will reduce the stigma associated with the condition (Dackis and O'Brien, 2005). They argue that highlighting the genetic basis of the disorder will lead to a greater acceptance of addiction as a real psychiatric disorder that requires medical treatment, rather than an immoral behavior that should be punished. There are conflicting views as to whether medicalization of addiction increases or decreases stigmatization (Buchman and Reiner, 2009). One view is that medicalization reduces stigmatization and discrimination of persons with addiction on the basis that they have not become addicted through moral weakness or of their own volition (Decamp and Sugarman, 2004). Another view is that medicalization increases stigma and discrimination because the genes that predispose to addiction are seen as a permanent (and irreversible) characteristic of the person (Berghmans et al., 2009). Research on the genetic basis of other psychiatric disorders suggests biological explanations may in fact harden people's attitudes toward the mentally ill, increasing stigmatization and social distance (Read and Harre, 2001; Buchman and Reiner, 2009). More research is needed to resolve this dispute.

Impacts on research and public policy priorities

A medicalized view of addiction may also influence levels of funding for research, preventative health, and treatment. Since the human genome project, our knowledge of genetic involvement in various common diseases has grown exponentially. However, there are concerns this may have inadvertently led to an underemphasis of the role of environmental factors in the etiology of common diseases (Evans et al., 2011). One possible consequence may be that even less priority is given to funding behavioral and psychological research on addiction (Midanik, 2006).

Midanik (2006) argues that the funding priorities for research commissioned by the National Institute on Alcohol Abuse and Alcoholism (NIAAA) in the United States over the last decade reflect an increased medicalization of alcohol-dependence research. She reports that investments in biomedical (including genetic and neuroscientific) research on alcoholism far exceeded all other categories of research during this period. For example, in 2003, research grants awarded in biomedical research on alcoholism represented approximately 80% of all research funding awarded by NIAAA that year. This is a problem, as NIAAA reportedly funds around 90% of all alcohol research in the world (Midanik, 2006). The National Institute on Drug Abuse (NIDA) has been reported to fund a similar percentage of biomedical research on other addictions (Vrecko, 2010).

This medicalization of research on alcohol dependence is not confined to government research funding. The Alcoholic Beverage Medical Research Foundation (ABMRF) is the largest independent not-for-profit foundation in North America that is dedicated to supporting research on the effects of alcohol on health and behavior and on the prevention of alcohol-related problems (The Foundation for Alcohol Research, 2008). The majority of its investment (58%) is in biomedical research, including a major research stream dedicated to alcoholism and genetics (Miller et al., 2012).

Critics of medicalization are also concerned it could undermine efforts to prevent harmful alcohol consumption and the development of alcoholism and nicotine dependence in the population. They fear that it will be used to justify an increased focus on interventions that address individual-level genetic and neurological factors while reducing the focus on those that aim to address the social and cultural determinants of disorders (e.g., taxes, reducing availability of alcohol, raising the minimum legal drinking age, and changes to legal blood alcohol concentration (BAC) levels for young adult drivers in the case of alcohol dependence; and taxes, plain packaging and bans on smoking in public places for nicotine dependence). If this occurred, it would be to the detriment of society, because the evidence shows that these interventions are more cost-effective ways of reducing the burden of disease attributable to these disorders than "high-risk" individual-level interventions that seek to address the biological factors that are thought to predispose to addiction (Laxminarayan et al., 2006; Campbell et al., 2009; Elder et al., 2010; Middleton et al., 2010).

Impacts on addiction treatment

Medicalization could also potentially affect the types of treatments for addiction that are made available or promoted in the medical community. For example, concerns have been raised that genetic research on alcoholism will reinforce beliefs that it is a biological disease that can only be addressed through individual-level treatment and be used by clinicians or the criminal justice system to enforce treatment in rehabilitation or judicial environments (Coors and Raymond, 2009). It may also encourage an overreliance on pharmacological interventions that seek to address the biological factors in severely dependent persons, while neglecting psychosocial and behavioral interventions that seek to address the underlying social determinants of addiction, such as poverty, lack of education, and social isolation (Kleiman, 1992). It has been shown that, in most cases, a combination of psychosocial and pharmacological interventions for alcohol and nicotine dependence produces the best outcomes (Lingford-Hughes et al., 2004; Weiss and Kueppenbender, 2006).

Pharmacogenetic research on addiction treatment may also influence the types of cessation treatments that are available. It may have the potential to rescue drugs that have been previously recalled owing to limited safety or efficacy (Garrison et al., 2008). However, investments in pharmacogenetics may have the potential to further stratify the market for medications. Pharmaceutical companies may be more inclined to invest in developing potential blockbuster drugs, that is, medicines that benefit the majority of patients with common diseases, than in developing medications which might provide a significant benefit for only a small number of patients with rarer diseases (See Nuffield Council on Bioethics, 2003 for a description of this issue).

Another possibility is that pharmacogenetic tests will be prematurely marketed to the public prior to validation of their effectiveness. This was the case with NicoTest, which was marketed to smokers over the Internet and doctors in the United Kingdom as guiding their choice of either nicotine replacement therapy or bupropion for smoking cessation before its clinical utility had been evaluated (GeneWatch UK, 2004; De Francesco, 2006). It has since been withdrawn from the market.

There is little evidence available to assess the seriousness of these concerns. We suggest they indicate some priorities for social and behavioral research on the impact of genetic research on social policy and public health responses to the harms caused by alcohol, tobacco, and other drug use.

Conclusion

Genetic research on addiction certainly has the potential to benefit public health. At present it seems unlikely that genetic research will lead to better prevention of addiction through population-level predictive screening. However, the potential for pharmacogenetic research to improve the treatment of addiction shows some promise. At this stage, more progress has been made in pharmacogenetic research on treatment for alcohol dependence than in pharmacogenetic research for smoking cessation. In particular, the *Asp40* allele of the *OPRM1* gene appears to predict differential response to naltrexone treatment for alcohol dependence. If it can be shown to cost-effectively predict treatment response in populations in whom the gene is less prevalent, it may well prove a good model for how pharmacogenetic testing could be applied to the treatment of addiction.

We must also be aware of the potential for genetic research on addiction to negatively impact public health if it is miscommunicated or misused and must take steps to prevent this from happening. Researchers, the media, clinicians, and the general public must responsibly communicate genetic research about addiction. This means clearly communicating the complex interactions between genetic, biological, social, and environmental factors involved in addiction. Doing so will help to prevent common misunderstandings about the role of genetics in addiction liability, and hopefully will help to prevent discrimination and stigmatization. A more concerted effort at improving the genetic literacy of the population could also help to achieve this.

Premature marketing of genetic research on addiction in the form of DTC genetic tests may cause harm to public health because the tests employed have no clinical validity or utility and results are not interpreted by a clinician. In the interests of protecting public health, these tests need to be regulated. Until they are, clinicians should advise clients against using these tests, or at the very least, advise them to be extremely skeptical of any results they generate.

Developments in genetic research on addiction are important, but must not be at the expense of investments in social, behavioral, and psychological research on addiction. Likewise, they must not be used to justify a reduced focus on interventions that address the social and cultural determinants of the disorder. Population health strategies such as increased taxation and reduced opportunities to smoke or drink alcohol are likely to remain more efficient preventive strategies by reducing cigarette smoking and risky alcohol use than are high-risk genomic medicine strategies such as genetic screening.

References

Anton, R. F., O'Maley, S. S., Ciraulo, D. A., et al. (2006). Combined pharmacotherapies and behavioral interventions for alcohol dependence: the COMBINE study: a randomized controlled trial. *The Journal of the American Medical Association*, 295, 2003–2017.

Audrain, J., Boyd, N. R., Roth, J., et al. (1997). Genetic susceptibility testing in smoking-cessation treatment: One-year outcomes of a randomized trial. *Addictive Behaviors*, 22, 741–751.

Babor, T., Miller, P., and Edwards, G. (2010). Vested interests, addiction research and public policy. *Addiction*, 105, 4–5.

BBC News (2004). "DNA test" to help smokers quit. *BBC News*. Available online at: http://news.bbc.co.uk/2/hi/health/4061137.stm [accessed March 13, 2012].

Bender, L., Silverman, L. M., Dinulos, M. B., Nickel, J., and Grody, W. W. (2010). Direct-to-consumer genotyping: are we ready for

a brave new world? *Clinical Chemistry*, 56, 1056–1060.

Berghmans, R., De Jong, J., Tibben, A., and De Wert, G. (2009). On the biomedicalization of alcoholism. *Theoretical Medical Bioethics*, 30, 311–321.

Berlin, I., Covey, L. S., Jiang, H., and Hamer, D. (2005). Lack of effect of D2 dopamine receptor taqI A polymorphism on smoking cessation. *Nicotine & Tobacco Research*, 7, 725–728.

Berrettini, W., Wileyto, E. P., Epstein, L., et al. (2007). Catechol-O-Methyltransferase (COMT) gene variants predict response to bupropion therapy for tobacco dependence. *Biological Psychiatry*, 61, 111–118.

Boffetta, P. and Hashibe, M. (2006). Alcohol and cancer. *Lancet Oncology*, 7, 149–156.

Buchman, D. and Reiner, P. B. (2009). Stigma and addiction: being and becoming. *American Journal of Bioethics*, 9, 18–19.

Campbell, C. A., Hahn, R. A., Elder, R., et al. (2009). The effectiveness of limiting alcohol outlet density as a means of reducing excessive alcohol consumption and alcohol-related harms. *American Journal of Preventative Medicine*, 37, 556–569.

Capella, J. N., Lerman, C., Romantan, A., and Baruh, L. (2005). News about genetics and smoking: Priming, family smoking history, and news story believability on inferences of genetic susceptibility to tobacco addiction. *Communication Research*, 32, 478–502.

Carlsten, C. and Burke, W. (2006). Potential for genetics to promote public health: Genetics research on smoking suggests caution about expectations. *Journal of the American Medical Association*, 296, 2480–2482.

Caulfield, T. (2011). Direct-to-consumer testing: if consumers are not anxious, why are policymakers? *Human Genetics*, 130, 23–25.

Chapman, S. and Mackenzie, R. (2010). The global research neglect of unassisted smoking cessation: causes and consequences. *PLoS Medicine*, 7, e1000216.

Christensen, K. D., Jayaratne, T. E., Roberts, J. S., Kardia, S. L., and Petty, E. M. (2010). Understandings of basic genetics in the United States: results from a national survey of black and white men and women. *Public Health Genomics*, 13, 467–476.

Clayton, D. G. (2009). Prediction and interaction in complex disease genetics: experience in type 1 diabetes. *PLoS Genetics*, 5, e1000540.

Coors, M. E. and Raymond, K. M. (2009). Substance use disorder genetic research: investigators and participants grapple with the ethical issues. *Psychiatric Genetics*, 19, 83–90.

Dackis, C. and O'Brien, C. (2005). Neurobiology of addiction: Treatment and public policy ramifications. *Nature Neuroscience*, 8, 1431–1436.

Dahl, J. P., Jepson, C. R., Wileyto, E. P., et al. (2006). Interaction between variation in the D2 dopamine receptor (*DRD2*) and the neuronal calcium sensor-1 (*FREQ*) genes in predicting response to nicotine replacement therapy for tobacco dependence. *Pharmacogenomics*, 6, 194–199.

David, S. P., Munafò, M. R., Murphy, M. F. G., Walton, R. T., and Johnstone, E. C. (2007). The serotonin transporter 5-*HTTLPR* polymorphism and treatment response to nicotine patch: Follow-up of a randomized controlled trial. *Nicotine & Tobacco Research*, 9, 225–231.

De Francesco, L. (2006). Genetic profiteering. *Nature Biotechnology*, 24, 888–890.

Decamp, M. and Sugarman, J. (2004). Ethics in population-based genetic research. *Accountability Research*, 11, 1–26.

Doran, C. M., Hall, W. D., Shakeshaft, A. P., Vos, T., and Cobiac, L. J. (2010). Alcohol policy reform in Australia: what can we learn from the evidence? *Medical Journal of Australia*, 192, 468–470.

Doyle, C. (2004). DNA test can identify "the smoker's gene". *The Telegraph*, December 3, 2004.

EGAPP (2009). Evaluation of genomic applications in practice and prevention. Available online at: www.egappreviews.org/ [accessed March 13, 2012].

Elder, R. W., Lawrence, B., Ferguson, A., et al. (2010). The effectiveness of tax policy interventions for reducing excessive alcohol consumption and related harms. *American Journal of Preventative Medicine*, 38, 217–229.

Evans, J. P., Meslin, E. M., Marteau, T. M., and Caulfield, T. (2011). Genomics. Deflating the genomic bubble. *Science*, 331, 861–862.

Garrison, L. P. Jr., Carlson, R. J., Carlson, J. J., et al. (2008). A review of public policy issues in promoting the development and commercialization of pharmacogenomic applications: challenges and implications. *Drug Metabolism Review*, 40, 377–401.

Gartner, C. E., Barendregt, J. J., and Hall, W. D. (2009). Multiple genetic tests for susceptibility to smoking do not outperform simple family history. *Addiction*, 104, 118–126.

Genetics & Public Policy Center (2010). DTC genetic testing companies. Available online at: www.dnapolicy.org/resources/ AlphabetizedDTCGeneticTesting Companies11.10. pdf [accessed March 13, 2012].

GeneWatch UK (2004). Three reasons not to buy the NicoTest genetic test. Available online at: www.genewatch.org/uploads/f03c6d66a9b354535738483c1c3d49e4/Nicotest_brief_final.pdf [accessed March 13, 2012].

Grucza, R. A., Wang, J. C., Stitzel, J. A., et al. (2008). A risk allele for nicotine dependence in *CHRNA5* is a protective allele for cocaine dependence. *Biological Psychiatry*, 64, 922–929.

Gundle, K. R., Dingel, M. J., and Koenig, B. A. (2010). "To prove this is the industry's best hope": big tobacco's support of research on the genetics of nicotine addiction. *Addiction*, 105, 974–983.

Gurwitz, D. and Manolopoulos, V. G. (2007). Personalized medicine. Comprehensive medicinal chemistry II. In D. J. Triggle and J. B. Taylor (eds.), *Comprehensive Medicinal Chemistry*, second edition. Amsterdam: Elsevier.

Haga, S. B., Khoury, M. J., and Burke, W. (2003). Genomic profiling to promote a healthy lifestyle: not ready for prime time. *Nature Genetics*, 34, 347–350.

Hall, W. D. (2005). British drinking: a suitable case for treatment? *British Medical Journal*, 331, 527–528.

Hall, W. D., Madden, P., and Lynskey, M. (2002). The genetics of tobacco use: methods, findings and policy implications. *Tobacco Control*, 11, 119–124.

Hall, W. D., Gartner, C. E., and Carter, A. (2008). The genetics of nicotine addiction liability: ethical and social policy implications. *Addiction*, 103, 350–359.

Hashibe, M., Mckay, J. D., Curado, M. P., et al. (2008). Multiple ADH genes are associated with upper aerodigestive cancers. *Nature Genetics*, 40, 707–709.

Hendershot, C. S., Otto, J. M., Collins, S. E., Liang, T., and Wall, T. L. (2010). Evaluation of a brief web-based genetic feedback intervention for reducing alcohol-related health risks associated with *ALDH2*. *Annals of Behavioral Medicine*, 40, 77–88.

Hoff, N., Evers-Casey, S., Weibel, S., Patkar, A., and Leone, F. (2005). Impact of genetic risk information on smokers' motivation to quit. In 11th Annual Meeting of the Society for Research on Nicotine and Tobacco, 2005, Prague, Czech Republic.

Hogarth, S. (2010). Myths, misconceptions and myopia: searching for clarity in the debate about the regulation of consumer genetics. *Public Health Genomics*, 13, 322–326.

Hughes, J. R. (2009). Smokers' beliefs about the inability to stop smoking. *Addictive Behavior*, 34, 1005–1009.

Hunter, D. J., Khoury, M. J., and Drazen, J. M. (2008). Letting the genome out of the bottle – will we get our wish? *New England Journal of Medicine*, 358, 105–107.

Ito, H., Matsuo, K., Wakai, K., et al. (2006). An intervention study of smoking cessation with feedback on genetic cancer susceptibility in Japan. *Preventive Medicine*, 42, 102–108.

Janssens, A. C., Aulchenko, Y. S., Elephante, S., et al. (2006). Predictive testing for complex diseases using multiple genes: fact or fiction? *Genetic Medicine*, 8, 395–400.

Johnson, B. A., Ait-Daoud, N., Seneviratne, C., et al. (2011). Pharmacogenetic approach at the serotonin transporter gene as a method of reducing the severity of alcohol drinking. *American Journal of Psychiatry*, 168, 265–275.

Johnstone, E. C., Yudkin, P., Griffiths, S. E., et al. (2004). The dopamine D2 receptor C32806T polymorphism (DRD2 Taq1A RFLP) exhibits no association with smoking behaviour in a healthy UK population. *Addiction Biology*, 9, 221–226

Khoury, M. J. (2003). Genetics and genomics in practice: the continuum from genetic disease to genetic information in health and disease. *Genetics in Medicine*, 5, 261–268.

Khoury, M. J., Thrasher, J. F., Burk, W., et al. (2000). Challenges in communicating genetics: a public health approach. *Genetics in Medicine*, 2, 198–202.

Khoury, M. J., Yang, Q., Gwinn, M., Little, J., and Flanders, W. D. (2004). An epidemiological assessment of genomic profiling for measuring susceptibility to common diseases and targeting interventions. *Genetics in Medicine*, 6, 38–47.

Kirchheiner, J., Fuhr, U., and Brockmoller, J. (2005). Pharmacogenetics-based therapeutic recommendations – ready for clinical practice? *Nature Review of Drug Discovery*, 4, 639–647.

Kleiman, M. (1992). *Against Excess: Towards a Drug Policy That Works*. New York: Basic Books.

Komiya, Y., Nakao, H., Kuroda, Y., et al. (2006). Application of aldehyde dehydrogenase 2 (*ALDH2*) genetic diagnosis in support of decreasing alcohol intake. *Journal of Occupational Health*, 48, 161–165.

Kuehn, B. M. (2009). Findings on alcohol dependence point to promising avenues for targeted therapies. *Journal of the American Medical Association*, 301, 1643–1645.

Laxminarayan, R., Mills, A. J., Breman, J. G., et al. (2006). Advancement of global health: key messages from the Disease Control Priorities Project. *Lancet*, 367, 1193–1208.

Lea, R. and Chambers, G. (2007). Monoamine oxidase, addiction, and the "warrior" gene hypothesis. *New Zealand Medical Journal*, 120, U2441.

Leader, A. E., Lerman, C., and Cappella, J. N. (2010). Nicotine vaccines: will smokers take a shot at quitting? *Nicotine Tobacco Research*, 12, 390–397.

Lee, A. M. and Tyndale, R. F. (2006). Drugs and genotypes: how pharmacogenetic information could improve smoking cessation treatment. *Journal of Psychopharmacology*, 20, 7–14.

Lerman, C., Glod, K., Audrain, J., et al. (1997). Incorporating biomarkers of exposure and genetic susceptibility into smoking cessation treatment: effects on smoking related cognitions, emotions and behavior change. *Health Psychology*, 16, 87–99.

Lerman, C., Shields, P. G., Wileyto, E. P., et al. (2003). Effects of dopamine transporter and receptor polymorphisms on smoking cessation in a bupropion clinical trial. *Health Psychology*, 22, 541–548.

Lerman, C., Wileyto, E. P., Patterson, F., et al. (2004). The functional mu opioid receptor (*OPRM1*) *Asn40Asp* variant predicts short-term response to nicotine replacement therapy in a clinical trial. *Pharmacogenomics*, 4, 184–192.

Lerman, C., Jepson, C., Wileyto, E. P., et al. (2006). Role of functional genetic variation in the dopamine D2 receptor (*DRD2*) in response to bupropion and nicotine replacement therapy for tobacco dependence: results of two randomized clinical trials. *Neuropsychopharmacology*, 31, 231–242.

Lingford-Hughes, A. R., Welch, S., and Nutt, D. J. (2004). Evidence-based guidelines for the pharmacological management of substance misuse, addiction and comorbidity: recommendations from the British Association for Psychopharmacology. *Journal of Psychopharmacology*, 18, 293–335.

Marteau, T. M. and Croyle, R. T. (1998). The new genetics. Psychological responses to genetic testing. *British Medical Journal*, 316, 693–696.

Marteau, T. M. and Weinman, J. (2006). Self-regulation and the behavioural response to DNA risk information: a theoretical analysis and framework for future research. *Social Science & Medicine*, 62, 1360–1368.

Marteau, T. M., Munafò, M. R., Prevost, A. T., et al. (2010). Impact of genetic feedback on adherence to nicotine replacement therapy: the personalised extra treatment (PET) trial. Baltimore. Society for Research on Nicotine and Tobacco Meeting.

McBride, C. M., Bepler, G., Lipkus, I. M., et al. (2002). Incorporating genetic susceptibility feedback into a smoking cessation program for African-American smokers with low income. *Cancer Epidemiology, Biomarkers and Prevention*, 11, 521–528.

McBride, C. M., Bowen, D., Brody, L. C., et al. (2010). Future health applications of genomics: priorities for communication, behavioral, and social sciences research. *American Journal of Preventive Medicine*, 38, 556–565.

McGuire, A. L. and Burke, W. (2008). An unwelcome side effect of direct-to-consumer personal genome testing: raiding the medical commons. *The Journal of the American Medical Association*, 300, 2669–2671.

Merikangas, K. R. and Risch, N. (2003). Genomic priorities and public health. *Science*, 302, 599–601.

Midanik, L. (ed.) (2006). *Biomedicalization of Alcohol Studies: Methodological Shifts and Institutional Challenges*. New Brunswick, NJ: Transaction Publishers.

Middleton, J. C., Hahn, R. A., Kuzara, J. L., et al. (2010). Effectiveness of policies maintaining or restricting days of alcohol sales on excessive alcohol consumption and related harms. *American Journal of Preventive Medicine*, 39, 575–589.

Miller, P., Carter, A., and De Groot, F. (2012). Investment and vested interests in neuroscience research of addiction: Why research ethics requires more than informed consent. In A. Carter, W. Hall and J. Illes (eds.), *Addiction Neuroethics: The Ethics of Addiction Research and Treatment*. New York: Elsevier.

Molster, C., Charles, T., Samanek, A., and O'Leary, P. (2009). Australian study on public knowledge of human genetics and health. *Public Health Genomics*, 12, 84–91.

Munafò, M. R., Johnstone, E. C., Wileyto, E. P., et al. (2006). Lack of association of *5-HTTLPR* genotype with smoking cessation in a nicotine replacement therapy randomized trial. *Cancer Epidemiology, Biomarkers and Prevention*, 15, 398–400.

Munafò, M. R., Elliot, K. M., Murphy, M. F. G., Walton, R. T., and Johnstone, E. C. (2007). Association of the mu-opioid receptor gene with smoking cessation. *Pharmacogenomics Journal*, 7, 353–361.

Ng, P. C., Murray, S. S., Levy, S., and Ventner, J. C. (2009). An agenda for personalized medicine. *Nature*, 461, 724–726.

Nuffield Council on Bioethics (2003). *Pharmacogenetics: Ethical Issues*. London: Nuffield Council on Bioethics.

Ooteman, W., Naassila, M., Koeter, M. W. J., et al. (2009). Predicting the effect of naltrexone and acamprosate in alcohol-dependent patients using genetic indicators. *Addiction Biology*, 14, 328–337.

Oslin, D. W., Berrettini, W, Kranzler, H. R., et al. (2003). A functional polymorphism of the mu-opioid receptor gene is associated with naltrexone response in alcohol-dependent patients. *Neuropsychopharmacology*, 28, 1546–1552.

Peto, J. (2001). Cancer epidemiology in the last century and the next decade. *Nature*, 411, 390–395.

Ray, L. A. and Hutchison, K. E. (2007). Effects of naltrexone on alcohol sensitivity and genetic moderators of medication response: a double-blind placebo-controlled study. *Archives of General Psychiatry*, 64, 1069–1077.

Ray, L. A., Miranda, R. Jr., Mackillop, J., et al. (2009). A preliminary pharmacogenetic investigation of adverse events from topiramate in heavy drinkers. *Experimental and Clinical Psychopharmacology*, 17, 122–129.

Read, J. and Harre, N. (2001). The role of biological and genetic causal beliefs in the stigmatisation of mental patients. *Journal of Mental Health*, 10, 223–235.

Sanderson, S. C., Humphries, S. E., and Hubbart, C. (2008). Psychological and behavioural impact of genetic testing smokers for lung cancer risk: a phase II exploratory trial. *Journal of Health Psychology*, 13, 481–494.

Senior, V., Marteau, T. M., and Weinman, J. (2000). Impact of genetic testing on causal models of heart disease and arthritis: an analogue study. *Psychology & Health*, 14, 1077–1088.

Shah, R. R. (2006). Can pharmacogenetics help rescue drugs withdrawn from the market? *Pharmacogenomics*, 7, 889–908.

Shields, A. E. and Lerman, C. (2008). Anticipating clinical integration of pharmacogenetic treatment strategies for addiction: are primary care physicians ready? *Clinical Pharmacological Therapies*, 83, 635–639.

Shields, A. E., Levy, D. E., Blumenthal, D., et al. (2008). Primary care physicians' willingness to offer a new genetic test to tailor smoking treatment, according to test characteristics. *Nicotine Tobacco Research*, 10, 1037–1045.

Spooner, C., Hall, W., and Lynskey, M. (2001). *The Structural Determinants of Youth Drug Use*. Canberra: Australian National Council on Drugs.

Taylor, S., Treloar, S., Barlow-Stewart, K., Stranger, M., and Otlowski, M. (2008). Investigating genetic discrimination in Australia: a large-scale survey of clinical genetics clients. *Clinical Genetics*, 74, 20–30.

The Foundation for Alcohol Research (2008). The Foundation for Alcohol Research. Available online at: www.abmrf.org [accessed March 13, 2012].

US Department of Health and Human Services (2000). *Healthy People 2010*. Washington, DC: US Department of Health and Human Services.

Udesky, L. (2010). The ethics of direct-to-consumer genetic testing. *Lancet*, 376, 1377–1378.

United States Government Accountability Office (2010). Direct-to-consumer genetic tests: misleading test results are further complicated by deceptive marketing and other questionable practices. Available online at: www.gao.gov/highlights/d10847thigh.pdf [accessed March 13, 2012].

Vrecko, S. (2010). Birth of a brain disease: science, the state and addiction neuropolitics. *History of the Human Sciences*, 23, 52–67.

Wang, J. C., Grucza, R., Cruchaga, C., et al. (2009). Genetic variation in the *CHRNA5* gene affects mRNA levels and is associated with risk for alcohol dependence. *Molecular Psychiatry*, 14, 501–510.

Weiss, R. D. and Kueppenbender, K. D. (2006). Combining psychosocial treatment with pharmacotherapy for alcohol dependence. *Journal of Clinical Psychopharmacology*, 26 Suppl 1, S37–42.

Wensley, D. and King, M. (2008). Scientific responsibility for the dissemination and interpretation of genetic research: lessons from the "warrior gene" controversy. *Journal of Medical Ethics*, 34, 507–509.

Willett, W. C. (2002). Balancing life-style and genomics research for disease prevention. *Science*, 296, 695–698.

Wray, N. R., Goddard, M. E., and Visscher, P. M. (2007). Prediction of individual genetic risk to disease from genome-wide association studies. *Genome Research*, 17, 1520–1528.

Wray, N. R., Yang, J., Goddard, M. E., and Visscher, P. M. (2010). The genetic interpretation of area under the ROC curve in genomic profiling. *PLoS Genet*, 6, e1000864.

Wright, A. J., Weinman, J., and Marteau, T. M. (2003). The impact of learning of a genetic predisposition to nicotine dependence: an analogue study. *Tobacco Control*, 12, 227–230.

Wright, C. F. and Gregory-Jones, S. (2010). Size of the direct-to-consumer genomic testing market. *Genetic Medicine*, 12, 594.

Chapter

12

Genetics, addiction, and stigma

Jo C. Phelan and Bruce G. Link

This chapter aims to further our understanding of how genetic research and genetic explanations of alcoholism and other addictions may affect the stigma that is attached to addictions. Because we found practically no empirical research directly addressing the connections among genetic causal attributions, stigma, and addictions, we approach the chapter in the following way. First, we review key conceptual models of stigma, which address three basic questions: (1) What is stigma? How can stigma be defined? (2) What are the dimensions of stigma? How does stigma vary depending on the characteristic that is stigmatized and the circumstances in which it is encountered? (3) Why do we stigmatize? How does stigmatization benefit the dominant nonstigmatized group? Second, we review existing conceptual and empirical work concerning the stigmatization of addictions, focusing primarily on alcohol and substance dependence, and we discuss addictions in relation to each of the general conceptual models of stigma.

Next, we focus on the implications of genetic explanations and understandings of addictions (or the "geneticization" of addictions) for stigma. Here we focus first on theories that have implications for the connection between genetic causal attributions and stigma, and then on empirical research that has addressed the connection between genetic attributions and stigma for characteristics such as mental illness, obesity, sexual orientation, anorexia, stuttering, and cancer. Finally, we use the theoretical models and empirical findings to construct predictions concerning the likely impact of genetic attributions for stigma related to addictions.

Conceptual models of stigma

What is stigma? How can stigma be defined?

The seminal work on stigma is Erving Goffman's *Stigma: Notes on the Management of Spoiled Identity* (1963). Goffman defines stigma as "the situation of the individual who is disqualified from full social acceptance" (Goffman, 1963: preface). Also, the stigmatized individual is "reduced in our mind from a whole and usual person to a tainted, discounted one" (Goffman, 1963: 3) by an attribute that is "deeply discrediting" (Goffman, 1963: 3). Goffman thus emphasizes two defining characteristics of stigma: social exclusion and status loss.

Subsequent to Goffman's (1963) conceptualization of stigma, the term has been used to describe what seem to be quite different concepts. It has been variously used to refer to the "mark" or "label" that is used as a social designation, to the linking of the label to negative

Genetic Research on Addiction, ed. Audrey R. Chapman. Published by Cambridge University Press.
© Cambridge University Press 2012.

stereotypes, and to the propensity to exclude or otherwise discriminate against the designated person. As a consequence of this variability in its usage, there has been confusion as to what the term means. In addition, dissatisfaction with the concept emerged in some circles for at least two reasons. First, the stigma concept was criticized for identifying an "attribute" or "mark" as residing in the person, as something the person possesses. The process of selecting and affixing labels was not taken to be as problematic as it should have been. In particular, too little attention had been focused on the identification of some characteristics for social salience from a vast range of possible characteristics that might have been selected instead. Second, too much emphasis had been placed on cognitive processes of category formation and stereotyping and too little on the prominent fact of discrimination and the influence of discrimination on the distribution of life chances.

In light of this confusion and controversy, Link and Phelan (2001) put forward a conceptualization of stigma that recognized the overlap between concepts such as stigma, labeling, stereotyping, and discrimination. The conceptualization they offered defined stigma in the relationship *between* interrelated components. They also responded to criticisms of the stigma concept by making the social selection of designations a prominent feature of their conceptualization, by incorporating discrimination into the concept, and by focusing on the importance of social, economic, and political power in the production of stigma. Link and Phelan describe their conceptualization as follows:

> In our conceptualization, stigma exists when the following interrelated components converge. In the first component, people distinguish and label human differences. In the second, dominant cultural beliefs link labeled persons to undesirable characteristics – to negative stereotypes. In the third, labeled persons are placed in distinct categories so as to accomplish some degree of separation of "us" from "them." In the fourth, labeled persons experience status loss and discrimination that lead to unequal outcomes. Stigmatization is entirely contingent on access to social, economic and political power that allows the identification of differentness, the construction of stereotypes, the separation of labeled persons into distinct categories and the full execution of disapproval, rejection, exclusion and discrimination. Thus we apply the term stigma when elements of labeling, stereotyping, separation, status loss and discrimination co-occur in a power situation that allows them to unfold. (Link and Phelan, 2001: 367)

Although a detailed exposition of each of these components is available elsewhere (Link and Phelan, 2001; Link et al., 2004), we provide a brief description of each component below.

Distinguishing and labeling differences

The vast majority of human differences, e.g., finger length or vegetable preferences, are not considered to be socially relevant. However, some differences, such as skin color and sexual preferences, are awarded a high degree of social salience in our time and place. Both the selection of salient characteristics and the creation of labels for them are social achievements that need to be understood as essential components of stigma.

Associating differences with negative attributes

In this component, the labeled difference is linked to negative stereotypes in such a manner that, for example, a person who has been hospitalized for mental illness is thought to represent a violence risk.

Separating "us" from "them"

A third aspect of the stigma process occurs when social labels connote a separation of "us" from "them." For example, certain ethnic or national groups (Morone, 1997), people with mental illness, or people with a different sexual orientation may be considered fundamentally different kinds of people from "us."

Emotional responses

From the vantage point of a stigmatizer, emotions of anger, irritation, anxiety, pity, and fear are likely. These emotions are important because they can be detected by the person who is stigmatized, thereby providing an important statement about a stigmatizer's response to them. Second, emotional responses may shape subsequent behavior toward the stigmatized person or group through processes identified by attribution theory (Weiner et al., 1988). From the vantage point of the person who is stigmatized, emotions of embarrassment, shame, fear, alienation, or anger are possible. Scheff (1998) has, for example, argued that the emotion of shame is central to stigma and that shaming processes can have powerful harmful consequences for stigmatized persons.

Status loss and discrimination

When people are labeled, set apart, and linked to undesirable characteristics, a rationale is constructed for devaluing, rejecting, and excluding them. This can occur in several ways.

Status loss

An almost immediate consequence of successful negative labeling and stereotyping is a general downward placement of a person in a status hierarchy. The person is connected to undesirable characteristics that reduce his or her status in the eyes of others. Research shows that external statuses, such as race and gender, shape status hierarchies within small groups of unacquainted persons, even though the external status has no bearing on proficiency at a task the group is asked to perform. Men and white people are more likely than women and black people to attain positions of power and prestige – they talk more frequently, have their ideas more readily accepted by others, and are more likely to be voted group leader (Berger et al., 1989). This implies that status loss has immediate consequences for a person's power and influence and thus his or her ability to achieve desired goals.

Discrimination

Link and Phelan (2001) conceptualize four broad mechanisms of discrimination as part of the stigma process: individual discrimination, discrimination that operates through the stigmatized individual, interactional discrimination, and structural discrimination.

Individual discrimination What usually comes to mind when thinking about discrimination is the classic model of individual prejudice and discrimination, in which Person A discriminates against Person B based on Person A's prejudicial attitudes or stereotypes connected to a label applied to Person B (Allport, 1954). For example, if, as in Page's experimental study (Page, 1996), a landlord learns about a history of psychiatric hospitalization and consequently denies that an advertised apartment is available, we would say that individual discrimination has occurred. This rather straightforward process doubtless occurs with considerable regularity, although it may often be hidden from the discriminated-against person; one rarely learns why one is turned down for a job, an apartment, or a date. We believe, however, that this relatively straightforward process represents the tip of the discrimination iceberg. Most discrimination, we argue, is extremely subtle in its manifestation if not in its consequences, and occurs without full awareness.

For example, Druss et al. (2000) has shown that people with schizophrenia are less likely to receive optimal treatment for heart disease even after controlling for the nature of the condition and availability of services. This is an example of individual discrimination, as it results from the behavior of individual physicians who make treatment decisions. Yet it is unlikely that the physicians are aware of their discriminatory behavior or the reasons for it. Comparing demographically similar samples of medical and psychiatric inpatients, Bromley and Cunningham (2004) found that, whereas the medical patients received gifts such as flowers, balloons, and chocolate, psychiatric patients generally received more practical gifts of toiletries, nonluxury foodstuffs, and tobacco. Again, this differential gift-giving behavior on the part of friends and family members is surely not deliberate or conscious; rather it reflects and reinforces societal attitudes about what it means to have a medical versus a psychiatric problem. Individual discrimination can have many sources, including community members, employers, mental health caregivers, family members, and friends (Wahl, 1999; Dickerson et al., 2002).

Discrimination that operates through the stigmatized individual Another form of discrimination that is subtle in its manifestation and insidious in its consequences operates within stigmatized individuals themselves (Prince and Prince, 2002; Freidl et al., 2003). As explained above, Link and colleagues (Link, 1982; Link, 1987; Link et al., 1989; Link et al. 1997) propose in their modified labeling theory that all people are exposed to common, ambient stereotypes about mental illness as part of socialization. If a person then develops a mental illness, these beliefs about how others will treat a person with mental illness become personally relevant (Link, 1982; Link et al., 1989). This process has been referred to as "internalized stigma" and is central to understanding the inner psychological harm caused by stigma (Corrigan, 1998; Corrigan and Watson, 2002). Internalized stigma consists of the devaluation, shame, secrecy, and withdrawal triggered by negative stereotypes one believes that others harbor (Corrigan, 1998).

Interactional discrimination A third type of discrimination emerges in the back and forth between individuals in interaction. A classic study that brings this form of discrimination to light was an experimental study conducted by Sibicky and Dovidio (1986). In the study, 68 male and 68 female introductory psychology students were randomly assigned in mixed-sex pairs to one of two conditions. In one condition, a "perceiver" (random assignment here as well) was led to believe that a "target" was recruited from the psychotherapy clinic at the college. In the other condition, the perceiver was led to believe that the individual was a fellow student in introductory psychology. In fact, the target was always recruited from the class, and targets and perceivers both were led to believe that the study was focusing on "the acquaintance process in social interaction." Each member of a pair completed a brief inventory of his or her courses, hobbies, and activities. Then the experimenter exchanged the inventories and provided the perceiver with the labeling information (student or therapy client). Subsequently the two engaged in a tape-recorded conversation that was later reliably evaluated by two raters blind to the experimental conditions. Even before meeting them, perceivers rated the therapy targets less favorably than the student targets. Moreover, the judges' ratings revealed that, in their interactions with therapy targets, perceivers were less open, secure, sensitive, and sincere. Finally, the results showed that the behavior of the labeled targets was adversely affected as well, even though they had no knowledge of the experimental manipulation. Thus, expectations associated with psychological therapy color subsequent interactions, actually calling out behaviors that confirm those expectations. An important lesson for stigma researchers is embedded in these studies of interactional discrimination – substantial differences in influence and social distance can occur even when it is difficult for participants to specify a discriminatory event that produced the unequal outcome.

Structural discrimination   Finally, structural discrimination occurs when social policy, laws, or other institutional practices disadvantage stigmatized groups cumulatively over time. Prominent examples are the policies of many health insurance companies that provide less coverage for psychiatric illnesses than they do for physical ones (Schulze and Angermeyer, 2003) or laws restricting the civil rights of people with mental illnesses (Corrigan et al., 2004). Structural discrimination need not involve direct or intentional discrimination by individuals in the immediate context (Corrigan et al., 2004); it can result from a practice or policy that is the residue of past intentional discrimination. For example, if a history of not-in-my-backyard (NIMBY) reactions have influenced the location of board-and-care homes over time so that they are situated in disorganized sections of the city where rates of crime, violence, pollution, and infectious disease are high, people with serious mental illness are more likely to be exposed to these noxious circumstances as a consequence. Again, although the unequal outcomes resulting from structural discrimination – unequal coverage for mental and physical health problems or undesirable location of board-and-care homes – may be readily apparent, the fact that these outcomes represent discrimination only becomes obvious upon reflection and analysis.

The dependence of stigma on power

A unique feature of Link and Phelan's (2001) conceptualization is the idea that stigma is entirely dependent on social, economic, and political power. Lower-power groups (e.g., psychiatric patients) may label, stereotype, and separate themselves from higher-power groups (e.g., psychiatrists). But in these cases, stigma as Link and Phelan define it does not exist, because the potentially stigmatizing groups do not have the social, cultural, economic, and political power to imbue their cognitions with serious discriminatory consequences.

What are the dimensions of stigma? How does stigma vary depending on the characteristic that is stigmatized and the circumstances in which it occurs?

Another useful conceptual scheme was developed by Jones et al. (1984) to describe key variations among stigmatizing conditions or, in their terminology, "marks." These authors identify six dimensions of stigmatizing marks that they considered to be most important in influencing the role of the mark in interpersonal interactions. *Concealability* refers to how obvious or detectable the characteristic is. Some marks, such as a facial scar, are unavoidably obvious in interpersonal interactions, while others, such as a prior history of mental illness or current diagnosis of cancer, may remain undetected. *Course* refers to how reversible the characteristic is. For example, short stature is not reversible, whereas smoking and substance abuse are. *Disruptiveness* is the extent to which a characteristic hinders, strains, and adds to the difficulty of interpersonal interactions. Concealed marks are not disruptive, whereas visible marks vary in terms of their disruptiveness. For example, stuttering makes appropriate interpersonal interaction pattern unpredictable and interferes with the communication process, whereas knowledge that a person is affected by HIV does not. *Aesthetics* refers to the extent to which a mark elicits an instinctive and affective reaction of disgust. Cleft palate and facial scarring are considered unaesthetic, whereas other stigmatized characteristics, such as being a child abuser, do not call out this dimension. *Origin* refers to how the characteristic came into being. Origin includes subdimensions of congenital versus noncongenital, when in the life course and how rapidly the mark developed, and the stigmatized individual's role in causing the mark. *Peril* refers to the extent to which the condition induces fear or perceived threat in others. The peril may involve threat of physical or verbal attack, physical contamination or contagion, or a "symbolic threat" to a person's beliefs, values, ideology, or worldview (Stangor and Crandall, 2000). Any stigmatized characteristic can be located at a point on each of these dimensions in terms of the objective situation, in terms of the perceptions of the stigmatized individual, and in terms of the perception of others. For example, many mental illnesses actually have a reversible course but are perceived as being incurable.

Why do we stigmatize?

Third, Phelan et al. (2008) provide a conceptual scheme addressing why particular characteristics become the object of stigma, and whether stigma serves a different function for different stigmatized characteristics. They propose three functions of stigma: (1) exploitation/domination (keeping people down); (2) enforcement of social norms (keeping people in); and (3) avoidance of disease (keeping people away).

Exploitation and domination

Some groups must have less power and fewer resources for dominant groups to have more. Some groups provide labor that is exploited by others or perform unpleasant or dangerous tasks that others prefer to avoid. Ideologies develop to legitimate and help perpetuate these inequalities (Marx and Engels, 1976; Jost and Banaji, 1994). Phelan et al. (2008) argue that exploitation and domination, along with their corresponding ideologies, are one basic function of stigma. Race is a clear example. Feagin describes how racism was "integral to the foundation of the United States" (Feagin, 2000: 2). "At the heart of the Constitution was protection of the property and wealth of the affluent bourgeoisie in the new nation" (Feagin, 2000: 10). Slavery was seen as an essential tool for maintaining this wealth, and discrimination was considered necessary. Ideologies that viewed African Americans as inferior, less worthy, and dangerous (i.e., stereotypes) developed to legitimate the discrimination (Morone, 1997). By this reasoning, Phelan et al. (2008) also consider stigmatization of people of low socioeconomic status, and ethnic minority groups to be rooted in exploitation and domination.

Enforcement of social norms

Societies also find it necessary to extract conformity with social norms. Phelan et al. (2008) propose that failure to comply with these norms, usually cast in terms of morality or character (Goffman, 1963; Morone, 1997), is a second ground for stigmatization. Here, the function of stigma may be to make the deviant conform and rejoin the in-group, as in reintegrative shaming (Braithwaite, 1989), or it may be to clarify for other group members the boundaries of acceptable behavior and identity and the consequences for nonconformity (Erikson, 1966). In either case, the goal is to increase conformity with norms. This type of stigma should only apply to behavior or identity perceived as voluntary. For example, although people with mental retardation may behave in deviant ways, Phelan et al. (2008) would not include it here, because the application of stigma cannot be expected to change the behavior. Examples of this form of stigma are numerous: non-normative sexual behavior or identities, such as homosexuality, polygamy, or (in some contexts) extramarital sex; political deviations; various forms of criminal behavior, such as theft, rape, or murder; substance abuse; smoking; perhaps obesity and some mental illnesses such as depression. This function of stigma is aligned with exploitation/domination in that the dominant group is influential in defining what is unacceptable. However, it differs importantly in that the dominant group does not, in any significant way, profit from the labor of the deviants.

Avoidance of disease

Many illnesses and disabilities are stigmatized, including mental illnesses, developmental disabilities, physical illnesses such as cancer, skin disorders, and AIDS, and physical disabilities and imperfections such as missing limbs, paralysis, blindness, and deafness. These for the most part do not seem to be stigmatized in order to exploit or dominate or in order to control behavior and enforce norms. Again, the dominant group does not profit in a significant way from the labor of people with these characteristics – in fact, people carrying this type of disease or disability labels often have trouble finding employment. Nor is society trying to control their behavior or set an example for others by subjecting them to stigmatization. Phelan et al. (2008) found this form of stigma difficult to explain in purely social or psychological terms, and consequently they turned to evolutionary psychology for a possible explanation.

Kurzban and Leary (2001) (also see Neuberg et al., 2000) argue that there are evolutionary pressures to avoid members of one's species who are infected by parasites. Parasites can lead to "deviations from the organism's normal (healthy) phenotype" (Kurzban and Leary, 2001: 197) such as asymmetry, marks, lesions, and discoloration; coughing, sneezing, and excretion of fluids; and behavioral anomalies due to damage to muscle-control systems. They argue that the advantage of avoiding disease "might have led to the evolution of systems that regard deviations from the local species-typical phenotype to be unattractive"; that systems might develop wherein people would "desire to avoid close proximity to potentially parasitized individuals"; and that "because of the possible cost of misses, the system should be biased toward false positives, and this bias might take the form of reacting to relatively scant evidence that someone is infested" (Kurzban and Leary, 2001: 198). Aesthetics, one of Jones et al.'s (1984) six dimensions of stigmatized "marks," are particularly relevant here. An evolutionary explanation for disease avoidance is consistent with humans' aesthetic preference for facial symmetry (Grammar and Thornhill, 1994), which develops early in life and across cultures (Johnson et al., 1991) and with Jones et al.'s observation that physical anomalies seem to "automatically elicit 'primitive' affective responses in the beholder" "not mediated by labels or causal attributions" (Jones et al., 1984: 226). Consistent with Kurzban and Leary's (2001) argument that disgust should be the primary emotion associated with parasite-avoidance stigma is the plethora of phrases to describe affective reactions to physical deviance, including "disgusting," "nauseating," "sickening," "repelling," "revolting," "gross," "makes you shudder," "loathsome," and "turns your stomach" (Jones et al., 1984). The evolutionary explanation applies most clearly to visible illnesses, deformities, and deviations in physical movements.

If "species-atypical phenotype" can be extended to illnesses that are not necessarily visible, such as cancer, and to psychological functioning that appears "diseased," such as psychosis, then the evolutionary model may apply broadly to stigmatized illnesses and disabilities. However, this broad application depends critically on the strength of bias toward false positives, which is unknown. Because evidence to connect many stigmatized illnesses to parasite avoidance is lacking, the evolutionary explanation must be considered provisional. According to this argument, the function of disease-avoidance stigma is rooted in our evolutionary past rather than in current social pressures. People may indeed consciously avoid others because they appear to be infected. However, the strong emotional reactions involved in this type of stigma, as well as its application to individuals who are not actually infected ("false positives"), are attributed to the disproportionate survival and procreation of individuals who exhibited extreme vigilance, resulting in exaggerated reactions in present-day humans. Thus, when we refer to the disease-avoidance function of stigma, we are referring to its past, not current, function.

Thus far, we have presented some major conceptual schemes applying to general stigma processes that are intended to encompass all types of stigmatized characteristics. Next we review empirical evidence relating to the stigmatization of addictions and consider addictions within the framework of each of the conceptual schemes reviewed above.

Stigma and addictions

The literature on stigma associated with addictions focuses largely on alcohol and, to a lesser extent, substance dependence and has most often been studied in comparison with stigma attached to other medical and mental disorders. This literature is much less extensive than that relating to stigma and mental illness. Schomerus et al. (2011) systematically reviewed results from representative population studies that examined stigma associated with alcoholism or alcohol dependence as well as stigma associated with non-substance-related mental disorders. Although alcohol dependence is defined as a psychiatric disorder, the reviewed studies found that alcohol-dependent persons were less likely to be seen as mentally ill, were held much more responsible for their condition, provoked more social rejection and negative emotions, and were at higher risk for structural discrimination (i.e., the public supported cutting funding for treatment) when compared with persons with substance-unrelated mental disorders. Only with regard to perceived dangerousness did schizophrenia approach the level of stigma attached to alcohol dependence. It is noteworthy that the level of stigma attached to addictions was usually found to be more extreme than that attached to schizophrenia, because schizophrenia is a severe and disruptive mental disorder that is considered to represent a classic and extreme example of stigmatization.

Many of the patterns found in Schomerus et al.'s review can be illustrated with Link et al.'s (1999) analysis of results from the General Social Survey, a survey of a nationally representative sample of American adults, which compared responses to individuals described in vignettes as having alcohol dependence, cocaine dependence, schizophrenia, or major depression. Link et al. (1999) found that only 49% of respondents considered alcohol dependence and 43% considered cocaine dependence to be a mental illness, compared with 69% for major depression and 88% for schizophrenia. On the question of personal responsibility, 51% considered alcohol dependence and 66% considered cocaine dependence somewhat or very likely to be caused by the vignette subject's own bad character, compared with 38% for major depression and 33% for schizophrenia. Further evidence on the strong tendency to blame addicted persons for their addictions comes from the United Kingdom and Germany. In two recent studies conducted in the United Kingdom, 60% and 54% of survey participants stated that alcohol-dependent persons are to blame for their problems, and 68% and 60% for drug-addicted persons, compared with 4–13% for depression, panic attacks, schizophrenia, and dementia (Crisp et al., 2000, 2005). In a German survey, 85% perceived alcohol-dependent persons to be responsible for their condition, versus 45% for myocardial infarction, 32% for diabetes, and 8–18% for Alzheimer's disease, schizophrenia, and depression (Schomerus et al., 2006).

Regarding perceived danger, Link et al. (1999) found that the cocaine-dependent vignette subject was seen as the most dangerous, with 87% of respondents indicating that the person was very or somewhat likely to do something violent toward other people, followed by 71% for alcohol dependence, 61% for schizophrenia, and 33% for major depression. Finally, to address the dimension of social rejection, Link et al. (1999) constructed a composite social distance score comprising willingness to move next door to the vignette subject, to spend an evening socializing, to make friends, to work closely with the person, and to have the person marry into the participant's family. Seventy percent of participants were generally unwilling to have contact with a person with alcohol dependence (that is, they scored above the midpoint – in the definitely to probably unwilling range – on the composite social distance scale) and 90% were unwilling to have contact with a person with cocaine dependence, compared with 63% unwilling for schizophrenia and 47% unwilling for major depression. Analyzing a more recent version of the same survey that excluded the cocaine dependence vignette, Pescosolido et al. (2010) found patterns of results similar to those of Link et al. (1999) when comparing public responses to schizophrenia, major depression, and alcohol dependence, although there were general changes between the first (1996) and second (2006) administrations of the survey. The tendency to identify each characteristic as a mental illness increased, as did the tendency to attribute the problem to genetics. Interestingly, only for alcohol dependence did the tendency to attribute the problem to the vignette person's bad character increase significantly over the 10-year period. More severe stigma for alcohol and substance abuse compared with non-substance-related mental disorders has also been found when the survey respondents are adolescents (Corrigan et al., 2005) and when the target of stigmatization is a family member of the substance-dependent person (Corrigan et al., 2006).

Armed with these empirical results, let us return to the conceptualizations of stigma with which we began this chapter and consider whether and how addictions fit within those definitions and characterizations of stigma.

Are addictions stigmatized?

Addictions fit Goffman's definition of a stigmatized characteristic, in that they are deeply discrediting and cause social rejection. Indeed, as documented above, social distance from persons with alcohol and substance abuse, as reported in social surveys, is more extreme than toward persons with schizophrenia (Schomerus et al., 2011).

Addictions entail each of Link and Phelan's interrelated components of stigma: social salience, labels, linking of labels with perceived negative characteristics, "us" and "them" distinctions, negative emotions, status loss, and discrimination.

Social salience

Unlike many other human differences, addictions seem to be bestowed with considerable social significance. That is, of all the facts one might wish to know about an individual, the presence of an addiction would probably be considered one of the most important.

Labels

Pejorative labels for people with addictions abound, for example: "addict," "wino," "boozer," "lush," "souse," and "junkie."

Linking of labels with perceived negative characteristics

These labels link the person in others' minds to negative personal characteristics. For example, as shown above, there is empirical support for the link between the addiction label and perceptions of danger and unpredictability (Schomerus et al., 2011). Dean and Rud (1984) found that among their undergraduate sample, "the overwhelming image [of a drug addict] was of a disoriented, unhealthy, thin, low-class, male 'hippie' with behavioral and skin problems who suffered from a disease" (Dean and Rud, 1984: 859).

"Us" and "them" distinctions

We know of no direct measures of "us" and "them" distinctions at this time, but it seems likely that many people would consider people with alcohol or substance addictions to belong to a somewhat separate category of persons, as would be the case for people with mental illness, or racial or sexual minority groups.

Negative emotions

Schomerus et al.'s (2011) review notes that addicted persons generally elicit more negative emotions, such as irritation, anger, repulsion, fear, and indifference, than do persons with mental disorders such as schizophrenia and depression (Angermeyer et al., 1992; Peluso and Blay, 2008a, 2008b).

Status loss

Status loss can be illustrated by contrasting the desirability of being seen entering an Alcoholics Anonymous meeting and entering an exclusive club or restaurant.

Discrimination

We have seen that social rejection, an important form of individual discrimination, can be severe for people with addictions (Schomerus et al., 2011). Discrimination might also operate through the stigmatized person, as when addicted persons limit their own social and economic opportunities by withdrawing from interaction with other people who are not addicted or through interactional discrimination, as when members of a group expect a person labeled with alcohol dependence to make less valuable contributions to the group. There is also evidence of public support for structural discrimination in the form of reducing funding for alcohol treatment (Beck et al., 2003; Matschinger and Angermeyer, 2004; Schomerus et al., 2006). Finally, Link and Phelan argue that stigma only exists when there is a power differential between stigmatizers and stigmatized that allows the stigmatizing group to effectively limit the life chances of the stigmatized group. In the case of addictions, power differentials enter in two ways. First, persons of lower social status are more likely to become addicted; second, addicted persons lose power as a result of their addictions. For both reasons, any clash between the wishes of nonaddicted and addicted groups is very likely to favor the former group.

Where do addictions fall along the dimensions of stigma?

Let us return to Jones et al.'s (1984) analysis of the dimensions of stigma and consider addictions within that framework. Regarding *course*, perceived and actual course diverge, and this divergence betrays the role of stigma. Despite the fact that addictions are most common in young adults and usually do not continue through the life course (Grant et al., 2004), we believe that addictions share with mental illness the characteristic of being "sticky" stigmas. That is, the expectation is that the person will always be an addict and that, even if they have not engaged in addictive behavior for many years, they may revert to addictive behavior at any time. In other words, addiction is seen as an essential, unchanging, characteristic of the person (Rothbart and Taylor, 1992). This idea in fact is embodied in the principles of Alcoholics Anonymous and related organizations. One study, however, found that presenting a pamphlet that described a person in remission reduced stigmatizing attitudes when the person was in remission from opiate or alcohol dependence to a greater degree than when the person was in remission from schizophrenia, suggesting that addictions may be seen as more reversible than schizophrenia (Luty et al., 2008).

The addicted person is also viewed as highly *perilous*. As noted above, in the General Social Survey, a vignette character with alcohol or cocaine dependence was seen as more likely to harm others than a vignette character with schizophrenia. We suspect that another form of peril attributed to addicted persons involves the joint perceptions that addictive behavior is initially voluntary ("onset controllable") and subsequently beyond one's control ("offset uncontrollable") (Corrigan, 2000). Thus an addicted person's greatest danger in others' eyes may be that associating with an addicted person will lure one down a negative pathway of addiction from which one can never return. The dimensions of *concealability* and *disruptiveness* are closely related. The concealability of addiction might be low and disruptiveness high when a person is actively using large amounts of alcohol or substances, but concealability should be relatively high and disruptiveness low in other circumstances. The dimension of *aesthetics* is also relevant to addictions. We believe persons with alcohol or drug dependence are stereotyped as dirty, poorly groomed and dressed, unattractive, and smelling of urine. Finally, regarding *origins*, as noted above, addictions are strongly perceived to be caused by the person's own character.

What functions are served by stigmatizing addictions?

Turning finally to Phelan et al.'s (2008) schema for the functions of stigma, it appears that norms enforcement would be the primary function of stigmatizing persons with addictions. Addiction is largely seen as being voluntary (Schomerus et al., 2011). The very term "addiction" suggests that an addicted person will face great difficulty, at the least, in overcoming the addictive behavior. Nevertheless, we believe the prevailing idea among the public is that people should be able to shake their addiction, or at the very least, are expected to try their utmost to shake it. Why are addictions something that society is motivated to denormalize and control? Several reasons seem likely. First, addiction to alcohol or drugs is costly and harmful to society in terms of impairing the addicted person's ability to fulfill social roles such as working, caring for children and maintaining other social relationships, and by causing injury through acts of violence or careless behavior such as impaired driving (Schomerus et al., 2011). As mentioned above, a grave perceived danger posed by addicted persons is their bad influence on others, enticing innocents to a life of depravity. As Erikson (1966) argues, by punishing or excluding deviants to demonstrate where the boundaries of acceptable behavior lie, social groups can help ensure that heretofore conforming people will not stray across the boundaries. Although persons with addictions have less power than others and will consequently have poorer life outcomes, it seems unlikely that exploitation or domination is the primary reason for stigmatizing persons with addiction. According to

Phelan et al. (2008), this type of stigmatization is directed toward groups, such as slaves and their progeny, who have been targeted as sources from whom labor or other benefits can be extracted without giving compensation that would be considered fair or usual for nonstigmatized groups. This does not appear to be the case with addicted persons as a group, and in fact, stereotypes of addicted persons as being inept and irresponsible would seem to make them poor candidates for exploitation. Likewise, disease avoidance would not seem to be a major function for stigmatizing addicted persons. Although in extreme cases, long-term alcohol addiction may cause one's face to become asymmetrical or marked in a way that might be consistent with parasite infection, this is relatively rare and cannot, we believe, be considered a major driver of addiction stigma.

Geneticization and stigma

This book is concerned with ethical issues raised by research on the genetic bases of addictions, and stigma is one such ethical concern. We focus on this issue in the remainder of this chapter. First, we address public beliefs regarding genetic causes of alcohol and substance dependence and trends in those beliefs. Next we discuss theoretical arguments about how genetic causal attributions might affect stigma. Because we are aware of no research directly addressing the relationship between genetic causal attributions and stigma for addictions, we will review empirical results concerning genetic attributions and stigma for other stigmatized characteristics and attempt to draw implications of this research for stigma associated with addictions.

Public beliefs in genetic causes of alcohol and substance dependence

It certainly seems that, in the wake of the Human Genome Project and subsequent research, genetic explanations for illness, personality, behavior, and every imaginable human characteristic are on the rise. The General Social Surveys conducted in 1996 and 2006 confirm this impression for alcohol dependence, schizophrenia, and major depression. Genetic attributions increased for all three disorders (from 61 to 71% for schizophrenia, 51 to 64% for major depression and 58 to 68% for alcohol dependence) (Pescosolido et al., 2010). Interestingly, only 27% endorsed genes as a cause of cocaine dependence in 1996 (Link et al., 1999), and no comparable data are available for 2006. In light of this increasing reliance on genetic explanations, it becomes important to ask what the consequences of genetic causal attributions are for stigma. Two theoretical perspectives are relevant, one of which suggests that genetic attributions should reduce stigma, and one of which suggests that genetic attributions should increase stigma.

Theories relating to genetic causal attributions and stigma

Attribution theory (Weiner, 1986, 1995) states that the attributions people make about the cause of a personal outcome influence emotions, expectancies, and behavior toward the individual affected by the outcome. One important application of the theory has been to stigmatized behaviors (Weiner et al., 1988; Corrigan, 2000). According to the theory, attribution of low causal responsibility for a stigmatized characteristic (e.g., brain dysfunction due to accidental injury rather than illicit drug abuse) is associated with less blame and more positive emotions – that is, pity rather than anger – which in turn lead to an inclination to help the person and a disinclination to punish (Reisenzein, 1986; Weiner et al., 1988; Rush, 1998; Corrigan et al., 2000).

Because one cannot be considered to have caused one's own genetic makeup, attribution theory suggests that genetic attributions should reduce the perceived causal responsibility and, consequently, the negative emotions and behaviors associated with a stigmatized characteristic. The destigmatizing potential of geneticization has been prominent in the arguments of activist groups such as the National Alliance for the Mentally Ill, as well as some gay rights activists (Whisman, 1996; Conrad, 1997; Johnson, 1989) and is well illustrated by the following quote: "A 'mental illness' is not caused by bad parenting and is not a character weakness… These illnesses are due to biochemical disturbances in the brain… The shame and fear once associated with cancer has largely been dispelled by accurate information and understanding. The same will happen for brain diseases – mental illnesses – once the facts are known" (National Alliance for the Mentally Ill of Oregon, 1997).

Less sanguine predictions concerning the effect of genetic causal attributions on stigma are generated by the concept of essentialism (Rothbart and Taylor, 1992) and the idea ("genetic essentialism") (Lippman, 1992; Nelkin and Lindee, 1995) that genetic understandings of human behavior and other characteristics increase the belief that those characteristics are an essential part of the person. In a genetic essentialist view, genes form the basis of our human and individual identities (i.e., "we are our genes") and are strongly deterministic of behavior, so that if one has genes associated with some behavior, that behavior will definitely occur and "is fixed and unchangeable" (Alper and Beckwith, 1993: 511). According to James Watson, "our fate is in our genes" (quoted in Jaroff, 1989). A genetic essentialist viewpoint suggests that genetic characteristics are irrevocably, or at least very firmly, attached to an individual and, by extension, to those with whom the person shares genes. Considerations of positively valued characteristics such as beauty or intelligence make it clear that genetic essentialism is not inherently stigmatizing. However, when applied to negatively valued qualities, genetic essentialism should exacerbate stigma via its influence on several perceptions: (1) that the person is fundamentally different from others; (2) that the problem is persistent and serious; and (3) that the problem is likely to occur in other family members. These perceptions in turn should increase negative behavioral orientations such as the endorsement of reproductive restrictions and social distance, particularly "associative" (Mehta and Farina, 1988) or "courtesy" stigma (Goffman, 1963), in which social distance is desired from the biological relatives of the stigmatized individual.

In sum, attribution theory predicts that geneticization will reduce stigma, whereas the idea of genetic essentialism predicts that stigma will be exacerbated. However, different outcomes are implied by the two theories. Attribution theory predicts stigma reduction via reduced blame, anger, and punishment and increased sympathy and helping. Genetic essentialism predicts stigma magnification via increased perceptions of differentness, and – indirectly through increased perceptions of seriousness, persistence, and risk to family members – via increased social distance and reproductive restriction. Thus, it is possible that both theories are correct and operate simultaneously.

Empirical evidence on genetic attributions and stigma

What is the evidence on the association between genetic attributions and stigma? In the next section, we review such evidence in relation to a variety of mental and physical illnesses.

First, we refer again to the General Social Surveys conducted in 1996 and 2006. We have already seen that genetic attributions increased over this period for alcohol dependence, as well as for schizophrenia and major depression. If such attributions led to destigmatization, we would expect that indicators of stigma would have declined over that same time period. However, there was no evidence whatsoever that stereotypes of violence and incompetence, or the willingness to interact with people with mental illnesses, changed for the better over the period between the studies (Pescosolido et al., 2010). This evidence challenges the idea that stigma will dissipate when the public is moved toward more medical and genetic views of mental illnesses, including addictions. This evidence is important because it assesses trends in beliefs over time at a population level. However, it does not allow an examination of whether genetic causal beliefs are related to stigmatizing attitudes for individuals. To provide this type of data, we located 17 studies that examined the association between genetic attributions and stigma-related outcomes for a variety of stigmatized characteristics (Eker, 1985; Piskur and Degelman, 1992; Menec and Perry, 1998; Martin et al., 2000; Phelan et al., 2002; Angermeyer et al., 2003; Teachman et al., 2003; Dietrich et al., 2004; Magliano et al., 2004; Phelan, 2005; Phelan et al., 2006; Breheny, 2007; Feldman and Crandall, 2007; Bennett et al., 2008; Jorm and Griffiths, 2008; Schnittker, 2008; Boyle et al., 2009). These focused primarily on mental illnesses ($N = 12$) and usually specifically on schizophrenia ($N = 11$) and/or major depression ($N = 9$). The most commonly studied stigma-related outcome was social distance ($N = 11$). Other outcomes included blame, perceived dangerousness, unpredictability and incompetence, emotions of anger and sympathy, and intentions to help, punish, or restrict reproduction. Nine of the studies employed experimental designs, randomly assigning research participants to be exposed to different causal statements. The eight nonexperimental studies assessed participants' causal beliefs and stigmatizing attitudes and measured the relationship between the two. Because our focus in this chapter is on genetic attributions, we included only studies that referred specifically to genetic causes of the characteristic in question. Accordingly, we excluded studies that referred to biological causal attributions more generally and studies that combined genetic and other biological causes (e.g., heredity and brain chemistry) in such a way that the effects of genetic explanations could not be assessed independently. In summarizing the results of these studies, we count each major outcome variable (e.g., social distance, fear), each stigmatized characteristic that was analyzed separately (e.g., schizophrenia, major depression), and each major subsample (e.g., different countries) as a separate result. Consequently, the number of results reported is greater than the number of studies. The results of these studies more often indicate a stigmatizing effect of genetic attributions than a destigmatizing effect, but the findings are far from consistent. Nineteen significant positive associations ($P < 0.05$) between genetic explanations and stigma, eight significant negative associations ($P < 0.05$), and twenty-eight nonsignificant associations were reported. The stigmatizing effects of genetic attributions varied by outcome, and we discuss the findings separately by outcome. First we discuss important general dimensions of stigma and then focus on outcomes pertinent to the two theoretical orientations relevant to geneticization and stigma.

Social distance

As noted, social distance is a central measure of stigmatization and was the most common outcome examined in the studies reviewed here. Social distance was generally a composite measure of willingness to have different forms of contact with the person or group in question (e.g., be friends, work with). Of 23 associations between genetic attribution and social distance evaluated, 7 were significantly positive, that is, genetic attribution was related to greater social distance; 4 were significantly negative; and 12 did not attain statistical significance.

Fear, danger, unpredictability

Emotions of fear and perceptions of danger and unpredictability are key aspects of stigma associated with mental illness. Of nine associations between these outcomes and genetic attribution that were evaluated, genetic attributions were significantly associated with greater stigma in five cases. The associations were nonsignificant in four cases, and there were no instances in which genetic attributions were associated with less fear or perception of danger or unpredictability.

General prejudice or bias

Three studies used general measures of prejudice – implicit bias against overweight people, prejudice against homosexuals and a variety of negative stereotypes about people who stutter. In two of these cases, genetic attribution was associated with less prejudice, and in one case, there was no significant association. No positive associations between genetic attributions and general prejudice were reported.

Outcomes related to attribution theory

Attribution theory makes predictions that are clearly relevant to genetic attributions, specifically that genetic explanations of a stigmatized characteristic should reduce blame, anger, and punishment, and increase pity and helping toward the stigmatized person or group. Thirteen associations were examined between these outcomes and genetic attribution. In four cases, results were significant and consistent with attribution theory. In nine cases, the associations were nonsignificant. There were no significant findings in the direction inconsistent with attribution theory.

Outcomes related to genetic essentialism

Here we discuss two groups of findings. One implication of genetic essentialism is that genetic attributions should increase the perceived seriousness and persistence of the stigmatized characteristic and increase perceived differentness of the stigmatized person. Of the six associations examined, genetic attribution was associated with greater perceived seriousness and persistence in four instances. Genetic attribution was not significantly related to persistence in another instance and was not associated with perceived differentness in the one case where differentness was examined. There were no findings that went significantly counter to essentialist predictions.

The second category of outcomes relevant to genetic essentialism is associative stigma affecting relatives of a stigmatized individual. In the studies reviewed, associative stigma was measured in terms of perceived risk that the relative would develop a mental illness and social distance from the relative. Four of four associations examined found that genetic attribution was associated with increased associative stigma.

In sum, the preponderance of results regarding general stigma outcomes suggested stigmatizing rather than destigmatizing effects of genetic attributions, but this pattern was by no means strong or dramatic. There were a considerable number of nonsignificant associations as well as a number of instances in which genetic attribution was associated with less stigma. Focusing on outcomes related to the two theoretical perspectives with specific relevance to genetic explanations for stigmatized characteristics, the number of relevant findings is small, but somewhat more consistent. Although we still find nonsignificant associations, all statistically significant findings are in the predicted direction. Clearly, the number of findings described here is too small to draw firm conclusions; nevertheless they are suggestive that genetic attributions may have opposite effects on stigma through the dual pathways of reducing blame and increasing genetic essentialism.

Implications for addictions

From our review of studies, we have concluded that the data are consistent with the idea that genetic attributions have dual positive and negative effects on stigma – increasing genetic essentialism (and consequently perceptions that the problem is serious and intractable, and desire for social distance from biological relatives) while simultaneously reducing blame (and consequently anger and the inclination to punish). The data are also consistent with the idea that genetic attributions may have somewhat stigmatizing effects in the key areas of social distance and perceived danger. We would expect that explaining addictions in genetic terms would have similar effects *if genetic causal explanations are communicated to and accepted by* the public. Here we point to one reason to expect that this condition may be difficult to achieve in the case of addictions. We have seen that people are strongly inclined to hold individuals accountable for their addictions (Schomerus et al., 2011). Thus, if the public is exposed to evidence or arguments that addictions have a genetic basis, two processes may occur that leave that strong belief in personal responsibility undisturbed. First, people do not always recall or believe what they are told. For example, Phelan (2005) found that 30% of participants in her vignette experiment either did not correctly recall or did not accept the causal explanation offered in the vignette. The same resistance is likely to exist when people are confronted with causal messages outside research contexts – for example, in the mass media or in medical settings. If prior causal beliefs are strongly held, as may be the case for addictions, they may be particularly difficult to supplant.

Second, causal understandings are complex and multifaceted. The General Social Survey results illustrate that research participants simultaneously endorse multiple causes of addictions. In 1996, 51% of participants endorsed (as very likely or somewhat likely causes) the person's own bad character as a cause of alcohol dependence, 63% endorsed a chemical imbalance in the brain, 66% endorsed the way the person was raised, 92% endorsed stressful circumstances, 60% endorsed genetic factors, and 9% endorsed God's will. For cocaine dependence, 66% of participants endorsed the person's own bad character, 48% endorsed a chemical imbalance in the brain, 42% endorsed the way the person was raised, 72% endorsed stressful circumstances, 27% endorsed genetic factors, and 6% endorsed God's will. Thus it is possible that an increased belief in genetic causes does not negate a belief in other causes, such as bad character. Consistent with this idea, the endorsement of genetics and of bad character as a cause of alcohol dependence both increased significantly between 1996 and 2006 (Pescosolido et al., 2010).

In this latter scenario, the possibility arises that an increasing prominence of messages attributing addictions to genetic factors may increase associative social distance via a "genetic essentialism" pathway, while leaving in place the negative outcomes of blame, anger, and punishment associated with attributions to personal responsibility via an "attribution theory" pathway.

Finally, we note the results of the only study reviewed above that specifically analyzed stigma associated with addictions. Schnittker (2008) found that genetic explanations were not significantly related to social distance or perceived dangerousness of an alcohol-dependent vignette subject, although genetic explanations were associated with greater perceived danger of a vignette subject with schizophrenia and with less social distance from a subject with major depression. This is only one study, but the findings raise the possibility that genetic attribution may be less important for stigma toward addictions than toward non-substance-related mental illnesses.

Conclusion

We conclude that addictions clearly fit within every major conceptualization of stigma, and research indicates that alcohol and substance dependence, specifically, are very highly stigmatized, even when compared with schizophrenia, another strongly stigmatized characteristic. Our conclusions are much less firm regarding the impact of genetic explanations on the stigma associated with addictions. Our review was based on a relatively small number of studies, and the results were somewhat inconsistent. Nevertheless, the preponderance of findings suggested that geneticization is more likely to increase than to decrease stigmatization when looking at major stigma outcomes of social distance and perceptions of danger. Somewhat more consistent results were found when we restricted focus to studies using outcomes relevant to attribution theory or genetic essentialism – the two theories that offer predictions relating to the association between genetic attributions and stigma. Here results suggested the possibility that genetic attributions simultaneously have positive effects, by reducing blame and anger and increasing pity, and negative effects, by increasing associative social distance affecting biological relatives. However, the number of studies is fairly small, and this notion is provisional.

We close with a strong call for research on the impact of genetic causal attributions on stigma associated with addictions. The confluence of several facts makes the need for such research particularly critical. First, the existing level of stigma directed at addicted persons is high – more extreme than for the most severe mental disorders. Therefore it is important to understand how this stigma might be reduced and what might exacerbate it. Second, the increasing focus on genetic explanations for many human characteristics including addictions makes it inevitable that the public will be increasingly exposed to the idea that addictions have a genetic basis. Third, the extreme degree to which addicted persons are held responsible for their addiction makes it difficult to predict the consequences of injecting into the public discourse the idea that addictions have a genetic basis. As suggested by the General Social Surveys results cited above, rather than replacing personal blame, increasing genetic explanations for addictions may be layered on top of personal blame, subjecting addicted persons and their families to the negative consequences associated with both personal and genetic explanations.

For researchers, practitioners, and advocates in the area of addictions, we suggest attentiveness to the issue of how genetic explanations may affect the stigma associated with addictions. Of course, neither research agendas nor public communications about research findings should be mainly driven by their impact on public perceptions. Our primary obligation is to report what our data suggest is the true state of affairs with regard to the causes of illnesses. But the causes of mental illnesses, addictions, and other stigmatized characteristics are complex and multifactorial, and so we are often in the position of choosing which causes to emphasize in communicating with affected individuals, families, and the public. In the area of mental illnesses, the idea has been prominent that biological and genetic explanations are destigmatizing. The research reviewed here makes it fairly clear that this is not true. Therefore, we caution against embarking on genetically based anti-stigma campaigns for mental illness. For the area of addictions, until research exists to clarify the effect of genetic explanations on stigma, we urge the same caution.

References

Allport, G. W. (1954). *The Nature of Prejudice*. Garden City, NJ: Doubleday.

Alper, J. S. and Beckwith, J. (1993). Genetic fatalism and social policy: The implications of behavior genetics research. *Yale Journal of Biology and Medicine*, 66, 511–524.

Angermeyer, M. C., Matschinger, H., and Siara, C. E. (1992). *Wissensbestande, Uberzeugugssysteme und Einstellungsmuster der Bevolkerung der Bunderpublik Deutschland bezuglich psychischer Erkrankyngen. Abschlussbericht*. Mannheim: Zentralinstitut fur Seelische Gesundheit.

Angermeyer, M. C., Matschinger, H., and Corrigan, P. W. (2003). Familiarity with mental illness and social distance from people with schizophrenia and major depression: Testing a model using data from a representative population survey. *Schizophrenia Research*, 69, 175–182.

Beck, M., Dietrich, S., Matschinger, H., et al. (2003). Alcoholism: Low standing with the public? Attitudes towards spending financial resources on medical care and research on alcoholism. *Alcohol and Alcoholism*, 38, 602–605.

Bennett, L., Thirlaway, K., and Murray, A. J. (2008). The stigmatising implications of presenting schizophrenia as a genetic disease. *Journal of Genetic Counseling*, 17, 550–559.

Berger, J., Fisek, M. H., and Norman, R. Z. (1989). The evolution of status expectations: A theoretical extension. In Joseph Berger, Morris Zelditch, Jr., and Bo Anderson (eds.), *Sociological Theories in Progress: New Formulations*. Newbury Park, CA: Sage, pp. 100–130.

Boyle, M. P., Blood, G. W., and Blood, I. M. (2009). Effects of perceived causality on perceptions of persons who stutter. *Journal of Fluence Disorders*, 34, 201–218.

Braithwaite, J. (1989). *Crime, Shame and Reintegration*. Cambridge, UK: Cambridge University Press.

Breheny, M. (2007). Genetic attribution for schizophrenia, depression, and skin cancer: Impact on social distance. *New Zealand Journal of Psychology*, 36, 154–160.

Bromley, J. S. and Cunningham, S. J. (2004). "You don't bring me flowers anymore": An investigation into experiences of stigma by psychiatric in-patients. *Psychiatric Bulletin*, 28, 371–374.

Conrad, P. (1997). Public eyes and private genes: Historical frames, news constructions, and social problems. *Social Problems*, 44, 139–154.

Corrigan, P. W. (1998). The impact of stigma on severe mental illness. *Cognitive and Behavioral Practice*, 5, 201–222.

Corrigan, P. W. (2000). Mental health stigma as social attribution: Implications for research methods and attitude change. *Clinical Psychology: Science and Practice*, 7, 48–67.

Corrigan, P. W. and Watson, A. C. (2002). The paradox of self-stigma and mental illness. *Clinical Psychology: Science and Practice*, 9, 35–53.

Corrigan, P. W., River, L. P., Lundin, R. K., et al. (2000). Stigmatizing attributions about mental illness. *Journal of Community Psychology*, 28, 91–102.

Corrigan, P. W, Markowitz, F. E., and Watson, A. C. (2004). Structural levels of mental illness stigma and discrimination. *Schizophrenia Bulletin*, 30, 481–491.

Corrigan, P. W., Lurie, B. D., Goldman, H. H., et al. (2005). How adolescents perceive the stigma of mental illness and alcohol abuse. *Psychiatric Services*, 56, 544–550.

Corrigan, P. W., Watson, A. C., and Miller, F. E. (2006). Blame, shame, and contamination: The impact of mental illness and drug dependence stigma on family members. *Journal of Family Psychology*, 20, 239–246.

Crisp, A. H., Gelder, M. G., Rix, S., et al. (2000). Stigmatisation of people with mental illness. *British Journal of Psychiatry*, 177, 4–7.

Crisp, A. H., Gelder, M. G., Goddard, E., et al. (2005). Stigmatization of people with mental illness: A follow-up study within the Changing Minds campaign of the Royal College of Psychiatrists. *World Psychiatry*, 4, 106–113.

Dean, J. C. and Rud, F. (1984). The drug addict and the stigma of addiction. *International Journal of the Addictions*, 19, 859–869.

Dickerson, F. B., Sommerville, J., Origoni, A. E., Ringel, N. B., and Parente, F. (2002). Experiences of stigma among outpatients with schizophrenia. *Schizophrenia Bulletin*, 28, 143–155.

Dietrich, S., Beck, M. Bujantugs, B., et al. (2004). The relationship between public causal beliefs and social distance toward mentally ill people. *Australia and New Zealand Journal of Psychiatry*, 38, 348–354.

Druss, B. G., Bradford, D. W., Rosenheck, R. A., Radford, M. J., and Krumholz, H. M. (2000). Mental disorders and the use of cardiovascular procedures after myocardial infarction. *Journal of the American Medical Association*, 283, 506–511.

Eker, D. (1985). Effect of type of cause on attitudes toward mental illness and relationships between the attitudes. *International Journal of Psychiatry*, 31, 243–251.

Erikson, K. T. (1966). *Wayward Puritans: A Study in the Sociology of Deviance*. New York: John Wiley & Sons.

Feagin, J. R. (2000). *Racist America: Roots, Current Realities, and Future Reparations*. New York: Routledge.

Feldman, D. B. and Crandall, C. S. (2007). Dimensions of mental illness stigma: What about mental illness causes social rejection? *Journal of Social and Clinical Psychology*, 26, 137–154.

Freidl, M., Lang, T., and Scherer, M. (2003). How psychiatric patients perceive the public's stereotype of mental illness. *Social Psychiatry and Psychiatric Epidemiology*, 38, 269–275.

Goffman, E. (1963). *Stigma: Notes on the Management of Spoiled Identity*. New York: Simon & Schuster.

Grammar, K. and Thornhill, R. (1994). Human (*Homo sapiens*) facial attractiveness and sexual selection: The role of symmetry and averageness. *Journal of Comparative Psychology*, 108, 223–242.

Grant, B. F., Dawson, D. A., Stinson, F. S., et al. (2004). The 12-month prevalence and trends in DSM-IV alcohol abuse and dependence: United States, 1991–1992 and 2001–2002. *Drug and Alcohol Dependence*, 74, 223–234.

Jaroff, L. (1989). The Gene Hunt. *Time*, March 20, 62–71.

Johnson, D. L. (1989). Schizophrenia as a brain disease: Implications for psychologists and families. *American Psychologist*, 44, 553–555.

Johnson, M. H., Dziurawiec, S., Ellis, H., and Morton, J. (1991). Newborns' preferential tracking of face-like stimuli and its subsequent decline. *Cognition*, 40, 1–19.

Jones, E., Farina, A., Hastorf, A., Markus, H, Miller, D. T., and Scott, R. (1984). *Social Stigma: The Psychology of Marked Relationships*. New York: Freeman.

Jorm, A. F. and Griffiths, K. M. (2008). The public's stigmatizing attitudes towards people with mental disorders: How important are biomedical conceptions? *Acta Psychiatrica Scandinavica*, 118, 315–321.

Jost, J. T. and Banaji, M. R. (1994). The role of stereotyping in system justification and the production of false consciousness. *British Journal of Social Psychology*, 33, 1–27.

Kurzban, R. and Leary, M. R. (2001). Evolutionary origins of stigmatization: the functions of social exclusion. *Psychological Bulletin*, 127, 87–208.

Link, B. G. (1982). Mental patient status, work, and income: An examination of the effects of a psychiatric label. *American Sociological Review*, 47, 202–215.

Link, B. G. (1987). Understanding labeling effects in the area of mental disorders: An assessment of the effects of expectations of rejection. *American Sociological Review*, 52, 96–112.

Link, B. G. and Phelan, J. C. (2001). Conceptualizing stigma. *Annual Review of Sociology*, 27, 363–385.

Link, B. G., Cullen, F. T., Struening, E., Shrout, P., and Dohrenwend, B. P. (1989). A modified labeling theory approach in the area of the mental disorders: An empirical assessment. *American Sociological Review*, 54, 400–423.

Link, B. G., Struening, E., Rahav, M., Phelan, J. C., and Nuttbrock, L. (1997). On stigma and its consequences: Evidence from a longitudinal study of men with dual diagnoses of mental illness and substance abuse. *Journal of Health and Social Behavior*, 38, 177–190.

Link, B. G., Phelan, J. C., Breshanan, M., Stueve, A., and Pescosolido, B. A. (1999). Public conceptions of mental illness: Labels, causes, dangerousness and social distance. *American Journal of Public Health*, 89, 1328–1333.

Link, B. G., Yang, L. H., Phelan, J. C., and Collins, P. Y. (2004). Measuring mental illness stigma. *Schizophrenia Bulletin*, 30, 511–542.

Lippman, A. (1992). Led (astray) by genetic maps: the cartography of the human genome and health care. *Social Science and Medicine*, 35, 1469–1476.

Luty, J., Rao, H., Arokiadass, S. M. R., Maducolileasow, J., and Sarkhel, A. (2008). The repentant sinner: Methods to reduce stigmatised attitudes toward mental illness. *Psychiatric Bulletin*, 32, 327–332.

Magliano, L., Fiorillo, A., De Rosa, C., Malangone, C., and Maj, M. (2004). Beliefs about schizophrenia in Italy: A comparative nationwide survey of the general public, mental health professionals, and patients' relatives. *Canadian Journal of Psychiatry*, 49, 322–330.

Martin, J. K., Pescosolido, B. A., and Tuch, S. A. (2000). Of fear and loathing: The role of "disturbing behavior," labels, and causal attributions in shaping public attitudes toward persons with mental illness. *Journal of Health and Social Behavior*, 41, 208–223.

Marx, K. and Engels, F. (1976). *The German Ideology*, third revised edition. Moscow: Progress Publishers.

Matschinger, H. and Angermeyer, M. (2004). The public's preferences concerning the allocation of financial resources to health care: Results from a representative population survey in Germany. *European Psychiatry*, 19, 478–482.

Mehta, S. I. and Farina, A. (1988). Associative stigma: Perceptions of the difficulties of college-aged children of stigmatized fathers. *Journal of Social and Clinical Psychology*, 7, 192–202.

Menec, V. H. and Perry, R. P. (1998). Reactions to stigmas among Canadian students: Testing attribution-affect-help judgment model. *Journal of Social Psychology*, 138, 443–453.

Morone, J. A. (1997). Enemies of the people: The moral dimension to public health. *Journal of Health Politics, Policy and Law*, 22, 993–1020.

National Alliance for the Mentally Ill of Oregon (1997). Available online at: www.nami. org/MSTemplate.cfm?site=NAMI_Oregon [accessed March 13, 2012].

Nelkin, D. and Lindee, M. S. (1995). *The DNA Mystique: The Gene as a Cultural Icon*. New York: Freeman.

Neuberg, S. L., Smith, D. M., and Asher, T. (2000). Why people stigmatize: toward a biocultural framework. In T. F. Heatherton, R. E. Kleck, M. R. Hebl, and J. G. Hull (eds.), *The Social Psychology of Stigma*. New York: Guilford Press, pp. 31–61.

Page, S. (1996). Effects of the mental illness label in 1993: Acceptance and rejection in the community. *Journal of Health and Social Policy*, 7, 61–68.

Peluso, E. T. P. and Blay, S. L. (2008a). Public perception of alcohol dependence. *Revista Brasileira de Psiquiatria*, 30, 19–24.

Peluso, E. T. P. and Blay, S. L. (2008b). Public perception of depression in the city of Sao Paulo. *Revista de Saúde Pública*, 42, 41–48.

Pescosolido, B. A., Martin, J. K., Long, J. S., et al. (2010). "A disease like any other"? A decade of change in public reactions to schizophrenia, depression, and alcohol dependence. *American Journal of Psychiatry*, 167, 1321–1330.

Phelan, J. C. (2005). Geneticization of deviant behavior and consequences for stigma: The case of mental illness. *Journal of Health and Social Behavior*, 46, 307–322.

Phelan, J. C., Cruz Rojas, R., and Reiff, M. (2002). Genes and stigma: the connection between perceived genetic etiology and attitudes and beliefs about mental illness. *Psychiatric Rehabilitation Skills*, 6, 159–185.

Phelan, J. C., Yang, L. H., and Cruz Rojas, R. (2006). Effects of attributing serious mental illnesses to genetic causes on orientations to treatment. *Psychiatric Services*, 57, 382–387.

Phelan, J. C., Link, B. G., and Dovidio, J. F. (2008). Stigma and discrimination: One animal or two? *Social Science and Medicine*, 67, 358–367.

Piskur, J. and Degelman, D. (1992). Effect of reading a summary of research about biological bases of homosexual orientation on attitudes toward homosexuals. *Psychological Reports*, 71, 1219–1225.

Prince, P. N. and Prince, C. R. (2002). Perceived stigma and community integration among clients of Assertive Community Treatment. *Psychiatric Rehabilitation Journal*, 25, 323–331.

Reisenzein, R. (1986). A structural equation analysis of Weiner's Attribution-affect Model of Helping Behavior. *Journal of Personality and Social Psychology*, 50, 1123–1133.

Rothbart, M. and Taylor, M. (1992). Category labels and social reality: Do we view social categories as natural kinds? In G. R. Semin and K. Fiedler (eds.), *Language, Interaction and Social Cognition*. London: Sage, pp. 13–36.

Rush, L. L. (1998). Affective reactions to multiple stigmas. *Journal of Social Psychology*, 138, 421–430.

Scheff, T. J. (1998). Shame in the labeling of mental illness. In P. Gilbert and B. Andrews (eds.), *Shame: Interpersonal Behavior, Psychopathology, and Culture*. New York: Oxford University Press.

Schnittker, J. (2008). An uncertain revolution: Why the rise of a genetic model of mental illness has not increased tolerance. *Social Science and Medicine*, 67, 1370–1381.

Schomerus, G., Matschinger, H., and Angermeyer, M. C. (2006). Alcoholism: Illness beliefs and resource allocation preferences of the public. *Drug and Alcohol Dependence*, 82, 204–210.

Schomerus, G., Lucht, M., Holzinger, A., Matschinger, H., Carta, M. G., and Angermeyer, M. C. (2011). The stigma of alcohol dependence compared with other mental disorders: A review of population studies. *Alcohol and Alcoholism*, 46, 105–112.

Schulze, B. and Angermeyer, M. C. (2003). Subjective experiences of stigma. A focus group study of schizophrenic patients, their relatives and mental health professionals. *Social Science & Medicine*, 56, 299–312.

Sibicky, M. and Dovidio, J. F. (1986). Stigma of psychological therapy: Stereotypes, interpersonal reactions, and the self-fulfilling prophecy. *Journal of Consulting and Clinical Psychology*, 33, 148–154.

Stangor, C. and Crandall, C. S. (2000). Threat and the social construction of stigma. In T. F. Heatherton, R. E. Kleck, M. R. Hebl, and J. G. Hall (eds.), *The Social Psychology of Stigma*. New York: Guilford Press, pp. 62–87.

Teachman, B. A., Gapinski, K. D., Brownell, K. D., Rawlins, M., and Jeyaram, S. (2003). Demonstrations of implicit anti-fat bias: The impact of providing causal information and evoking empathy. *Health Psychology*, 22, 68–78.

Wahl, O. F. (1999). Mental health consumers' experience of stigma. *Schizophrenia Bulletin*, 25, 467–478.

Weiner, B. (1986). *Attributional Theory of Motivation and Emotion*. New York: Springer-Verlag.

Weiner, B. (1995). *Judgements of Responsibility: A Foundation for a Theory of Social Conduct*. New York: Guilford Press.

Weiner, B., Perry, R. P., and Magnusson, J. (1988). An attributional analysis of reactions to stigmas. *Journal of Personality and Social Psychology*, 55, 738–748.

Whisman, V. (1996). *Queer by Choice: Lesbians, Gay Men, and the Politics of Identity*. New York: Routledge.

Chapter

13

Lay beliefs about genetic influences on the development of alcoholism: Implications for prevention

Toby Jayaratne, Alicia Giordimaina, and Amy Gaviglio

Medical researchers say they have pinpointed for the first time a gene that may make people prone to alcoholism, adding weight to the belief that alcoholism is a disease and not a weakness.
(Coleman, 1990, appearing in the San Jose Mercury News)

Medical science has increasingly focused attention on the identification of genes associated with the development of a range of diseases and characteristics (Collins and McKusick, 2001; Guttmacher et al., 2001). One goal of this research is to identify, primarily by means of genetic testing, individuals at increased risk for various conditions in order to target preventive interventions (Kardia and Wang, 2005; Omenn, 2005). As part of this effort, it is thought that individuals who understand they are at higher risk due to their genetic makeup may be motivated to engage in preventive behaviors (Gable et al., 2007). However, research is equivocal with regard to the type of effect genetic explanations have on such attitudes. Although several studies suggest genetic explanations can result in greater motivation to reduce risk (Frosch et al., 2005; Chao et al., 2008; Sanderson et al., 2008), some scholars argue that, conversely, genetic explanations can result in fatalistic attitudes toward prevention (Alper and Beckwith, 1993; Macintyre, 1995) that may impede risk-reduction efforts. Both these potential effects of the use of genetic explanations have important implications for preventive behaviors. In this chapter, however, we do not examine the cause-and-effect relationship between genetic explanations for alcoholism and the motivation to engage in preventive behaviors directly. Instead, we take a step back to illuminate and explore the potential links between genetic explanations and illness representations that potentially influence such motivation, and we speculate how these links might function to influence preventive behavior. We focus on three research questions: (1) To what extent does the lay public employ genetic factors to explain the development of alcoholism?; (2) What do genetic explanations for alcoholism imply in terms of the perceived stability and controllability of developing this condition?; and (3) To what extent do risk perceptions for alcoholism predict the use of genetic explanations?

The foundation for our work derives from an extensive theoretical and empirical literature on attributions and lay theories (Weiner, 1986; Dweck et al., 1993; Campbell and

Genetic Research on Addiction, ed. Audrey R. Chapman. Published by Cambridge University Press.
© Cambridge University Press 2012.

Sedikides, 1999). Viewed through these frames, we propose that genetic explanations are appealing to some individuals because they tend to imply that the development of alcoholism is stable and uncontrollable. Such a perspective can shift blame for the development of this condition from the individual to the gene, and therefore can serve as a psychological coping mechanism that, from the point of view of the individual, reduces perceived threat and preserves self-integrity.

Our investigation is based on an analysis of data collected as part of a pilot study assessing the lay public's use of genetic explanations for alcohol problems. This study also assessed beliefs about genetic influences on diabetes, which are not reported here. It is important to note that our emphasis on prevention (as opposed to treatment) necessitated the inclusion of respondents who identified themselves as *not* having an alcohol problem and *not* having been diagnosed with diabetes. While recognizing the preliminary nature of this study, we suggest that our findings will have particular value in laying the groundwork for future research that more fully addresses the specific issues we raise here.

The extent to which genetic factors are thought to influence alcoholism

At different points in time, alcoholism has variously been categorized in the scholarly literature as a moral weakness (moral model), a psychological disorder (psychological model), or a biological disease (medical model). These models help shape lay perceptions of alcoholism and prevention, including acceptance of genetic explanations. Genetic explanations are situated within the medical model, which supports the argument that alcoholism is a disease originating in the biology of an individual (Kincaid and Sullivan, 2010). The competition between models has a complex history (reviewed in Keller, 1976; Schneider, 1978), but the medical model of alcoholism has dominated among health-care professionals since its endorsement from the American Medical Association in 1956 (American Medical Association, 1956; Kloss and Lisman, 2003).

Given the health-care community's advocacy for the medical model, and given that Americans generally have high regard for medical authority, one might expect that the American public is fairly accepting of the medical model of alcoholism. However, evidence of which model of alcoholism currently dominates among the lay public is complicated by conflicting survey results. Although most national opinion polls of American adults from the 1970s and 1980s found support for the medical model (Gallup Organization, 1988), data from the 1990s up to 1999 suggests that, despite the public's continual approval of this model, the psychological model is becoming increasingly popular (National Mental Health Association, 1996; Harvard School of Public Health, 1999). Whether this difference is a reflection of an actual shift in opinion or contrasting research methodologies has not been examined, and there is too little evidence from the past two decades to confirm a trend. Regardless, the medical community's historical advocacy for the disease concept of alcoholism, and evidence that many Americans have employed this model in the recent past, probably means that the medical model of alcoholism is culturally salient to the lay public.

The burgeoning field of genetic research has attracted much popular media attention (e.g., Elmer-Dewitt et al., 1994; also see Nelkin and Lindee, 1995), exposing the public to headlines touting the potential benefits of genetic science and making genetic factors an easily accessible explanation for various human conditions. Although many scientists and scholars have expressed concern about how such research is reported and interpreted (e.g., see Lewontin et al., 1984; Moore, 2001; Allen, 2005), surveys suggest that the American public has generally been optimistic about genetic research and its benefits (Virginia Commonwealth University Center for Public Policy, 2004; Priest, 2006; Kruger and Jayaratne, 2008). This sympathetic perspective probably reflects the general value of, and faith in, science among the large majority of Americans (Miller, 2004; National Science Board, 2010).

Included among genetic claims in the popular press are research reports promoting the genetic basis for addiction, including alcoholism (Sherman, 2006; Associated Press, 2008; Reuters, 2008). The view that alcoholism has a genetic basis is consistent with the medical model (Conrad, 2008; Kincaid and Sullivan, 2010), as both perspectives tend to imply that the origins of alcoholism are physical, alluding to the existence of a concrete and essential cause.

To what extent does this translate into the lay public's use of genetic explanations for alcoholism? Only a few polls and surveys have examined Americans' opinions on this issue. A national poll conducted in 1997 indicated that only 20% of Americans believed genes played *no* part in alcoholism (US News & World Report and Bozell Worldwide, 1997). By contrast, 33% said that alcoholism was either mostly or completely "determined by heredity and genes." Creeden et al. reported in 2000 that 77% of respondents in a telephone survey said that genetics has "a lot" or "some" effect on a person's likelihood of developing alcoholism. A study based on the 2006 General Social Survey found that 68% of Americans attributed alcohol dependence to genetic factors (Pescosolido et al., 2010), an increase of 10% compared with the same question in the 1996 General Social Survey. Evidence from these studies suggests that genetic explanations for alcoholism have been growing in popularity. Based on these findings and on the frequency of recent media coverage of genetic science, we posit that a sizable percentage of individuals will invoke genetic factors to explain the development of alcoholism.

The extent to which genetic explanations imply the stability and uncontrollability of alcoholism

Our understanding of the lay public's use of genetic explanations is informed by research in social psychology, and primarily attribution theory, which is concerned with people's beliefs about the causes of their own and others' characteristics and behaviors. This research literature documents the existence of various perceived *causal dimensions* that underlie explanations and that are associated with a range of relevant attitudinal and behavioral outcomes (Weiner, 1986; Försterling, 2001). For the purpose of understanding genetic explanations for alcoholism, the most relevant causal dimensions are stability and uncontrollability (Anderson and Riger, 1991). Specifically, we propose that the use of genetic explanations for alcoholism tends to imply that this condition is perceived as stable and uncontrollable. This common interpretation of genetic effects, more generally, is reflected in the popular media (Scott, 1993; MSNBC, 2008), in film (Kirby, 2000), in scholarship on social and ethical issues in genetic research (e.g., Andrews, 1999), and in advocacy for social policy (Human Rights Campaign, 2005). Such interpretations have also been found in studies of correlates of genetic explanations (Haslam et al., 2000; Keller, 2005; Jayaratne et al., 2009). Although genes are physically internal to the individual, and internal factors are typically seen as controllable, genes can function *psychologically* as external agents because they are commonly thought to imply uncontrollability. In sum, both research on the public's use of genetic explanations and popular culture suggest that the stronger the belief in genes as causal factors in alcoholism, the greater the perception of the stability and uncontrollability of this condition.

The effect of perceived risk for developing alcoholism on genetic explanations

In addressing our third research question, we suggest that genetic explanations may help individuals cope with a perceived risk for developing alcoholism because genetics tends to imply that the cause of a condition is not controllable. As noted above, genetic explanations can exonerate individuals by shifting blame for an undesirable condition from the person to the gene, thus serving as a psychological coping mechanism (Monterosso et al., 2005). There are at least two situations in which genetic explanations might be particularly attractive for individuals dealing with risk: (1) when they sense that the behavior required to reduce their risk is difficult; and (2) when they experience threat to their self-image owing to stigmas associated with a condition. Both of these situations can apply to alcoholism (abstaining from alcohol consumption can be challenging and significant stigma is attached to individuals with alcohol problems). We therefore anticipate that perceived risk of alcoholism will positively predict the use of genetic explanations for the development of this condition.

Method

Sample

For this study, we first conducted a short telephone screening interview in 2007 with 419 adults randomly selected from telephone directories in southeastern Michigan. Individuals who identified themselves as nonalcoholic[1] were invited to participate in the survey. Three hundred and forty-four respondents agreed to participate (82%) and were sent a survey either by mail or email, based on their stated preference. The final sample included 192 respondents who completed the survey (response rate of 46% based on all respondents contacted). Participants ranged in age from 22 to 90, were mostly female, and had higher incomes and education levels than the general population. The large majority of respondents self-identified as non-Hispanic White, with small numbers indicating membership in minority ethnic groups. Table 13.1 presents a description of the sample.

Measures

The survey assessed beliefs about and experiences with alcoholism, general health attitudes, and several demographic factors. Below we describe the measures employed in our analyses, including several control variables.

Genetic explanations for alcoholism

We constructed the *Genetic Explanations for Alcoholism* scale by obtaining the mean of two questions: "How much do you think the development of alcoholism problems is influenced by a person's genes or genetic makeup?" (answer options: 1 = not at all, 2 = a little, 3 = some, 4 = a fair amount, 5 = a lot, 6 = almost completely) and "Whether a person develops an alcohol problem is due to the genes they get from their mother or father" (answer options:

---

[1] Individuals were also excluded if they indicated that they had diabetes, as explained previously.

Table 13.1 Demographic characteristics of respondents ($N = 192$)

	Percent
Gender	
Men	27
Women	73
Education	
Less than 12th grade	2
Graduated high school (GED)	19
Some college	36
Bachelor's degree	26
Advanced degree	17
Ethnicity	
Asian American	1
Black or African American	8
Hispanic	2
Asian Indian	2
Native American	4
White, non-Hispanic	82
Multiracial/multiethnic	1
	Mean
Age	54 (SD = 15.5)
	Median (in dollars)
Yearly income range	60 000–69 999

1 = strongly disagree, 2 = disagree, 3 = slightly disagree, 4 = slightly agree, 5 = agree, 6 = strongly agree). The resulting scale (see Figure 13.1) ranged from 1 (genes have less influence) to 6 (genes have more influence) ($M = 3.52$, SD = 1.15, $\alpha = 0.79$).

Alcoholism stable/uncontrollable

The *Alcoholism Stable/Uncontrollable* scale was constructed by obtaining a mean of three items: "There is not much a person can do to control whether they develop alcoholism," "Alcohol problems are likely to be permanent, rather than temporary," and "Once someone develops an alcohol problem they will have the condition for the rest of their life." Respondents answered these items using the same 6-point agree/disagree scale mentioned above. The resulting scale ranged from 1 (alcoholism less stable/uncontrollable) to 6 (alcoholism more stable/uncontrollable) ($M = 3.15$, SD = 0.99, $\alpha = 0.63$).

Perceived risk

This three-item *Perceived Risk* scale assessed the respondent's belief in their own personal risk for developing alcoholism. One item asked, "In your opinion, how likely is it that you will ever develop alcoholism during your lifetime?" (Answer options: 1 = not at all likely, 2 = not too likely, 3 = somewhat likely, 4 = very likely, 5 = I am sure I will develop an alcohol

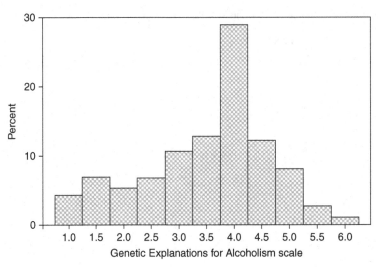

Figure 13.1. Percent distribution on the Genetic Explanations for Alcoholism scale (*N* = 187). Higher scores indicate greater belief that genes influence the development of alcoholism.

problem). Two additional 6-point agree/disagree statements read as "I will never develop an alcohol problem (reversed)" and "I believe I am more likely than the average person to develop alcoholism during my lifetime." The three items were standardized and then averaged (*M* = 1.91, SD = 1.00, α = 0.71). The scale ranged from 1 (low perceived risk) to 6 (high perceived risk).

Family history

We assessed family history of alcoholism by asking the respondent to list all of their blood relatives who had an alcohol problem. Based on their answers we constructed a *Family History* scale that took into account both the number of blood relatives and the degree of relationship to the respondent. The measure includes the following categories: 0 = no relatives, 1 = any third-degree relatives, 2 = one second-degree relative, 3 = two or more second-degree relatives, 4 = one first-degree relative, 5 = two or more first-degree relatives (higher codes have priority over lower codes). Higher scores thus indicate a stronger family history of alcoholism than lower scores.

Alcohol consumption

Respondents indicated how often in a typical week they consume alcohol and how much they tend to drink each time. The *Alcohol Consumption* scale was scored either 0 (no alcohol consumption), 1 (low: one drink per day or two drinks per day but less than once a week), or 2 (moderate/high: two or more drinks per day and more than once a week).

Health fatalism

The *Health Fatalism* scale was constructed by obtaining the mean of two 6-point agree/disagree items: "Even when I take care of myself, it's easy to get sick" and "No matter what I do, I'm likely to get sick." The scale ranged from 1 (less fatalistic) to 6 (more fatalistic) (*M* = 2.94, SD = 1.09, α = 0.65).

Table 13.2 Distribution on the Genetic Explanations for the Development of Alcoholism scale items

How much do you think the development of alcohol problems is influenced by a person's genes or genetic makeup? [a]	Percent
Not at all	8
A little	11
Some	22
A fair amount	37
A lot	20
Almost completely	2
Whether a person develops an alcohol problem is due to the genes they get from their mother or father [b]	
Strongly disagree	11
Disagree	15
Slightly disagree	11
Slightly agree	45
Agree	14
Strongly agree	4

[a] $N = 192$;
[b] $N = 187$.

Age, education, and gender

The respondent's age, education level, and gender were assessed through self-reporting. Higher scores on these variables indicate greater age, higher education, and female gender, respectively.

Results

The extent to which genetic factors are used to explain the development of alcoholism

Table 13.2 shows that a majority of respondents on both genetic explanation items indicated that genes influence the development of alcoholism. For example, 63% of respondents agreed with the statement, "Whether a person develops an alcohol problem is due to the genes they get from their mother or father." On the question, "How much do you think the development of alcoholism is influenced by a person's genes or genetic makeup?", 59% of respondents reported that genes had at least a "fair amount" of influence on alcoholism. Only 19% of respondents reported that genes had little or no influence.

To assess the extent to which genetic explanations for alcoholism are used across population subgroups, we examined whether such beliefs differed by gender, age, or education. We found that genetic explanations for alcoholism were not significantly correlated with either age [$r (181) = -0.01$] or education level [$r (184) = 0.05$] and did not differ significantly by gender [$t (183) = -1.63$]. These results suggest that genetic explanations for alcoholism are distributed across a wide segment of the population.

Table 13.3 Predicting alcoholism to be stable/uncontrollable

	B	SEB	β
Genetic explanations for alcoholism	0.263	0.071	0.289***
Family history	0.046	0.038	0.092
Health fatalism	0.099	0.073	0.107
Alcohol consumption	0.061	0.112	0.043
Age	0.013	0.005	0.201*
Education	0.056	0.056	0.084
Gender	−0.004	0.187	−0.002
Adjusted R^2	0.104 $F(7,151) = 3.625$**		

$N = 160$; *$p < 0.05$, ***$p < 0.001$ (two-tailed).

The effect of genetic explanations on beliefs about the stability/uncontrollability of alcoholism

We examined the effect of genetic explanations for alcoholism on perceived stability/uncontrollability of the condition, controlling for the effects of family history, fatalism, alcohol consumption, age, education, and gender. The results, shown in Table 13.3, demonstrate that, with other variables held constant, use of genetic explanations for alcoholism is a significant predictor of the belief that alcoholism is a stable and uncontrollable condition. Specifically, greater belief in genetic influence is associated with the perception of alcoholism as relatively stable and uncontrollable. In addition to this effect, older respondents, compared with younger respondents, tended to report the development of alcoholism as relatively stable and uncontrollable.

The effect of perceived risk of developing alcoholism on genetic explanations for alcoholism

To assess the extent to which perceived risk of developing alcoholism is associated with genetic explanations, we examined a predictive model, regressing genetic explanations on perceived risk and five control variables (family history, health fatalism, age, education, and gender). Alcohol consumption was not included in this regression because of concerns about multicollinearity between this variable and perceived risk for alcoholism [$r(168) = 0.38, p < 0.001$]. Results, shown in Table 13.4, indicate that perceived risk is a significant predictor of genetic explanations for alcoholism. Specifically, with other variables held constant, the more the perceived risk, the greater the reported influence of genes. We also found that female gender and higher education were associated with greater belief in the influence of genes. Finally, a marginally significant effect of health fatalism indicated that fatalistic attitudes were associated with greater perceived influence of genes.

Discussion

Recent coverage of the genetic basis of addiction in the popular media (e.g., Sherman, 2006; Associated Press, 2008; Reuters, 2008) makes understanding how the lay public interprets

Table 13.4 Predicting genetic explanations for alcoholism

	B	SEB	β
Perceived risk	0.376	0.085	0.327***
Family history	−0.001	0.041	−0.002
Health fatalism	0.140	0.075	0.136†
Age	0.000	0.006	0.000
Education	0.122	0.059	0.163*
Gender	0.567	0.185	0.224**
Adjusted R^2	0.121 $F_{(6,169)}$ = 4.997***		

N = 176; *p < 0.05, **p < 0.01, ***p < 0.001 (two-tailed); †marginally significant p = 0.07.

and utilizes such information a pressing need. Our work addresses three interrelated issues within this domain: (1) the prevalence of genetic explanations for the development of alcoholism; (2) the extent to which genetic explanations for alcoholism imply the stability and uncontrollability of developing alcoholism; and (3) the use of genetic explanations among those who perceive personal risk for developing alcoholism.

Prevalence of genetic explanations for alcoholism

Owing to the heavy media coverage of genetic research (see Nelkin and Lindee, 1995) and results of public opinion polls (e.g., US News & World Report/Bozell Worldwide, 1997; Pescosolido et al., 2010), we expected a sizable portion of respondents in our survey would endorse genetic explanations for alcoholism. We found that a substantial majority reported that genes have at least "some" influence, with only a small percentage reporting no influence at all. We also found that a wide spectrum of individuals across age, education, and gender groups report genetic explanations for alcoholism, suggesting that such causal beliefs have broad appeal. We interpret this appeal as reflecting, in part, popular culture's portrayal of addiction as a biological disease (e.g., Sherman, 2006), which is consistent with the medical model of alcoholism. Additionally, American cultural perspectives tend to favor dispositional and essentialist views of individual differences (Fiske and Taylor, 1991; Nisbett, 2004; Bastian and Haslam, 2006). Such views suggest, for example, that there is something inherently different between people categorized as "alcoholic" and "not alcoholic" – an essential factor that defines and identifies these groups (see Haslam et al., 2000; Gelman, 2003). In this way, both genetic explanations and the medical model imply that the origins of addiction are situated physically, as a concrete essence, within the individual.

Although most respondents in our study reported that genes influence the development of alcoholism, very few indicated that genes were completely responsible for the condition. This suggests that many believe alcoholism to be multifactorial, a finding that is consistent with other research on the public's causal beliefs for a range of characteristics (see Jayaratne et al., 2009; Condit, 2010). We speculate that it is psychologically advantageous for individuals to have access to multiple causal frameworks, so that particular explanations can be invoked situationally.

Despite the evidence for the public's use of genetic explanations for alcoholism, there are important reasons why some individuals might want to steer clear of such causal accounts.

As described above, genetic explanations can function to decrease individual blame for behaviors that are seen as undesirable (Jayaratne et al., 2006). Avoiding such explanations will tend to implicate either the individual (as having chosen the behavior, implying the moral model) or the environment (implying a psychological model). For example, people who have suffered because of another's alcoholism (e.g., victims of a drunken driver) may feel better by focusing blame on that individual. Similarly, parents of alcoholics may prefer to blame the "bad crowd" with whom their child associated, rather than feel they are responsible for passing on their "alcoholism" genes. Additionally, American culture encourages a belief in individual responsibility and free will (Sarkissian et al., 2010), commonly thought to be antithetical to determinism, thus possibly mitigating the use of genetic explanations.

Genetic explanations and beliefs about the control and stability of alcoholism

Our second research question investigates how people interpret genetic influences – specifically whether such beliefs imply the stability and uncontrollability of the development of alcoholism. We anticipated that the use of genetic explanations would indicate a belief that such development is not malleable and not subject to control by the individual. Previous research (Jayaratne et al., 2009) and popular media portrayals (Nelkin and Lindee, 1995) suggest an inverse association between genetic factors and personal choice. Indeed, conditions that are subject to choice (manipulated) must necessarily be perceived as both malleable and controllable to some extent.

Tests of our predictive model support these expectations. Genetic explanations for the development of alcoholism were associated with stronger perceptions of stability and uncontrollability. In this way, genetic explanations may shift responsibility away from the individual, owing to a tendency to see genes as ultimate causes and deterministic (Keller, 2005). This viewpoint is at odds with scientific opinion, which emphasizes the importance of complex gene–environment interactions rather than the reductionist "nature versus nurture" approach that is more commonly found in public discourse (Moore, 2001). The discrepancy between scientific and lay interpretations may be attributable, in part, to the limited comprehension of genetic science in the population (Marteau and Senior, 1997; Lanie et al., 2004; Libman and Arslanian, 2007) and the strength of folk beliefs about inheritance (Finkler, 2001).

Genetic explanations for alcoholism and the medical model stand in stark contrast to the moral model, which holds an individual responsible for "choosing" to engage in such culturally deviant behavior. Historically, the shift from the moral model to the medical model was seen to be advantageous because "…it lifts a large burden of irrational guilt from both patient and family" (Blume, 1983: 16). Although we recognize this apparent benefit, which is primarily psychological, it is an open question as to whether this viewpoint promotes or inhibits preventive attitudes and behaviors – an issue we address below.

Genetic explanations among those who perceive risk of developing alcoholism

Research in social psychology and health behavior suggests that individuals who perceive they are at risk for developing conditions they consider highly undesirable are likely to take action to decrease the threat that such situations pose (Cameron and Leventhal, 2003).

Although not all risks are perceived to be threatening, the strong stigma associated with alcoholism (Pescosolido et al., 2010) means that a propensity for alcoholism probably represents a serious threat to one's self-image. Thus, individuals who perceive their risk of alcoholism to be high should be motivated to decrease this threat by employing any number of psychological or behavioral coping tactics. Behavioral coping is likely to mean decreasing or eliminating alcohol use, a response that may be particularly difficult for those who perceive higher risk due to their greater levels of alcohol use. As an alternative strategy, shifting blame or responsibility to an "external" factor may be an easier method of decreasing perceived threat. We therefore expected that risk perceptions for the development of alcoholism would predict endorsement of genetic causal factors. We found support for this hypothesis; as respondents' perceived risk for alcoholism increased, so did their belief in the influence of genetic factors on the development of alcoholism.

In addition to this association, we found that those with higher education levels were more likely to endorse genetic explanations, compared to those with less education. This result is consistent with research by Kruger and Jayaratne (2008), which showed that greater education was associated with more favorable views of genetic research. The association between genetic beliefs or attitudes and education may be attributable to increased exposure to genetic science in the classroom or to a greater understanding of news reports of genetic research among those with higher levels of education. In addition, we found that women were more likely than men to use genetic explanations. This result may be due to the fact that alcoholism-associated stigma is asymmetrically gendered. Alcoholism is more common in men (Keyes et al., 2008), is linked to masculine gender stereotypes (e.g., Lemle and Mishkind, 1989; Lyons and Willott, 2008), and women perceive that *society* disapproves of drunkenness in females more than males (reviewed in Nolen-Hoeksema, 2004). Women who have higher perceived risk for alcoholism may report genetic explanations more than men because they fear a higher level of stigmatization. We caution, however, that given the small number of men surveyed ($n = 27$), these findings ought to be confirmed in a larger sample.

Although our results suggest a link between genetic explanations and *psychological* coping, it is also likely that, for some individuals, behavioral change (e.g., reducing or eliminating alcohol intake) could result from their belief that they are genetically predisposed to alcoholism. In terms of alcohol prevention, risk perceptions that result in behavioral change are clearly a more favorable outcome than merely coping psychologically. This raises a question about who uses which strategy for dealing with risk. In our study, however, this question could not be examined because we did not assess the respondent's preferred strategy or their actual or intended behavioral change if they felt they were at risk. To more fully understand the relationships between perceived risk, genetic explanations, psychological coping strategies, and behavioral change it will be helpful to collect longitudinal data to explore causal relationships and to assess complex models that untangle these relationships.

The role of health fatalism

An alternative approach that informs these issues is to ask if fatalistic health beliefs contribute to the likelihood of using genetic explanations. Fatalistic attitudes are generally pessimistic, deterministic beliefs about one's future health that undermines self-efficacy for disease prevention and health promotion behaviors (Straughan and Seow, 1998). A fatalist will tend to believe that the outcome of their health is fixed and that they cannot do

Table 13.5 Predicting genetic explanations for alcoholism among those with low and high health fatalism

	Low health fatalism[a]			High health fatalism[b]		
	B	SEB	β	B	SEB	β
Perceived risk	0.260	0.166	0.191	0.520	0.125	0.471***
Family history	0.006	0.067	0.010	0.026	0.067	0.045
Education	0.077	0.092	0.093	0.213	0.090	0.281*
Gender	0.279	0.316	0.099	0.845	0.291	0.341**
Adjusted R^2	−0.001 $F_{(4,77)} = 0.974$			0.242 $F_{(4,58)} = 6.947$***		

[a] $n = 82$; [b] $n = 63$; * $p < 0.05$, ** $p < 0.01$, *** $p < 0.001$ (two-tailed).

much, if anything, to alter that outcome. Thus, fatalism shares with genetic explanations the tendency to view outcomes as stable and uncontrollable. However, although genetic explanations may or may not increase preventive action, fatalism has been correlated with decreased uptake for medical screens and tests, decreased preventive health behaviors, and a higher rate of risky behaviors (Hardeman et al., 1997; Straughan and Seow, 1998; Yi et al., 2010). Therefore, we wondered if the effect of perceived risk on genetic explanations is stronger among those who hold fatalistic attitudes toward health than those with a more optimistic view. We reasoned that genetic explanations might be particularly appealing to those who perceive risk *and* who hold fatalistic beliefs. Additionally, fatalism may increase the perceived threat associated with risk of alcoholism (owing to the implied lack of control of such risk), which as noted above, was associated with use of genetic explanations. Most importantly, a strong link between perceived risk and genetic explanations among those who hold fatalistic attitudes gives credence to the possibility that, at least among this group of individuals, genetic explanations contribute to a decreased likelihood of preventive attitudes and behaviors.

To test for this possibility, we conducted an additional analysis examining the effect of perceived risk on genetic explanations separately for those with high health fatalism (M = 3.5 to 6.0, n = 66) and for those with low health fatalism (M = 1.0 to 2.5, n = 86), based on their score on the 6-point *Health Fatalism* scale. We excluded respondents who scored in the middle category (M = 3.0, n = 37), due to the likelihood that their fatalism beliefs were not as clearly defined.[2] To adjust for the smaller subsample size in each group (compared with the previous analysis), a nonsignificant predictor (age) was removed from the new regressions. The results, shown in Table 13.5, support our expectations. Among the low health fatalism group the overall regression model was not significant. Among those with high health fatalism, we found a highly significant effect of perceived risk on genetic explanations.

These findings suggest that genetic explanations may be particularly useful as a coping mechanism among individuals who perceive a risk of alcoholism *and* who hold fatalistic views about health. Among those with lower health fatalism, it is likely that factors other

---

[2] In consideration of the number of predictors in the regression, we attempted to keep the *n* for the high and low health fatalism groups as large and evenly balanced as possible.

than those in our model may better predict the use of genetic explanations. Speculating from the viewpoint of social psychological theory, genetic explanations may serve as part of the larger pattern of fatalistic thinking about health in general (Mirowsky and Ross, 1990). In this way, health fatalists may already be using coping methods that shift responsibility for health outcomes away from themselves and onto external factors (e.g., fate and luck). Such speculation implies a direct link between health fatalism and the use of genetic explanations, an association shown to be marginally significant ($p = 0.07$) in the model predicting genetic explanations (see Table 13.4).

Limitations and future research

It is important to note several limitations to our work and point out how future research can advance some of the theories we address in our study. First are issues concerning the sample. Respondents in this study represent only a small segment of Americans (both geographically and in terms of those self-identified as nonalcoholic and nondiabetic). Thus, the opinions that were expressed may not reflect the broader range of views held across the larger population. Additionally, owing to our focus on prevention, we only included respondents who were not self-reported as having an alcoholism problem. Individuals who self-identify as alcoholic may hold distinct beliefs about the role of genetics. Studies on this population are likely to be fruitful because they can potentially inform alcoholism treatment efforts.

Second, the cross-sectional design of this study meant we could not assess the direction of causal relationships between the major constructs. For data analyses, we conceptualized the effect of genetic explanations on beliefs about stability/uncontrollability in order to understand what is implied when people use such explanations. We examined the effect of perceived risk on the use of genetic explanations to answer our question about how those who perceive risk might employ such explanations. However, it is likely that genetic explanations are bidirectionally associated with both beliefs about stability/controllability and perceived risk, and it would be valuable to know whether genetic explanations function primarily as a cause or a result in their relationship with such constructs.

Finally, the wording of our questions raises issues that should be addressed in future research. First, our genetic explanation and stability/uncontrollability items assessed beliefs about people in general. We deemed such questions conceptually easier for the respondents to answer than if we asked about the respondent's beliefs on a personal level (e.g., their own genetic influence and ability to control their own development of alcoholism). This contrasts with how we asked about risk, which reflected the respondent's personal assessment (*"your risk to develop alcohol problems"*). It would be important for future investigators to take a dual approach, measuring beliefs both at the population and personal level to more fully explore which of these offer the best fit in models exploring the effect of genetic explanations on preventive attitudes and behaviors. Second, our questions about genetic influence ask specifically about the "development of alcohol problems" because of our interest in alcohol prevention. Such wording emphasizes how genes affect the *origins* of alcoholism, in contrast to *recovery* from alcoholism. Although it is unclear to what extent our findings in this study are applicable to issues of rehabilitation and treatment, we speculate that the conceptual foundation of our work should also apply in this context, given the need for individuals with alcohol problems to cope with this undesirable condition.

Conclusions and implications for alcohol prevention

The results from this study have particular relevance to alcoholism prevention because, although respondents did not self-identify as having alcoholism, those respondents at higher subjective risk were also at higher risk objectively, based on their reported alcohol consumption. Thus, our findings are likely to apply to those who are objectively at risk for alcoholism. In such individuals, the use of genetic explanations may function as a psychological coping strategy, a process that may well be enhanced if individuals also hold fatalistic beliefs about health. This method of coping, however, may have negative consequences for behavioral risk reduction. Individuals who feel control over outcomes are more motivated to engage in preventive behaviors compared with those who feel less control (Lewis and Daltroy, 1990; Mirowsky and Ross, 1990; Roesch and Weiner, 2001). If the use of genetic explanations for alcoholism tends to decrease an individual's sense of control over the development of alcoholism, then it may diminish an individual's effort to decrease their risk more effectively. Although one potential avenue of intervention would be to manipulate beliefs about the relative importance of genetic contribution to alcoholism or the relationship between genetic explanations and uncontrollability, our findings related to fatalism complicate the matter. Because the use of genetic explanations may be part of the individual's larger fatalistic coping schema, interventions may need to address the individual's broader attitudes toward health and be sensitive to the problems presented by trying to remove or alter a psychological coping strategy.

In conclusion, we stress the significance of two issues that have a bearing on the arguments we have made in this chapter. First, moving genetic research from benchside to bedside is a slow process. Science moves with relative trepidation compared with the media, who are freer to publicize simplified, sometimes sensational, accounts of genetic discovery and their future applications. Genetic explanations for a disease or condition often become available to the public far in advance of clinical utility, if ever clinical utility is achieved or was even intended at all. Therefore, the relationship between the lay public's use of genetic explanations and preventive attitudes becomes relevant to behavioral prevention efforts long before patients reach the physician's office. This issue takes on added significance when preliminary genetic research fails to be replicated or is disconfirmed (Allen, 2005), as this news does not always filter down to the public.

Second, we contend that current debates about whether lay use of genetic explanations act to increase or decrease preventive behaviors do not often include discussion of the complexity and causal relationships involved in such potential effects. Although our analysis was clearly limited in these ways owing to the preliminary nature of this study, the most fruitful path of investigation for future research should take into account these issues, as well as the plethora of situational factors and individual cognitive styles that influence how individuals deal with perceived and actual risk. Genetic explanations can play many and varied roles in such processes. We believe that research in this domain can best be advanced by identifying such roles and their part in encouraging attitudes and behaviors that promote and sustain health and well-being.

Acknowledgment

We thank Jillian Tietjen and Lesli Kiedrowski for their assistance in the preparation of this chapter and appreciate comments on the manuscript from Elizabeth Robinson. We also acknowledge the data collection efforts of Daniela Lopez and Thuan Dang.

References

Allen, A. (2005). The disappointment gene: Why genetics is so far a boondoggle. Available online at: www.slate.com/id/2128292/ [accessed March 13, 2012].

Alper, J. S. and Beckwith, J. (1993). Genetic fatalism and social policy: The implications of behavior genetics research. *Yale Journal of Biology and Medicine*, 66, 511–524.

American Medical Association (1956). Report of the board of trustees: Hospitalization of patients with alcoholism. *Journal of the American Medical Association*, 162, 750.

Anderson, C. A. and Riger, A. L. (1991). A controllability attributional model of problems in living – Dimensional and situational interactions in the prediction of depression and loneliness. *Social Cognition*, 9, 149–181.

Andrews, L. B. (1999). Predicting and punishing antisocial acts: How the criminal justice system might use behavioral genetics. In R. A. Carson and M. A. Rothstein (eds.), *Behavioral Genetics: The Clash of Culture and Biology*. Baltimore, MD: Johns Hopkins University Press.

Associated Press (2008). Can't quit smoking? Blame your genes. Available online at: www.msnbc.msn.com/id/23919596/ns/health-addictions/t/cant-quit-smoking-blame-your-genes/ [accessed March 13, 2012].

Bastian, B. and Haslam, N. (2006). Psychological essentialism and stereotype endorsement. *Journal of Experimental Social Psychology*, 42, 228–235.

Blume, S. B. (1983). *The Disease Concept of Alcoholism Today*. Minneapolis, MN: Johnson Institute.

Cameron, L. D. and Leventhal, H. (2003). *The Self-Regulation of Health and Illness Behaviour*. London: Routledge.

Campbell, W. K. and Sedikides, C. (1999). Self-threat magnifies the self-serving bias: A meta-analytic integration. *Review of General Psychology*, 3, 23–43.

Chao, S., Roberts, J. S., Marteau, T. M., et al. (2008). Health behavior changes after genetic risk assessment for Alzheimer disease: The REVEAL Study. *Alzheimer Disease and Associated Disorders*, 22, 94–97.

Coleman, B. C. (1990). Researchers say they have identified gene linked to alcoholism. *Associated Press*, April 17, 1990.

Collins, F. S. and McKusick, V. A. (2001). Implications of the Human Genome Project for medical science. *JAMA: Journal of the American Medical Association*, 285, 540–544.

Condit, C. (2010). Public understandings of genetics and health. *Clinical Genetics*, 77, 1–9.

Conrad, P. (2008). A mirage of genes. In Conrad, Peter (ed.), *The Sociology of Health & Illness: Critical Perspectives*, eighth edition. New York: Worth Publishers.

Creeden, T. M., Manowitz, P., Hamer, R. M., and Ballou, J. (2000). The belief in the role of genetics in the development of alcoholism. *Journal of Genetic Counseling*, 9, 538–539.

Dweck, C., Hong, Y.-Y., and Chiu, C.-Y. (1993). Implicit theories: Individual differences in the likelihood and meaning of dispositional inference. *Personality and Social Psychology Bulletin*, 19, 644–656.

Elmer-Dewitt, P., Bjerklie, D., Dorfman, A., and Gorman, C. (1994). The genetic revolution. *Time*, 144, 32–40.

Finkler, K. (2001). The kin of the gene: The medicalization of family and kinship in American society. *Current Anthropology*, 42, 235–263.

Fiske, S. T. and Taylor, S. E. (1991). *Social Cognition*. New York: McGraw-Hill.

Försterling, F. (2001). *Attribution: An Introduction to Theories, Research, and Applications*. Philadelphia: Psychology Press.

Frosch, D. L., Mello, P., and Lerman, C. (2005). Behavioral consequences of testing for obesity risk. *Cancer Epidemiology, Biomarkers & Prevention*, 14, 1485–1489.

Gable, D., Sanderson, S. C., and Humphries, S. E. (2007). Genotypes, obesity and type 2 diabetes – can genetic information motivate weight loss? A review. *Clinical Chemistry and Laboratory Medicine*, 45, 301–308.

Gallup Organization (1988). *Gallup Poll # 1988–870 Government/1988 Presidential Election*. Washington, DC: Gallup Organization.

Gelman, S. A. (2003). *The Essential Child: Origins of Essentialism in Everyday Thought*. New York: Oxford University Press.

Guttmacher, A. E., Jenkins, J., and Uhlmann, W. R. (2001). Genomic medicine: who will practice it? A call to open arms. *American Journal of Medical Genetics*, 106, 216–222.

Hardeman, W., Pierro, A., and Mannetti, L. (1997). Determinants of intentions to practise safe sex among 16–25 year-olds. *Journal of Community & Applied Social Psychology*, 7, 345–360.

Harvard School of Public Health (1999). Illicit drugs and alcohol treatment survey. Boston, MA: Harvard School of Public Health.

Haslam, N. N., Rothschild, L., and Ernst, D. (2000). Essentialist beliefs about social categories. *British Journal of Social Psychology*, 39, 113–127.

Human Rights Campaign (2005). New research suggests genetic basis to sexual orientation. Available online at: www.hrc.org/press-releases/entry/new-research-suggests-genetic-basis-to-sexual-orientation [accessed March 13, 2012].

Jayaratne, T. E., Ybarra, O., Sheldon, J. P., et al. (2006). White Americans' genetic lay theories of race differences and sexual orientation: Their relationship with prejudice toward Blacks, and gay men and lesbians. *Group Processes & Intergroup Relations*, 9, 77–94.

Jayaratne, T. E., Gelman, S. A., Feldbaum, M., et al. (2009). The perennial debate: Nature, nurture, or choice? Black and White Americans' explanations for individual differences. *Review of General Psychology*, 13, 24–33.

Kardia, S. L. R. and Wang, C. (2005). The role of health education and behavior in public health genetics. *Health Education & Behavior*, 32, 583–588.

Keller, J. (2005). In genes we trust: The biological component of psychological essentialism and its relationship to mechanisms of motivated social cognition. *Journal of Personality and Social Psychology*, 88, 686–702.

Keller, M. (1976). The disease concept of alcoholism revisited. *Journal of Studies on Alcohol*, 37, 1694–1717.

Keyes, K. M., Grant, B. F., and Hasin, D. S. (2008). Evidence for a closing gender gap in alcohol use, abuse, and dependence in the United States population. *Drug and Alcohol Dependence*, 93, 21–29.

Kincaid, H. and Sullivan, J. A. (2010). Medical models of addiction. In D. Ross, H. Kincaid, D. Spurrett, and P. Collins (eds.) *What is Addiction?* Cambridge, MA: MIT Press.

Kirby, D. A. (2000). The new eugenics in cinema: Genetic determinism and gene therapy in "GATTACA." *Science Fiction Studies*, 27, 193–215.

Kloss, J. D. and Lisman, S. A. (2003). Clinician attributions and disease model perspectives of mentally ill, chemically addicted patients: a preliminary investigation. *Substance Use & Misuse*, 38, 2097–2107.

Kruger, D. J. and Jayaratne, T. E. (2008). Who supports genetic research? Demographic factors associated with beliefs on risks and benefits. Annual Meeting of the American Public Health Association, San Diego, CA.

Lanie, A. D., Jayaratne, T. E., Sheldon, J. P., et al. (2004). Exploring the public understanding of basic genetic concepts. *Journal of Genetic Counseling*, 13, 305–320.

Lemle, R. and Mishkind, M. E. (1989). Alcohol and masculinity. *Journal of Substance Abuse Treatment*, 6, 213–222.

Lewis, F. M. and Daltroy, L. H. (1990). How causal explanations influence health behavior: Attribution theory. In K. Glanz, F. M. Lewis, and B. K. Rimer (eds.), *Health Behavior and Health Education: Theory, Research, and Practice*. San Francisco: Jossey-Bass Publishers.

Lewontin, R. C., Rose, S., and Kamin, L. J. (1984). *Not in Our Genes: Biology, Ideology, and Human Nature*. New York: Pantheon Books.

Libman, I. M. and Arslanian, S. A. (2007). Prevention and treatment of type 2 diabetes in youth. *Hormone Research*, 67, 22–34.

Lyons, A. and Willott, S. (2008). Alcohol consumption, gender identities and women's changing social positions. *Sex Roles*, 59, 694–712.

Macintyre, S. (1995). The public understanding of science or the scientific understanding of the public? A review of the social context of the "new genetics". *Public Understanding of Science*, 4, 223–232.

Marteau, T. M. and Senior, V. (1997). Illness representations after the Human Genome Project: The perceived role of genes in causing illness. In K. J. Petrie and J. Weinman (eds.), *Perceptions of Health and Illness: Current Research and Applications*. Amsterdam: Harwood Academic Publishers.

Miller, J. D. (2004). Public understanding of, and attitudes toward, scientific research: What we know and what we need to know. *Public Understanding of Science*, 13, 273–294.

Mirowsky, J. and Ross, C. E. (1990). Control or defense? Depression and the sense of control over good and bad outcomes. *Journal of Health and Social Behavior*, 31, 71–86.

Monterosso, J., Royzman, E. B., and Schwartz, B. (2005). Explaining away responsibility: Effects of scientific explanation on perceived culpability. *Ethics & Behavior*, 15, 139–158.

Moore, D. S. (2001). *The Dependent Gene: The Fallacy of Nature/Nurture*. New York: Times Books.

MSNBC (2008). Can't quit smoking? Blame your genes. Available online at: www.msnbc. msn.com/id/23919596/ [accessed March 13, 2012].

National Mental Health Association (1996). *Clinical Depression and its Treatment Survey*. Los Angeles: Wirthlin Group.

National Science Board (2010). *Science and Engineering Indicators 2010*. Arlington, VA: National Science Foundation.

Nelkin, D. and Lindee, M. S. (1995). *The DNA Mystique: The Gene as a Cultural Icon*. New York: Freeman.

Nisbett, R. E. (2004). *The Geography of Thought: How Asians and Westerners Think Differently … and Why*. New York: Free Press.

Nolen-Hoeksema, S. (2004). Gender differences in risk factors and consequences for alcohol use and problems. *Clinical Psychology Review*, 24, 981–1010.

Omenn, G. S. (2005). Genomics and public health. *Issues in Science and Technology*, 21, 42–48.

Pescosolido, B. A., Martin, J. K., Long, J. S., et al. (2010). "A disease like any other"? A decade of change in public reactions to schizophrenia, depression, and alcohol dependence. *American Journal of Psychiatry*, 167, 1321–1330.

Priest, S. H. (2006). The public opinion climate for gene technologies in Canada and the United States: Competing voices, contrasting frames. *Public Understanding of Science*, 15, 55–71.

Reuters (2008). Drug addiction genes identified. Available online at: www.reuters.com/ article/2008/01/08/us-drugs-china-addiction-idUSHKG24467620080108 [accessed March 13, 2012].

Roesch, S. C. and Weiner, B. (2001). A meta-analytic review of coping with illness: Do causal attributions matter? *Journal of Psychosomatic Research*, 50, 205–219.

Sanderson, S. C., Humphries, S. E., Hubbart, C., et al. (2008). Psychological and behavioural impact of genetic testing smokers for lung cancer risk. *Journal of Health Psychology*, 13, 481–494.

Sarkissian, H., Chatterjee, A., De Brigard, F., et al. (2010). Is belief in free will a cultural universal? *Mind & Language*, 25, 346–358.

Schneider, J. W. (1978). Deviant drinking as disease – alcoholism as a social accomplishment. *Social Problems*, 25, 361–372.

Scott, J. (1993). The latest parenting debate. *Los Angeles Times*, December 8, p. E1.

Sherman, W. (2006). Test targets addiction gene. *New York Daily News*, February 12, p. 28.

Straughan, P. T. and Seow, A. (1998). Fatalism reconceptualized: A concept to predict health screening behavior. *Journal of Gender, Culture, and Health*, 2, 85–100.

US News & World Report and Bozell Worldwide (1997). Available online at: www.ropercenter.uconn.edu/data_access/ipoll/ipoll.html [accessed March 13, 2012].

Virginia Commonwealth University Center for Public Policy (2004). Virginia Commonwealth University Poll # 2004-LIFE: VCU Life Sciences Survey, 2004. Storrs, CT: Roper Center for Public Opinion Research.

Weiner, B. (1986). *An Attributional Theory of Motivation and Emotion*. New York: Springer-Verlag.

Yi, H., Sandfort, T. G. M. and Shidlo, A. (2010). Effects of disengagement coping with HIV risk on unprotected sex among HIV-negative gay men in New York City. *Health Psychology*, 29, 205–214.

Chapter

14

Personalizing risk: How behavior genetics research into addiction makes the political personal

Jonathan M. Kaplan

Introduction: Addiction, genetics, and the disease model

Addiction is both economically costly and contributes significantly to excess morbidity and mortality (see e.g., Merikangas and Risch, 2003). Although estimates of the total costs of addictive behaviors are by necessity imprecise and subject to much debate, in the United States alone, estimates of economic costs of around half a trillion dollars a year are frequently cited (see Rice, 1999), along with more than half a million excess deaths in the United States per year (see, e.g., Minino and Smith, 2001; MMWR, 2008).

Given these high costs, and the difficulties in successfully treating addictions (see, e.g., Sellman, 2009 and citations therein), there is obvious interest in learning more about the etiology of addiction, with the aim of reducing the costs – both in terms of human suffering and financial costs – of addiction. Studies of the genetic contributions and/or susceptibility to addiction are usually framed as part of this project of ameliorating the costs of addiction. The idea is that if the underlying genetic factors associated with addictive behaviors can be elucidated, then targeted interventions (such as individually tailored pharmaceuticals and/ or more focused psychological/therapeutic help) might provide a low(er) cost method of reducing the frequency and impact of addictive behaviors. Alternatively, broad population screening might permit people with particular susceptibilities to addictive behaviors or to particular kinds of addiction (e.g., alcohol) to be warned of their particular risk, and to change their behaviors accordingly. The following examples are illustrative of the tone of much published research on this topic.

> Understanding the genetic basic of alcoholism is a crucial step for the development of efficient pre-vention strategies and personalized treatments. For this purpose, it is important to identify genes predisposing individuals to alcoholism, genes moderating consequences of alcohol exposure, clin-ical course and treatment response, mechanisms through which genes exert their effects on behavior and interactions of genes with other genes and with environmental factors. (Ducci and Goldman, 2008)
>
> Employing the power of genetic studies … will enhance research on etiology, treatment, and prevention for these complex diseases. (Berrettini et al., 2004)
>
> [The] public health impact of gene discovery for the addictions is potentially very large … this goal [the integration of genotypes into diagnosis] is particularly timely given the enormous public-health impact of addictions and the potential power of precisely and inexpensively defined geno-types associated with these heritable diseases. (Goldman et al., 2005)

Genetic Research on Addiction, ed. Audrey R. Chapman. Published by Cambridge University Press.
© Cambridge University Press 2012.

Of course, understanding vulnerability can lead to the best possible "treatment", which is prevention of the development of addictive disorders … the role of genes is unfolding and should influence the development of more effective biological treatments … In the area of addiction we have already begun to knock on the door of genomic medicine … Systematic probing as discussed by Schumann using animal models, genetics, brain imaging and other measures may well allow us to predict in advance which patients are most likely to respond to which treatment. (O'Brien, 2007)

As the above suggest, much of the contemporary research into the genetics of addiction/addictive behaviors has focused on attempting to understand individual variation in addiction or susceptibility to addiction or addictive behaviors. That is, the research has focused on which distinct features of this person, or this person's experiences, led him or her to become an addict. Why, in other words, did *this* person and not *that* person become addicted? What risk factors account for some people becoming addicts rather than others? What identifies people at high risk for being addicts? Research into the genetics of addiction generally attempts to answer this question by finding genetic correlates to addiction and/or addictive behaviors – that is, by finding alleles (variants of genes) that are more common in addicts than in nonaddicts, and, ideally, by finding plausible biochemical pathways that would result in these different alleles being associated with different risks of addiction.

While there are technical and ethical challenges to both conducting such research and interpreting the results of that research (for a discussion, see Kaplan, 2006; see Munafò, 2009b for discussion of addiction research in particular; see Ioannidis et al., 2001 for a review of the difficulties inherent in genetic association studies more generally), it is rather the stated goals of genomic approaches to understanding addiction, and the difficulties that these approaches have in achieving those goals, on which this chapter will focus. The difficulty is that there is a disconnection between studying the causes of individual variation in addiction (which particular risk factors are associated with this person and not that person becoming an addict) and working to reduce the harms associated with addiction. Seriously reducing the economic costs and human suffering associated with addiction probably requires more than an attention to the details of individual addicts or to those people particularly susceptible to addiction. Indeed, it is likely that an attention to this kind of individual variation – including genetic variation – can have at best a relatively minor impact on the overall costs, both economic and health-related, of addiction and addictive behaviors.

In fact, seriously reducing the costs associated with addiction probably requires attention to the broader social environment in which addiction takes place. Both rates of addiction and the harms associated with addiction vary significantly between social environments – for example, there is substantial variation in the rates of addiction and the associated harms between different countries, between locales within countries (including rural/urban divides), and between racial/ethnic groups. Rather than looking for the correlates to addiction within a particular social environment (within a particular country or locale, for example), looking toward the differences that emerge in different social environments – that is, the differences *between* populations – might well reveal the causes of the differences in rates and costs of addiction between those social environments. Often, this kind of analysis reveals that attempting to modify the broad social environment has more potential for harm and cost reduction than does a focus on high-risk individuals within a particular social environment (see below and Rose, 1985).

However, the difficulty with interventions aimed at population differences is that they require a kind of "political will" that is strikingly absent from current social and political policymaking and discourse. The kinds of changes that a focus on between-population vari-ation suggests often include public policies that influence the costs and availability of particu-lar substances (e.g., cigarettes, alcohol), or activities (gambling); in many cases, entrenched industry interests and extant taxation schemes make serious changes to these policies dif-ficult to implement. Perhaps even more problematically, between-population variation is often associated with such seemingly intractable social and political issues as poverty/deprivation, income distribution, and social opportunities. Although it might be true that one reason to oppose, for example, tax policies that result in more unequal distributions of income and wealth is that such unequal income and wealth distributions are associated with higher addiction rates and costs (see below), it would seem that in the United States the pol-itical will is missing even to think seriously about addressing these kinds of inequality.

Given this, there are reasons to worry that genetic research into addiction susceptibil-ity might result in an increased focus on the individual as the proper locus of research, and that the "cause" of addiction might come to be increasingly seen as something internal to the individual addicts. Indeed, in this sense, the move toward explanations of addiction at the genetic level might be seen as an extension of the disease model of addiction and addict-ive behavior (see Edwards, 2010 for a discussion). While the disease model itself has had a tendency to shift the focus to the individual, the search for "susceptibility" genes suggests a move to treating addiction as a *genetic* disease, and hence a disease with roots internal to the individual and ever less connected to the social environment.

It is likely that researchers into the genetics of individual variations in addiction suscep-tibility are being sincere when they state that one of their goals is to find ways of amelior-ating the suffering associated with addiction. But as a way of addressing that suffering, an approach that focuses on the causes of individual variation within a social environment is rather weak. More worrisome, such research is not only likely to fail to seriously reduce the harms associated with addiction, but it is likely to keep the focus of policy discussions and decision making on the individual addicts themselves. By focusing on the individual varia-tions, these approaches provide a way of shifting blame back to the individual addicts. Even if the addicts' *genes* make them more susceptible, by locating the causes of their addictions within the bodies of the addicts themselves, these approaches keep the focus on the individ-uals and away from the broader social environment. If the social environment is not a locus of explanation, changes in the social environment that might be efficacious will not even be considered: the focus will stay away from the broad social and political policy choices that get made and create the environments in which addiction and its associated harms take place. Although it might, in the end, be politically impossible to shift US policy to one that favors more economic equality, for example, if the broad risks associated with the current policy remain hidden (behind discoveries centered on individual variation), the discussion itself becomes impossible.

Explaining human behaviors: Addiction as an example

There are multiple different questions that can be asked about any biological trait, includ-ing the behaviors of biological entities. If asked "what explains this trait?" the answer will depend on exactly what it is about the trait one wants explained. The options include at least the following:

(1) Ontogeny: How does the trait develop? That is: How does the trait in question arise in the development of the individual organism? Developmental accounts can include, for

example, analyses of cell differentiation and the genetic pathways employed, as well as following particular kinds of environmental inputs.

(2) Phylogeny: What explains the presence of the trait in the population (at whatever level it is present)? Historically, how did the trait first emerge, how and why did it spread in the population, and, if it is being actively maintained in the population now, what is the mechanism that is maintaining it? These accounts are *evolutionary* in nature – they attempt to explain, from the perspective of the evolutionary history of the type of organism, how the traits in question came to be. Sometimes this will involve *selective* accounts (fitness variations), sometimes it will involve "phylogenetic inertia," sometimes drift, etc.

(3) Individual variation: If the trait varies between individuals within a population, what explains the *variability* of the trait in that population? Why do different individuals have different versions of the trait, or why do some individuals have the trait and not others? Generally speaking, many – if not most – analyses of individual variation within a population approach the question via an "analysis of variance" and attempt to partition the variation in the population between potential variables causally associated with that variation (often these causes are roughly divided into genetic, environmental, and interactive causes of various sorts). For example, in humans, *most* variation in eye color is the result of genetic variation, whereas *most* variation in finger number is the result of environmental variation (traumatic amputations account for most of the variation in finger number in humans!).

(4) Population variation: If the frequency or form of the trait varies between populations, what explains the variation of that trait between populations? Why do different populations, for example, have different proportions of individuals that have the trait in question, etc.? Here, the question is about why a particular trait is more common in one population than another. Again, this question is usually approached via an analysis of variance, but the variance to be explained is the variance between *populations* rather than individuals within a population.

Although these questions are not strictly independent of one another, each demands attention to a different (but not unique) set of variables, and to different sorts of details; in general each requires different kinds of evidence to answer. Understanding the "genetic contribution" to a trait may involve attempting to answer any (or all!) of the above questions, but what that "genetic contribution" involves, and how it can be tested or explored, is often very different. In Box 14.1, these four questions are explored for two different traits: lactase persistence and nicotine addiction. Lactase persistence is a fairly-well-understood trait – in some populations (those with a history of dairy farming), lactase continues to be produced after infancy, permitting the digestion of lactose (in milk). Most mammals cannot effectively digest milk after infancy, and the nonpersistence of lactase was the "original" state for humans; lactase persistence became prevalent in some populations because it is confers a strong selective advantage. The details in the case of nicotine addiction remain less well established, but nevertheless separating out the different questions provides a sense of the diversity of possible approaches to the seemly straightforward question "What explains nicotine addiction?"

Much of the current genomic research into addictions has focused on individual variation (mainly trying to answer the third kind of question noted above). By contrast, much of the extensive work into the neurobiology of addiction and addictive behaviors has focused

Box 14.1 Different questions, different fields, different evidence: Two examples

Questions/cases	Field/evidence	Lactase persistence[a]	Nicotine addiction[b]
Ontogeny: How does the trait develop?	Developmental biology, including molecular and cellular biology	Change in the promoter region associated with gene expression keeps lactase production high throughout life.	Nicotine addiction develops primarily with self-administration of nicotine, via the effects of nicotine on the (evolutionarily highly conserved) nicotinic acetylcholine receptors (nAChRs).
Phylogeny: What explains the presence of the trait in the population (at whatever level it is present)?	Evolutionary biology; analysis of related species, fitness consequences of the trait in various environments, etc.	History of dairy farming. Populations with a history of dairy farming acquired lactase persistence because of the adaptive advantages of being able to consume dairy foods. It is maintained in populations that consume dairy owing to its continued adaptive significance (different populations have different mutations associated with continued gene expression, revealing that the trait arose independently multiple times in different populations).	The nAChRs are part of a highly conserved (ancient) set of receptors involved in neurotransmission. The nAChRs play functional roles in various tissues in organisms in the Bilateria phylum. Given this, addiction to nicotine can occur with exposure to (self-administered) nicotine, with tobacco use being the primary mechanism in humans.
Individual variation: If the trait varies between individuals within a population, what explains the variability of the trait in that population?	Analysis of variance, quantitative genetics, developmental biology, environmental field work (including, e.g., sociology in humans), ethology	Individual variation in lactose tolerance (lactase persistence) within populations tends to be the result of recent *migration* from other populations. There is some variation within populations due to mutation, etc., but it is not highly significant.	Within different populations, different factors are associated with the probability of an individual's smoking and becoming addicted to nicotine; these include gender, socioeconomic status, etc. In addition to environmental influences, there is some evidence that different variants of the nAChRs may play a role, and there is the possibility of other sorts of genetic variations (say, those associated with impulse control in particular environments, etc.) playing a role as well.

Box 14.1 (*cont.*)

Questions/cases	Field/evidence	Lactase persistence[a]	Nicotine addiction[b]
Population variation: Why do different populations have different proportions of individuals that have the trait in question, for example?	Population genetics, environmental field work, ethology, evolutionary biology including fitness differences associated with different environments, etc.	Rates of lactase persistence vary substantially between populations, based on whether that population has an (evolutionary) history of dairy farming.	Broadly environmental/ social factors, such as tobacco accessibility (including price), social acceptability of smoking, etc., account for much of the variation. Although it is possible that genetic differences between populations might contribute to the different rates of addiction, it seems unlikely that this is a major factor in the different population rates.

[a] See, e.g., Ingram and Swallow, 2007; Ingram et al., 2009.
[b] See, e.g., Mineur and Picciotto, 2008; Benowitz, 2010.

Box 14.2 Epigenetic mechanisms and addiction/addictive behaviors

"Epigenetics," in its most general sense, refers to heritable nongenetic variation; more often, it is used to refer to heritable changes in gene expression. The two most commonly cited examples are *DNA methylation* and changes in the *chromatin structure*. The addition (or removal) of *methyl groups* to DNA modifies gene expression (generally, but not always, methylated genes are "downregulated" or silenced); these changes can be environmentally caused and are partially heritable. Similarly, modifications to the chromatin structure (the physical structure of the DNA and associated proteins) can influence which genes are accessible for transcription and are (partially) heritable. (See Rakyan and Beck, 2006 and citations therein for a review.)

Epigenetic changes can therefore be a part of answering questions about the ontogeny of traits (the first question noted above – how a particular trait develops in an individual organism) as well as about the causes of individual variations in traits (the third question noted above); indeed, in some cases, epigenetic variation might even be part of addressing variation between populations (the fourth question noted above), and might be implicated in certain selective scenarios (and hence relevant to the phylogeny of traits!).

If addiction can modify gene expression, either through modifying methylation or chromatin structure, those changes might explain the stability of addiction (how difficult it is to change addiction/addictive behaviors; see, e.g., Holder, 2009; Sellman, 2009) and the heritability of addiction (see, e.g., Ball, 2007; Agrawal and Lynskey, 2008). There is some compelling evidence that epigenetic effects are implicated in the first of these, but evidence for the second remains merely suggestive. (See Renthal and Nestler, 2008 and citations therein for reviews.) Nevertheless, the possibility of epigenetic inheritance in the case of addiction should not be dismissed.

on the development of addiction (the first kind of question noted above). Although research into the neurobiology of addiction has led to fascinating insights, it is also, as Kalant notes, unlikely to be of much help elucidating the unique nature of addiction (as opposed to, e.g., nonaddictive drug dependence) (Kalant, 2010; see also Carter and Hall, 2010). The mechanisms underlying the neurobiology of addiction would seem to be diverse and ubiquitous, involved in many "normal" functions as well as addiction (Kalant, 2010; for a summary of some of the diverse functions of nicotinic acetylcholine receptors, see Egleton et al., 2008 and citations therein). Likewise, we should expect that the genes involved in those processes are similarly diverse in both their form and their expression. Although there are some promising early results on changes in gene expression associated with addiction/addictive behaviors (see Box 14.2), these have yet to garner significant public attention. In both cases, the failure of these research programs to capture the public attention probably emerges from their addressing a variant of the question "What explains addiction?," which is perceived to be less exciting than explanations that address the causes of individual variation. They do not, in other words, address the kinds of individual risk factors that the public has come to expect from "explanations" of human behavior genetics, or from human epidemiology more generally.

Instead, significant public attention accrues primarily to research associated with explaining individual variations in addiction/addictive behavior; this is true both of genes that are supposed to predispose one to becoming addicted to particular substances and genes that are supposed to predispose one to addictions more generally. For example, consider the following newspaper and magazine headlines:

"Gene keeps some from nicotine addiction, study says." (*New York Times*, 1998)
"Gene linked to addiction, cancer." (*Sydney Morning Herald*, 2008)
"Gene glitch tied to youth smoking addiction." (Fox News, 2004)
"Genes influence smoking addiction: study." (ABC Science, 2010)
"Coffee addiction 'in your genes.'" (Briggs, 2011)
"Addictive personality? You might be a leader." (Linden, 2011)
"Marijuana, alcohol addiction may share genes." (Thomas, 2009)
"Drug addiction could be down to your genes." (Highfield, 2007)
"Gene may protect against alcoholism." (*Los Angeles Times*, 2010)

In each case, the focus is on explaining why some individuals, but not others, are addicts. In some cases, the issue is a specific substance and a specific gene somehow associated with this substance. For example, the article "Gene glitch tied to youth smoking addiction" states that the risk of addiction was "especially high for those [seventh graders] with an inactive CYP2A6 gene" and that this may be because the inactive version of the gene makes "people more vulnerable to nicotine" (Fox News, 2004). The article claiming that coffee addiction is "in your genes" states that "genetic factors could explain why some people consume large amounts of coffee" and that the "two stretches of DNA linked with high caffeine consumption contain two genes thought highly likely to be involved in the way the body processes caffeine" (Briggs, 2011, reporting for the BBC). In other cases, the claims surround not genes specifically involved with particular substances, but rather with personality traits (or general biological pathways) that predispose one to addiction more generally. So for example, the article "Addictive personality? You might be a leader" posits that genetic factors associated with being a "compulsive risk taker" and with "a high degree of novelty-seeking behavior" may partially account for both one's risk of addiction and for behavioral traits associated with engaging in successful high-risk work (Linden, 2011, reporting for the *New York Times*).

Of course, addiction to particular substances is impossible in the absence of the substance; addiction, by its very nature, depends on the environmental availability of the stimulus. But as Lachman (2006) notes, most people who try particular addictive substances or activities do not become dependent: "although initial use of an addictive substance is a necessary step in the development of dependence, clearly such use is not sufficient to cause it" (Lachman, 2006: 134). Lachman asks "what converts a casual drug or alcohol user into an addict, or an occasional gambler into a compulsive one?" This question might be about the mechanisms that underlie addiction in general – one might be asking which developmental processes are associated with people becoming addicts. The difference between addicts and nonaddicts would be cashed out in terms of the particular processes they have undergone, rather than in terms of their preexisting risks. This would focus attention on the first and second questions noted above – on ontogeny and phylogeny. But Lachman's approach to this question instead moves in a very different direction; Lachman notes that a "substantial body of evidence from family, twin, and adoption studies indicates that a genetic component underlies all addiction disorders" (Lachman, 2006: 134), and proceeds to place his focus directly back on attempts to explain individual variations. This is the approach taken by most review articles on the genetics of addiction, as well: the focus is always on the question of individual variation (see, e.g., Agrawal and Lynskey, 2008; Ball, 2007). The interest is in individual variation within a particular social environment rather than on the way the trait develops or on the ways in which the trait varies *between* populations.

The focus on explanations for individual variations within particular (social) environments is hardly unique to research on addiction genetics, or addiction more generally. Indeed, the same pattern can be seen in research into other human behaviors generally seen as troublesome, or even as merely interesting. Longino, for example, has explored the different levels of "uptake," in both the popular media and in further research publications, that different kinds of explanatory projects wrapped up in human behavior receive. She notes that research privileging explanations that focus on *individual differences* (rather than *population differences*) tends to get more uptake in the media (Longino, in press; see also Longino, 2003) and, further, that genetic research is seen as advancing the goal of explaining (and, eventually, manipulating) those differences. So for example, she writes that in the popular media "biologically/genetically oriented research [is] represented as eventually producing results, in contrast to environmental research [which is] represented as terminally inconclusive" and that any criticism of the claims made regarding genes "is presented as but a tempering of claims, rather than as representing an alternative framework for research" (Longino, in press). Longino argues that researchers interested in the genetics of behavior tend to conceptualize behavior "as individual behavior" and take "difference and variation among individuals" as their explanatory target, with "research focused on population/ecological issues" making "no appearance" (Longino, in press).

So, for example, research into the biological and genetic correlates to individual variation in violence/violent behavior has historically had, and continues to have, more "uptake" in both the popular press and the academic literatures than has research into the broader social correlates to violence and violent behavior. Consider, for example, Caspi et al.'s (2002) work on gene-by-environment interactions in the production of violent behavior. Famously, Caspi et al. found that male children born with one variant of the *MAOA* gene (more precisely, the shorter rather than longer promoter region) had a higher risk of committing violent crimes as adults, but *only* if they also grew up in households with significant violence (households with serious domestic violence) (Caspi et al., 2002). Children with the short version of the promoter were *not* at higher risk if their households were not violent. Children with *either* version were at higher risk in violent households than in nonviolent households, but the risk was much greater for children with the short version. Headlines reporting this research ranged from the relatively cautious "Scientists identify gene that may trigger violence in abused children," to the rather bolder "Genetic link to cycle of violence identified," through to the rather absurd "Beware the aggression gene" (*Milwaukee Journal Sentinel*, 2002).

But while many of these sources dutifully reported that the small fraction (about 12%) of men in the study who had both the short *MAOA* gene variant *and* a history of abuse as children were responsible for almost half of the violent crimes, the disparity between the levels of violent crimes cross-culturally (and especially cross-nationally) was less well reported (see below for more on this issue). This is not surprising; Caspi et al. ended their article with the claim that their "findings could inform the development of future pharmacological treatments" (Caspi et al., 2002: 853). Whereas Caspi et al. were ostensibly focused on the ways that different genes interacted with different environments in the production of human behaviors, the focus shifts rapidly to *biochemical* intervention and away from environmental intervention. As Longino notes, despite Caspi et al.'s research's supposed focus on "integrative" biology and the *interaction* between genes and environment, in fact the model they offer "is treated as an insight into how a specific gene works" rather than as the beginning of a truly integrative approach to the development of particular traits (Longino, in press).

Changing behaviors: Individuals and populations in the modification of human behaviors

For studies of human behaviors that are subject to social disapproval, the companion to *explaining* the behaviors in question is *controlling* them. And indeed, both research articles and media reports on the genetics of addictive behaviors follow this pattern; *explaining* addiction is seen as the first step in *preventing* or *curing* addiction. From research articles, claims like the following are common:

> An increased understanding of the mechanisms of nicotine addiction has led to the development of novel medications (e.g., varenicline) that act on specific nicotinic receptor subtypes. The development of other drugs that act on nicotinic receptors and other mediators of nicotine addiction is likely to further enhance the effectiveness of smoking-cessation pharmacotherapy. (Benowitz, 2010)
>
> Applied genomic research has a role to play in … [identifying] biologic targets for intervention such as drugs and vaccines. Although most clinical applications of genomics are not ready for widespread use, there is an increasing need to develop, evaluate, and integrate genomic tools into clinical and public health research. (Khoury et al., 2005)
>
> Future [addiction] research must also find a role for genotypes, either as guides to new therapeutic targets or as predictors for treatment and prevention, in natural populations of patients and individuals at risk where the efficacy of new tools can objectively be defined and integrated into multidimensional management. (Goldman et al., 2005)

In these cases, the expressed hope is that research that attempts to explain the individual *variations* in addiction (why some people become addicts and not others) will also be useful for developing *interventions* that can be applied in individual cases. This line is followed in the news media as well. For example, in a 2007 article in *The Telegraph*, Highfield reports that Dalley said of his research into the genetics of traits that predispose one to addiction that it "may provide important new leads in the search for improved therapies for compulsive brain disorders" (Highfield, 2007). And, capitalizing on the idea that knowing one's *risk* of acquiring an addiction might change one's behaviors, Roan argued, in an article in the *Los Angeles Times*, that genes associated with variations in alcohol metabolism "might be used in the future to give people, especially young people who have not yet started to drink, an idea of their odds of developing alcohol problems" (Roan, 2010).

In "Do we need genomic research for the prevention of common diseases with environmental causes?" Khoury et al. (2005) argue that although population-based approaches aimed at modifying the environmental risk factors for common diseases might be effective, this focus should not detract from a focus on individual treatment. They write for example that "although we know that smoking and drugs cause disease, they also cause addiction, undermining interventions focused exclusively on the causative environmental agents ... new knowledge derived from applied genomic research could lead to new pharmacologic and behavioral methods of combating addiction to tobacco and drugs" (Khoury et al., 2005: 800).

Over a quarter of a century ago, Rose argued that strategies to address population health were likely to be very different than those that addressed individual health, and that population-based approaches had the potential to impact population health in ways that individual approaches could not (Rose, 1985). Khoury et al. acknowledge Rose's basic point, but argue that "both high-risk approaches to prevention (those targeted toward high-risk subgroups) and population approaches to prevention will be needed" to address common diseases, and that since "individual" and "population" approaches are not in competition, "we should strive to develop, validate, and integrate applied genomic tools in our public health research agenda" (Khoury et al., 2005: 804). But this misses what Rose regarded as the "radical" aspect of a population focus – namely, that by focusing on *between* rather than *within* population variation, far more variability is revealed. Rose writes that:

> There is hardly a disease whose incidence rate does not vary widely, either over time or between populations at the same time. This means that these causes of incidence rates, unknown though they are, are not inevitable. It is possible to live without them, and if we knew what they were it might be possible to control them. (Rose, 1985: 34)

Although the ostensible focus of Khoury et al. is, again, the need for an integrative approach, the focus remains on variations within particular cultures, and on high-risk individuals and high-risk environments. There may be no competition *in principle* between those approaches focused on individual risk and those approaches focused on the variations in population-level incidence, but *in practice* the individual-based approach easily becomes the "default" in these cases.

Consider again the claim by Caspi et al. noted above, that their findings regarding the interaction between abusive home environments and particular alleles in the production of violent adults "could inform the development of future pharmacological treatments" (Caspi et al., 2002: 853). Perhaps it could. But the idea of identifying high-risk children – those with both the shorter MAOA promoter variant *and* who are exposed to serious domestic abuse in their homes – and addressing that risk *by drugging the children* seems, on the face of it, insane. Given that whichever gene variant the children had, being exposed to serious domestic abuse *raised* the probability of their becoming violent adults, "treating" the problem by changing the MAOA levels would have *less* of an impact, *ceteris paribus*, than changing the level of violence in the household. And of course, preventing domestic violence is a worthy goal *whatever* effects it has on the children's chances of becoming violent adults!

Even leaving aside Caspi et al.'s particular findings and recommendations, the focus on the individual as the locus of intervention would seem to be, in the case of violence, deeply and obviously misguided. The refrain from researchers into the biological correlates of violence is that, cross-culturally, a small fraction (6–12%) of the young men commit a large fraction (50–70%) of the violent crimes; but while that may be true, the *rates* of violent crime vary between cultures by more than an order of magnitude. (For a discussion, see Kaplan, 2007 and citations therein.) Consider, for example, the difference in violent crime rate between the countries of southern Africa (with over 30 homicides per 100 000 per year) and those in western Europe (with less than 3 homicides per 100 000 per year) (see GBAV, 2008). Surely, if one is interested in ameliorating the burdens associated with violent crime, these profound differences in rates *between* cultures represents a greater potential source of change than does a focus on some large set of supposedly high-risk individuals (this, again, is what Rose refers to as the "radical" aspect of population health; Rose, 1985).

It is reasonable to suggest that the case is similar for addiction. For example, rates of nicotine addiction follow (roughly) the rates of smoking, and as the percentage of smokers in the population drops, so too do the number of addicted smokers. In the United States, the prevalence of smoking dropped from a high of over 40% in 1965 to around 20% in 2010 (see Levy et al., 2010: 1253), and the average number of cigarettes smoked per person per year dropped from a high of over 4300 per person in the mid-1960s to around 2300 per person by 1999 (Gale et al., 2010); it goes without saying, one hopes, that the distribution of genes associated with nicotine addiction did not change that rapidly in the United States. Higher cigarette prices (via taxation), changing media messages, and "clean air laws" (smoking ban in workplaces and other public areas) resulted in fewer people initiating smoking, more people trying to quit, and in smokers reducing the average number of cigarettes smoked per day. There are good reasons to think that further reductions in smoking (and nicotine addiction) rates could be achieved with further population-based policy changes along the same lines (see Levy et al., 2007 and citations therein), independently of the genetics involved in individual variation.

More generally, rates of addiction vary with socioeconomic status (within societies) and with the overall degree of social inequality within a society (between societies). People who are at the lower end of the socioeconomic scale are more likely to be addicts (more likely to be addicted smokers, illegal drug users, problem gamblers, etc.) than people at the upper end of the socioeconomic scale, and people within societies that are more unequal are more likely to be addicts than people who live in societies that are more equal (see, e.g., Wilkinson and Marmot, 2003; Room, 2005; Baumann et al., 2007). There are two immediate lessons to be drawn from this. First, individual genotyping for addiction risk or tailored pharmaceutical intervention is unlikely to have a profound effect on addiction rates, given that the people most at risk are the least likely to be in a position to access new medical technologies. That is, as the poor within a society are generally the least likely to have access to the latest medical technologies, high-technology targeted approaches are most likely to miss the very people who suffer the most from addictive disorders. Second, approaches that treat the individual as the proper focus for addiction prevention and amelioration will miss those variables associated with the most dramatic differences in addiction rates. One is unlikely to pay attention to cross-cultural variability and the associated different levels of harm in different cultures if one is focused on the causes of individual variation *within* particular cultures or social environments.

The individualization and internalization of addiction as disease

There is nothing inherently wrong with research that investigates individual variations in addiction; indeed, as Khoury et al. (2005) forcefully argue, research into individual variation in human behaviors can be a valuable research tool. But such research is not without its risks. A focus on what makes *this* individual more susceptible to addiction than *that* individual can make the individual out to be the (only) proper locus of explanation and intervention. If it is individuals who are at risk of addiction because of (in part) their particular genetic (and other) endowments, it is natural to focus on those "at-risk" individuals, rather than the broader social environment, when thinking about addiction.

That this kind of individualization of risk can be problematic with respect to public policy is perhaps most obviously seen in the case of gambling addiction/pathological gambling. Despite ongoing arguments regarding whether non-substance-abuse-based disorders should count as "addictions" (see, e.g., Petry, 2006; Potenza, 2008), studies of the genetics of gambling addiction make the same sorts of claims as studies of other addictive behaviors, both with respect to their findings and the reasons for pursuing the research. For example, Lobo and Kennedy state that "results from family and genetic investigations corroborate further the importance of understanding the biological underpinnings of PG [pathological gambling] in the development of more specific treatment and prevention strategies" (Lobo and Kennedy, 2009). Again, the focus is on individual variation – why some people but not others "exposed" to gambling develop problems (become addicted), with an emphasis on which factors *internal* to the person in question determine that person's risk of being a pathological gambler.

The idea that the pathological gambler is a type of person – that one's risk of becoming a pathological gambler is determined mainly or at least in large part by one's particular circumstances, including one's genetic endowments – feeds into the idea that pathological gamblers are simply an inevitable part of gambling's existence. In an interview on *60 Minutes*, Pennsylvania Governor Ed Rendell repeats the refrain that the proximity of gambling opportunities does not create new problem gamblers, and that given that problem gamblers will be problem gamblers (and lose their money) whatever Pennsylvania does, it is better that the money lost by Pennsylvanians stays in Pennsylvania. When Lesley Stahl asks him if he is concerned that the easy availability of gambling in Pennsylvania has resulted in more people becoming problem gamblers, he responds with visible annoyance that "You don't listen. Anyone who has that bent would be doing it in other places had Pennsylvania not legalized gambling" (CBS News, 2011). This is essentially the line taken by the American Gaming Association (AGA); for example, Frank Fahrenkopf, the AGA's President, argues that problem gamblers constitute "somewhere between 1–5% of the population" and that they are "people who can't help themselves and will go in and gamble away their money" (Koughan, 1997). Later, Fahrenkopf takes the internalization route quite directly when he argues that "despite the exponential growth of the gaming industry during the past 30 years, the prevalence rate of pathological gambling has held steady. Approximately 1 percent of the population suffers from pathological gambling, and an additional 2 percent have problems gambling" (Fahrenkopf, 2010). If the availability of gambling created problem gamblers,

Fahrenkopf implies, the prevalence rate of pathological gambling should be increasing along with the growth of the gaming industry.

These quite plausible-sounding arguments regarding the prevalence rates suggested by Fahrenkopf and others, combined with idea that there is something about the individuals that makes those people become problem gamblers, are what allows people like Governor Rendell to claim that creating new opportunities to gamble does not create new problem gamblers, but rather simply results in problem gamblers gambling in one location (or on one kind of game) rather than another. It suggests that any attempt to address problem gambling must address those particular problem gamblers (or people at a high risk of becoming problem gamblers), because, given the impossibility of completely eliminating gambling opportunities, no other approach could reasonably be expected to reduce the prevalence of problem gambling. Of course, it also permits cities and states to support gambling as a revenue source without having to acknowledge that their actions might create problem gamblers where none were before.

This reasoning fails to take into account several lines of evidence. The prevalence of problem gambling does seem to depend critically on the availability of (particular kinds of) gambling opportunities. Perhaps the most famous example comes from the 14-week period in 1994 when video lotteries, which had been widespread, were unavailable in South Dakota (the South Dakota courts having declared them illegal), before a voter referendum reinstated them (see Carr et al., 1996). During that time, other forms of gambling remained available ("regular" lotteries, "scratch ticket" lotteries, and Native American casinos all remained legally available). However, South Dakota agencies treating problematic gambling reported a sharp drop in both inquiries and the number of gamblers actually treated during that period, with a return to higher numbers after the video lottery games were reinstated (Carr et al., 1996: 31). There is also considerable evidence that proximity to particular kinds of gambling opportunities *does* influence the chances that a person will engage in problematic gambling behavior and/or become a pathological gambler. The National Gambling Impact Study found that pathological gambling risk roughly doubles within 50 miles of gambling facilities, and that "some of the greatest increases in the number of problem and pathological gamblers shown in these repeated surveys came over periods of expanded gambling opportunities in the states studied" (NGIS, 1999; see also Reith and The Scottish Centre for Social Research, 2006 for similar results in the context of Scotland; on more multidimensional approaches to opportunity, see for example Thomas et al., 2011). How the results of these studies jibe, or fail to jibe, with the data on the relative stability of problem gambling rates in the United States as a whole is an interesting problem; the suggestion that the relative stability of problem gambling rates in US surveys is an artifact of the survey methodology and the ways in which the gaming industry has so far grown should not be dismissed.

It is not obvious what policy implications, if any, should be drawn from these more social (or "ecological," see, e.g., Welte et al., 2006) accounts of gambling addiction, including the substantial evidence that gambling availability influences the rate of problem gambling. However, it *is* obvious that these more multidimensional accounts point toward *more options* for policymakers than do strictly individual accounts. If problem gambling is seen to be the result only of features internal to the problem gambler, rules limiting the kinds of gambling available and/or the locations of availability will simply not be considered; if problem gambling is considered a multidimensional problem in which particular kinds of games and availability will come together with individuals to produce particular kinds and numbers of problem gamblers, such changes will at least be seen as possible responses. Whether modifying the availability of (kinds of) gambling opportunities would have benefits that outweigh the costs is of course debatable and, indeed, should be a matter for policymakers and public debate; however, a view of gambling addiction as caused by something *internal to the addict* cuts off that debate before it can start.

A similar scenario may be playing out now with respect to nicotine addiction. The tobacco industry, having been forced to admit to the serious health impacts of tobacco use, would seem to be poised to argue that nicotine is not addictive *per se*, but rather is only addictive for those people who are genetically predisposed to be nicotine addicts. For most people, smoking would be a "choice," but for those genetically predisposed to addiction, it would be the result of a genetic disease; in neither case would tobacco companies be to blame (or liable) for people's smoking habits. Gundle et al. (2010) argue that as early as the mid-1970s tobacco industry public relations and legal teams had considered actively pursuing the idea that nicotine might be addictive for *some* people genetically predisposed to nicotine addiction, but nonaddictive for everyone else; Gundle et al. argue that the primary reason the tobacco industry did not actively pursue that argument was that the industry was still officially denying that nicotine was addictive *at all* and did not want to be seen to be supporting research that might undermine that official position (Gundle et al., 2010: 976–978). However, given that the addictive nature of nicotine is now well established, Gundle et al. argue that research pointing toward nicotine addiction as a feature of particular individuals with particular genetic traits, rather than a feature of the nicotine itself, could be useful to the tobacco industry for both legal defenses and, perhaps more importantly, for advertising to future smokers (Gundle et al., 2010: 979). "The tobacco industry can argue that the genetic revolution, including genetic research not funded by the industry, is confirming what they have long known: that a crucial component of nicotine addiction is genetic and that there is a small number of people who should not smoke, but for the vast majority of people cigarettes are a product that can be used in a responsible and voluntary way" (Gundle et al., 2010: 979). Genetic tests could be marketed, and the idea is that those people who are less susceptible to nicotine addiction could "safely" choose to smoke, as they would be able to control the quantity and style of their smoking, and that they would be able to quit any time they chose.

This is not a message that most researchers interested in improving public health could possibly approve of; increased rates of tobacco use would be problematic from a public health standpoint, even if those people *most* susceptible to nicotine addiction were somehow alerted to their special risk and were able to avoid smoking. Indeed, Gundle et al. argue that the "tobacco industry's agenda in promoting the notion of 'addiction-free' smokers is at odds with goals of genetic researchers who hope to understand more clearly the biology of addiction or provide new and better targeted therapies for tobacco dependence," and that research focused on finding genetic variation between individuals in how susceptible they are to nicotine addiction is in danger of being "co-opted" by the tobacco industry (Gundle et al., 2010: 979). But research that is focused on each potential smoker's individual risk, and on developing new treatments for individual smokers, is easy to co-opt. The idea behind such research, after all, is that individuals who are particularly susceptible to nicotine addiction can be targeted for particular interventions, including being warned of their particular susceptibility; those who are already addicted can be targeted with specific pharmacological treatments aimed at the particular pathways that make them addicts. In principle, this would address the goal of ameliorating the harms of smoking, a goal shared by many researchers. And of course, this position aligns nicely with a position that makes smoking – or at least nicotine addiction – out to be a matter of factors that are internal to the addict, a view that the tobacco industry might very well find useful.

Although it might be possible to target high-risk individuals for intervention, the goal of using these screening techniques and associated interventions to actually improve population health (that is, to have a meaningful impact on the costs and harms associated with tobacco use) will remain unrealized in the vast majority of those cases in which smoking remains a major health concern. One problem is that the very people who suffer most from tobacco-related illnesses and other attendant costs are the least likely to benefit from individualized high-technological approaches; these include particular subpopulations within societies (usually the poor, but also the disenfranchised more generally) as well as, for example, developing nations. Again, one of the lessons of a public health approach to improving population health is that individual interventions aimed at "high-risk" individuals *rarely* have a measurable impact on population health (Rose, 1985; see Frohlich and Potvin, 2008 and citations therein for a more contemporary review). In this case, given that the people currently most at risk (Cokkinides et al., 2009) from smoking-related illnesses are those who are least likely to have access to personalized medicine (such as personal genetic-pharmacological and genome-based medicines, etc.), the ability of these approaches based on individual risk to make a substantial difference should seem even more dubious (for further discussion of these related difficulties, see e.g., Hall et al., 2008; for skepticism regarding the clinical utility of genetic testing for addiction more generally, see Munafò, 2009a). On the other hand, reducing the harms of nicotine addiction and smoking via policy shifts is likely to be efficacious and requires no new technologies or discoveries, and it can be implemented at a variety of different levels of social organization (see e.g., Levy et al., 2007; Cokkinides et al., 2009; Levy et al., 2010; but see Holder, 2009 for a more cautious appraisal of the success of current public programs).

Conclusions: Thinking about risk

Human behavioral genetics can highlight the roles that people's different genetic endowments play in behaviors that vary within particular social environments. Research on the genetics of addiction/addictive behaviors has tended to follow this path, focusing on the genetics of the different levels of risk for addiction or addictive behaviors associated with different individuals. Although the hype surrounding the possibility of using genetic discoveries to develop new treatments has so far outpaced the reality, there can be little doubt that most researchers in this area are driven by a sincere desire to understand addiction and work toward ameliorating the harms associated with addiction and addictive behaviors (see, e.g., Smith et al., 2005; O'Brien, 2007).

However, in thinking through the results of contemporary genetics research into addiction, we should remain mindful of the lessons of public health approaches to improving the health of populations. Even if we find genes that "predispose" particular people to addiction (either to particular addictions or to addictions in general) within a particular social environment, those genes may or may not be associated with an increased risk of addiction in a different social environment, and even if they are so associated, the risk of addiction in different social environments may be very different indeed. It may turn out that if we want to reduce the harms associated with addiction and addictive behavior, looking to the reasons that rates of addictive behaviors vary *between* populations will reveal more effective possible interventions than will attention to individual variation. Indeed, even where rates of addiction may be similar in different social environments, the harms associated with those addictions may be very different in those different social environments, and attention to those kinds of differences may point toward effective interventions that can lessen the harms associated with the addictions (see, e.g., Stegmayr et al., 2005 on "snus" use and nicotine addiction in Sweden).

Human behavioral genetics is fraught with difficulties, but the potential for it to generate real insights should not be dismissed. But these insights, focused as they so often are on explaining individual variation within societies, are not guaranteed to be useful – indeed, they may not even be *likely* to be useful – for making major improvements in population health, or for significantly reducing the costs and harms associated with addiction. And the excitement surrounding the insights of human behavioral genetics on addiction must not be permitted to distract us from aggressively pursuing research into the public health aspects of addiction and addictive behaviors. Although it is often unclear that there is the political will to pursue the kinds of population-based strategies for harm reduction that public health approaches give us good reason to believe would be effective, such research at least invites consideration of those sorts of policies.

References

ABC Science (2010). Genes influence smoking addiction: study. April 26, 2010. Available online at: www.abc.net.au/science/articles/2010/04/26/2882597.htm [accessed March 9, 2012].

Agrawal, A. and Lynskey, M. T. (2008). Are there genetic influences on addiction: Evidence from family, adoption and twin studies. *Addiction*, 103, 1069–1081.

Ball, D. (2007). Addiction science and its genetics. *Addiction*, 103, 360–367.

Baumann, M., Spitz, E., Guillemin, F., et al. (2007). Associations of social and material deprivation with tobacco, alcohol, and psychotropic drug use, and gender: A population-based study. *International Journal of Health Geographics*, 6, 50.

Benowitz, N. L. (2010). Nicotine addiction. *New England Journal of Medicine*, 362, 2295–2303.

Berrettini, W., Bierut, L., Crowley, T. J., et al. (2004). Setting priorities for genomic research. *Science*, 304, 1445–1446.

Briggs, H. (2011). Coffee addiction "in your genes". BBC News, April 8, 2011. Available online at: www.bbc.co.uk/news/health-12992374 [accessed March 9, 2012].

Carr, R. D., Buchkoski, J. E., Kofoed, L., and Morgan, T. J. (1996). "Video lottery" and treatment for pathological gambling. A natural experiment in South Dakota. *South Dakota Journal of Medicine*, 49, 30–32.

Carter, A. and Hall, W. D. (2010). The need for more explanatory humility in addiction neurobiology. *Addiction*, 105, 790–796.

Caspi, A., McClay, J., Moffitt, T. E., et al. (2002). Role of genotype in the cycle of violence in maltreated children. *Science*, 297, 851–854.

CBS News (2011). Slot machines: The big gamble. *60 Minutes*. January 10, 2011. Available online at: www.cbsnews.com/video/watch/?id=7228424n [accessed March 9, 2012].

Cokkinides, V., Bandi, P., McMahon, C., et al. (2009). Tobacco control in the United States: Recent progress and opportunities. *CA Cancer Journal for Clinicians*, 59, 352–365.

Ducci, F. and Goldman, D. (2008). Genetic approaches to addiction: genes and alcohol. *Addiction*, 103, 1414–1428.

Edwards, G. (2010). The trouble with drink: Why ideas matter. *Addiction*, 105, 797–804.

Egleton, R. D., Brown, K. C., and Dasgupta, P. (2008). Nicotinic acetylcholine receptors: Multiple roles in proliferation and inhibition of apoptosis. *Trends in Pharmacological Sciences*, 29, 151–158.

Fahrenkopf, Jr., F. J. (2010). Gambling disorders: A new understanding, a new definition. Published by Global Gaming Business. Available online at: www.americangaming. org/newsroom/op-eds/gambling-disorders-new-understanding-new-definition [accessed March 13, 2012].

Fox News (2004). Gene glitch tied to youth smoking addiction. Published November 24, 2004. Available online at: www.foxnews. com/story/0,2933,139484,00.html [accessed March 9, 2012].

Frohlich, K. L. and Potvin, L. (2008). Government, politics, and law: Transcending the known in public health practice. *American Journal of Public Health*, 98, 216–221.

Gale, H. F. Jr., Foreman, L., and Capehart, T. (2010). *Tobacco and the Economy: Farms, jobs, and communities.* Economic Research Service, US Department of Agriculture, Agricultural Economic Report No. 789. Available online at: www.ers.usda.gov/ publications/aer789/ [accessed March 13, 2012].

GBAV (2008). The global burden of armed violence. Geneva Declaration Secretariat, Geneva. Available online at: www. genevadeclaration.org/fileadmin/docs/ Global-Burden-of-Armed-Violence-full-report.pdf [accessed March 5, 2012].

Goldman, D., Oroszi, G., and Ducci, F. (2005). The genetics of addictions: uncovering the genes. *Nature Reviews Genetics*, 6, 521–532.

Gundle, K. R., Dingel, M. J., and Koenig, B. A. (2010). Vested interests in addiction research and policy "to prove this is the industry's best hope": big tobacco's support of research on the genetics of nicotine addiction. *Addiction*, 105, 974–983.

Hall, W. D., Gartner, C. E., and Carter, A. (2008). The genetics of nicotine addiction liability: ethical and social policy implications. *Addiction*, 103, 350–359.

Highfield, R. (2007). Drug addiction could be down to your genes. *The Telegraph*. March 2, 2007. Available online at: www.telegraph. co.uk/news/uknews/1544336/Drug-addiction-could-be-down-to-your-genes. html [accessed March 13, 2012].

Holder, H. (2009). Prevention programs in the 21st century: what we do not discuss in public. *Addiction*, 105, 578–581.

Ingram, C. J. E. and Swallow, D. M. (2007). Population genetics of lactase persistence and lactose intolerance. In *Encyclopedia of the Life Sciences.* Chichester, UK: John Wiley & Sons.

Ingram, C. J. E., Mulcare, C. A., Itan, Y. Thomas, M. G., and Swallow, D. M. (2009). Lactose digestion and the evolutionary genetics of lactase persistence. *Human Genetics*, 124, 579–591.

Ioannidis, J. P. A., Ntzani, E. E., Trikalinos, T. A., and Contopoulos-Ioannidis, D. G. (2001). Replication validity of genetic association studies. *Nature Genetics*, 29, 306–309.

Kalant, H. (2010). What neurobiology cannot tell us about addiction. *Addiction*, 105, 780–789.

Kaplan, J. (2006). Misinformation, misrepresentation, and misuse of human behavioral genetics research. *Law and Contemporary Problems*, 69, 47–80.

Kaplan, J. (2007). Violence and public health: Exploring the relationship between biological perspectives on violent behavior and public health approaches to violence prevention. In H. Kincaid and J. Mckitrick (eds.), *Establishing Medical Reality.* Dordrecht: Springer, pp. 199–214.

Khoury, M. J., Davis, R., Gwinn, M., Lindegren, M. L., and Yoon, P. (2005). Do we need genomic research for the prevention of common diseases with environmental causes? *American Journal of Epidemiology*, 161, 799–805.

Koughan, M. (1997). Easy money. Frontline. June 10, 1997. Available online at: www.pbs. org/wgbh/pages/frontline/shows/gamble/ [accessed March 9, 2012].

Lachman, H. M. (2006). An overview of the genetics of substance use disorders. *Current Psychiatry Reports*, 8, 133–143.

Levy, D. T., Hyland, A., Higbee, C., Remer, L., and Compton, C. (2007). The role of public policies in reducing smoking prevalence in California: Results from the California Tobacco Policy Simulation Model. *Health Policy*, 82, 167–185.

Levy, D. T., Mabry, P. L., Graham, A. L., Orleans, C. T., and Abrams, D. B. (2010). Exploring scenarios to dramatically reduce smoking prevalence: A simulation model of the three-part cessation process. *American Journal of Public Health*, 100, 1253–1259.

Linden, D. J. (2011). Addictive personality? You might be a leader. *New York Times*, July 24, 2011, p. SR4.

Lobo, D. S. S. and Kennedy, J. L. (2009). Genetic aspects of pathological gambling: a complex disorder with shared genetic vulnerabilities. *Addiction*, 104, 1454–1465.

Longino, H. (2003). Behavior as affliction: Common frameworks of behavior genetics and its rivals. In L. S. Parker and R. A. Ankeny (eds.), *Mutating Concepts, Evolving Disciplines: Genetics, Medicine, and Society*. Amsterdam, Netherlands: Kluwer Academic Publishers, pp. 165–187.

Longino, H. (in press). *Understanding the Sciences of Human Behavior* (working title). Forthcoming from the University of Chicago Press. Quotes are from a lecture at the Konrad Lorenz Institute's workshop on "The Roles of Theory in Biology" June, 2011.

Los Angeles Times (2010). Gene may protect against alcoholism. Published on October 20, 2010. Available online at: http://articles.latimes.com/2010/oct/20/news/la-heb-alcohol-gene-20101020 [accessed March 9, 2012].

Merikangas, K. and Risch, N. (2003). Genomic priorities and public health. *Science*, 302, 599–601.

Milwaukee Journal Sentinel (2002). Beware the aggression gene. Published on August 15, 2002, 18A.

Mineur, Y. S. and Picciotto, M. R. (2008). Genetics of nicotinic acetylcholine receptors: relevance to nicotine addiction. *Biochemical Pharmacology*, 75, 323–333.

Minino, A.M. and Smith, B. L. (2001). Deaths: Preliminary data for 2000. *National Vital Statistics Reports 49*. Hyattsville, MD: National Center for Health Statistics.

MMWR (2008). Smoking – attributable mortality, years of potential life lost, and productivity losses – United States, 2000–2004. The Centers for Disease Control and Prevention *Morbidity and Mortality Weekly Report*, 57, November 14, 2008.

Munafò, M. R. (2009a). The clinical utility of genetic tests. *Addiction*, 104, 127–128.

Munafò, M. R. (2009b). Reliability and replicability of genetic association studies. *Addiction*, 104, 1439–1440.

New York Times (1998). Gene keeps some from nicotine addiction, study says. Published on June 25, 1998. Available online at: www.nytimes.com/1998/06/25/us/gene-keeps-some-from-nicotine-addiction-study-says.html [accessed March 9, 2012].

NGIS (1999). National Gambling Impact Study Commission final report, chapter 4: Problem and pathological gambling. Available online at: http://govinfo.library.unt.edu/ngisc/reports/fullrpt.html [accessed March 9, 2012].

O'Brien, C. (2007). Commentary: Treatment of addiction in the era of genomic medicine. *Addiction*, 102, 1696–1700.

Petry, N. M. (2006). Should the scope of addictive behaviors be broadened to include pathological gambling? *Addiction*, 101(S1), 152–160.

Potenza, M. N. (2008). The neurobiology of pathological gambling and drug addiction: an overview and new findings. *Philosophical Transactions of the Royal Society B: Biological Sciences*, 363, 3181–3189.

Rakyan, V. K. and Beck, S. (2006). Epigenetic variation and inheritance in mammals. *Current Opinion in Genetics & Development*, 16, 573–577.

Reith, G. and The Scottish Centre for Social Research. (2006). Research on the social impacts of gambling: final report. Available online at: www.scotland.gov.uk/Publications/2006/08/17134534/0 [accessed March 9, 2012].

Renthal, W. and Nestler, E. J. (2008). Epigenetic mechanisms in drug addiction. *Trends in Molecular Medicine*, 14, 341–350.

Rice, D. P. (1999). Economic costs of substance abuse, 1995. *Proceedings of the Association of American Physicians*, 111, 119–125.

Roan, S. (2010). Gene may protect against alcoholism. *Los Angeles Times*, October 20, 2010. Available online at: http://articles.latimes.com/2010/oct/20/news/la-heb-alcohol-gene-20101020 [accessed March 12, 2012].

Room, R. (2005). Stigma, social inequality and alcohol and drug use. *Drug and Alcohol Review*, 24, 143–155.

Rose, G. (1985). Sick individuals and sick populations. *International Journal of Epidemiology*, 14, 32–38.

Sellman, D. (2009). The 10 most important things known about addiction. *Addiction*, 105, 6–13.

Smith, G. D., Ebrahim S., Lewis S., et al. (2005). Genetic epidemiology and public health: Hope, hype, and future prospects. *Lancet*, 366, 1484–1498.

Stegmayr, B., Eliasson, M., and Rodu, B. (2005). The decline of smoking in Northern Sweden. *Scandinavian Journal of Public Health*, 33, 321–324.

Sydney Morning Herald (2008). Gene linked to addiction, cancer. Published on April 3, 2008. Available online at: www.smh.com.au/news/science/gene-linked-to-addiction-cancer/2008/04/02/1206851016947.html [accessed March 9, 2012].

Thomas, A. C., Bates, G., Moore, S., et al. (2011). Gambling and the multidimensionality of accessibility: More than just proximity to venues. *International Journal of Mental Health and Addiction*, 9, 88–101.

Thomas, J. (2009). Marijuana, alcohol addiction may share genes. *Bloomberg Businessweek*, December 18, 2009. Available online at: www.businessweek.com/lifestyle/content/healthday/634259.html [accessed March 13, 2012].

Welte, J. W., Wieczorek, W. F., Barnes, G. M., and Tidwell, M-C. O. (2006). Multiple risk factors for frequent and problem gambling: Individual, social, and ecological. *Journal of Applied Social Psychology*, 36, 1548–1568.

Wilkinson, R. and Marmot, M. (eds.) (2003). *Social Determinants of Health: The Solid Facts*, 2nd edition. Geneva: World Health Organization.

15

Summary and recommendations: Ethical guidance for genetic research on addiction and its translation into public policy

Audrey R. Chapman, Jonathan M. Kaplan, and
Adrian Carter

The contributions to this volume identify ethical considerations implicated in genetic research on addiction and their translation into public policy. This chapter draws conclusions and proposes specific recommendations to guide research practice and help shape policy development based on this analysis. It should be noted that the views expressed in the summary and recommendations represent the views of the three authors of this chapter and may not necessarily be those of the authors of the rest of the chapters in this volume. The guidance is organized into four sections: (1) conceptualizing addiction; (2) the limitations of behavioral genetics in general and addiction genetics in particular; (3) research ethics; and (4) the translation and interpretation of addiction genetics research.

Conceptualizing addiction

The manner in which addiction is conceptualized has been a controversial topic, with implications for the treatment of affected individuals and for social policy. Addiction is usually thought of as comprising a combination of three characteristics: physical dependence (e.g., physical symptoms of withdrawal and tolerance), psychological dependence (e.g., drug cravings), and harmful use. Most addicts will exhibit all three, but the manner in which they are manifested at different points can vary significantly. For example, it is possible to be addicted to largely nonharmful substances, i.e., caffeine. There are also forms of addiction that do not entail significant physical dependence: pathological gambling, for instance, is a harmful pattern of gambling that primarily involves psychological dependence. Conversely, substances may be used in ways that cause considerable acute physical and social harm in the absence of either psychological or physical dependence (e.g., alcohol-induced violence, drunk driving). It is also possible to develop a physical dependence to a substance in the absence of psychological dependency. For example, the administration of opiates by a physician or other third party, often in the treatment of pain, may lead to physical dependence (e.g., tolerance to the pharmacological effects of opiates necessitating increasing doses to maintain the same analgesic effects or adverse withdrawal symptoms following abrupt cessation of opiates), but no psychological dependence (i.e., no psychological need to use a drug post-detoxification).

There are three basic models that are used to explain or understand addiction: the moral, biomedical, and psychological models. Each contributes important insights into the nature

Genetic Research on Addiction, ed. Audrey R. Chapman. Published by Cambridge University Press.
© Cambridge University Press 2012.

of addiction. Of the three, the biomedical model, broadly conceived, provides the fullest explanation of addiction and is the best supported by scientific research. Informed by neuroscience research and brain-imaging studies, the biomedical approach associates an addicted person's drug-seeking behavior with changes in the structure and function of the brain caused by chronic substance use. The biomedical model does not necessarily entail a reductive genetic or neuro-essentialist conception of addiction that fails to take into account the importance of social, environmental, and cultural factors. Nor does it imply that individuals with an addiction lack any control over their decision making and therefore should not be considered morally accountable for their behavior. Regardless of perspectives about the nature of addiction, most ethicists, even those who acknowledge that addiction at a minimum involves a partial impairment of decision-making capacity, still concur that individuals with addictions should be held responsible (see Chapter 1).

Limitations of behavioral genetics (in general) and addiction genetics (in particular)

Methodological issues (see Chapters 1 and 2)

We are still a long way from identifying the individual genetic differences that contribute to the development of any form of substance dependence. For example, the susceptibility alleles for alcohol dependence identified to date account for only a fraction of the heritability estimated from twin and adoption genetic studies. The inability to identify commonly occurring susceptibility alleles strongly predictive of addiction risk has been a major challenge. Alcohol dependence is a complex, multifactorial polygenic disorder, and the evidence to date indicates that it is unlikely that one or even a small number of genes will be identified that explain all the variance in its heritability. The pathways by which genes contribute to behaviors are convoluted and multifactorial. Complex disorders, such as susceptibility to addictions, appear to be shaped by multiple alleles (variant forms of a gene) from the same or different groups of genes, each contributing a small effect, that dynamically interact with each other and with environmental factors. Because gene–environment interaction studies vary significantly in the measures, methods, and sample sizes used, it is difficult to draw conclusions or to replicate them.

Applications of addiction genetics

Population health (see Chapter 11)

- Because candidate alleles have small effect sizes and lack replication, any attempts to use these in predictive genetic screening are likely to have limited specificity (the number of negative cases of the disorder that are correctly identified) and sensitivity (the number of positive cases of the disorder that are correctly identified).
- Whole population screening seems unlikely to be cost-effective under any reasonably likely circumstances. We are probably looking at many genes, each with small effects. There may be complicated multiple gene–gene and gene–environmental interactions that are difficult to identify in genome-wide studies, and disease liability may also be affected by epigenetic modifications (environmentally induced changes in DNA that regulate gene expression). Most people will probably have "modest" risk.

Box 15.1 Testing individuals for alleles associated with addiction

- Genetic testing of individuals for alleles associated with addiction is not currently ready for clinical use.
- It is unlikely to ever be of much clinical use (exception: pharmacogenetics; see below).
- Commercial testing products (of tests that are not ready for clinical use and/or of very limited clinical use) should be vigorously resisted. If permitted, these testing products should be regulated for accuracy of the information and reliability of the laboratories doing the analysis.

- Population screening for nicotine and alcohol dependence would also be prohibitively expensive, owing to the extremely high numbers of people who would need to be screened to detect one "high-risk" case.
- In general, improvements in population health are unlikely to emerge from genetic research into addiction.
- It is possible that there are racial differences in the distribution of the alleles that contribute to susceptibility to specific forms of addiction. Nevertheless, it is unlikely that these differences will be important to health outcomes.
- Given the potential for racist misuse of results, extreme care is necessary in reporting results or designing studies involving race and addiction genetics.

Individual health

- The complexity of unraveling the genetic contributions to alcohol dependence and other forms of addiction precludes any likelihood that genetic research will be able to contribute to predictive genetic screening or pharmacogenetic testing to inform treatment selection of addictive disorders in the near future (see Box 15.1).
- There is more hope of the potential application of genetic information for pharmacogenetics than of predictive screening that will enable physicians to more effectively tailor treatments to individual patients and improve treatment outcomes. However, the alleles identified so far are prevalent only in very limited populations and virtually nonexistent in others. One example is the alleles that influence response to naltrexone, a drug that inhibits alcohol-induced opioid activity, found in 15–18% of Caucasians and absent in the Asian and African American population. More research is needed to demonstrate the utility and cost-effectiveness of genetic testing for pharmacogenetic applications before it is introduced into clinical use.
- More research is necessary on how clinicians will make use of and communicate risk information about genetic liability for addiction.
- More research is also necessary on how individuals will make use of risk information provided by clinicians.

Research ethics

Risks of research participation

Research on the genetic contribution to addiction exposes subjects, their families, and broader social communities to a variety of types of risk. In general, there are two groups of risks related to conducting genetic research on substance-use disorders: risks that arise by virtue of studying participants who have substance-use disorders, and risks that arise specifically from the study of genetic material.

Risks to subjects

- Because substance-use disorders are so highly stigmatizing, genetic research related to addiction has significant implications for the individual research participant.
- Subjects in a study of the genetics of alcohol dependence or other forms of addiction could experience stigma, discrimination, and loss of opportunities just from being identified as participants. Those who are identified as carrying specific genes associated with addiction or dependence could experience additional and more concrete harms regardless of whether they are symptomatic or not (see Chapter 7).
- Individuals with substance-use disorders have impaired decisional capacity and often come from poor socioeconomic environments and should therefore be considered to be vulnerable. However no clear, inherent vulnerability appears to preclude their participation in genetic studies related to addiction as long as standard research protections (i.e., informed consent, reasonable incentives, and institutional oversight) are in place (see Chapter 3).
- Research protocols that provide participants with their drugs of choice carry particular risks, but this is a rare design for genetic research (see Chapter 3).
- Risks to subjects include the loss of privacy and the loss of control of sensitive personal information.
- The possibility of discrimination from others accessing genetic information is a general risk. There have been concerns that insurers may learn of the results of genetic testing and deny coverage to at-risk persons or that employers with access to genetic information may use the data to make decisions about hiring, firing, and promoting people.
- The 2008 Genetic Information Nondiscrimination Act (GINA) (US) provides some protections for presymptomatic individuals. It bars health insurers from using genetic information from presymptomatic individuals to make underwriting decisions for health insurance and prohibits employers from obtaining or using genetic information to make decisions about hiring and firing. However, the scope of GINA does not extend to life, disability, or long-term care insurance.
- Given the sensitivity of genetic research on addiction and the possibility that research subjects may experience stigmatization, it is important that research data be fully de-identified and protected.
- Genetic explanations may encourage those with substance-use disorders to view themselves fatalistically as having an unavoidable and uncontrollable problem (see Chapter 13). There is also some evidence that genetic attributions may increase social stigma (see Chapter 12).
- Pharmacogenetic research may expose participants to adverse reactions from the drugs being tested.
- Genetic research exposes participants to risks related to incidental research findings, such as information related to misattributed paternity.
- The risks to individuals whose samples or information are stored in biobank repositories will depend on: whether the information is identified or de-identified; whether informed consent was obtained, and if so whether it was limited or general; whether the research is on a sensitive topic; and what kinds of oversight exist (see Chapter 6).

- Enrolling children from high-risk families in research on the genetics of addictive disorders poses a number of significant and unique ethical challenges for researchers related to recruitment issues, obtaining consent or assent from the children, potential exploitation by researchers, and exploitation by parents (the addicts themselves) (see Chapter 5).

Risks to relatives and groups

- Like other forms of genetic research, genetic research on addiction expands the ambit of risks and potential harms from the individual participant to family members who potentially share their genetic heritage. Family members may also suffer from the social stigma and psychological burden of knowing they or other family members are at a genetically increased risk of addiction.
- Recruitment procedures for children may lead to inadvertent disclosure of familial risk.
- If ethnic and racial groups or other communities with different allele frequencies associated with addictive behaviors are discovered, this will increase the risk of discrimination and stigmatization of those populations.

Recruitment

- Addicts in general should be treated as a potentially vulnerable population, but that does not mean that, simply by virtue of being addicts, they are incapable of giving meaningful informed consent. Autonomy in all areas of an addict's life is not automatically undermined by the addiction.
- It is important to assess potential candidates individually for their ability to provide meaningful informed consent.
- Many substance abusers have situation factors that may present issues that affect the autonomy of their decisions to participate. Researchers often recruit substance abusers from settings that are implicitly "coercive," such as inpatient units, detoxification facilities, and prisons. Clients from these settings may perceive, correctly or incorrectly, that their treatment may be compromised by choosing not to participate (see Chapter 4).
- In multisite research settings, recruitment and consent should be performed as consistently as possible, both for ethical and scientific reasons (i.e., the reliability of the data).
- Individuals recruited should be representative of the population of interest in terms of their social and economic standing (e.g., criminal background, race/ethnicity, gender).
- As in other types of research, methods used for recruitment must be nonexploitative. The population of interest should not be based on who will be the easiest to manipulate into participation.
- Assessment of potential research subjects should include their need for clinical services. If a need is identified, the candidates should be informed about available treatment services. It is also important to make clear that the study is not a substitute for seeking treatment.
- Assessment of the ability to provide meaningful informed consent should exclude both those who are intoxicated and those experiencing withdrawal.
- It is appropriate to provide fair compensation for incurred expenses, time, and inconvenience. There is currently no evidence that reasonable compensation increases the use of drugs and alcohol.
- When offering compensation, it is important to keep in mind that the low levels of educational attainment, high rates of unemployment, low income levels, and generally

lower socioeconomic status that are characteristic of many substance abusers may make them more susceptible to excessive monetary influence (see Chapter 4). Excessively large inducements that may be coercive should be avoided.

- To reduce the influence of incentives and the possibility that cash payments could be used to purchase alcohol or drugs, it may be preferable to compensate participants with gift cards and other nonmonetary items or services (see Chapter 3).

Special issues related to the recruitment of children (see Chapter 5)

- The burden to protect minors participating in genetic research is high because children do not typically have the legal authority to make informed decisions on their own. There is the risk that children will be pressured by their families to participate in the research. Additionally, children have a particular difficulty in understanding the right of refusal.
- Research with asymptomatic minors of addicted parents may increase the perception that they are at risk for future addiction or problematic in other ways (see Chapter 5).
- As children with a substance-abusing parent are at greater risk for child abuse and neglect, researchers studying genetic risk must have clear procedures for responding to issues that arise related to the well-being of the children (e.g., disclosure of abuse to third parties). Such procedures must be specified during the informed consent process (see below).
- Because of the greater risks of exploitation, special safeguards may be needed when recruiting children in the custody of the child welfare system, such as appointing an independent advocate to protect their interests.
- Incentive payments to parents to encourage the participation of children are unacceptable because of the risk that it may induce them to coerce their children to participate. Additional payments to participants in research for the inclusion of children should also be discouraged.
- Payment may be made to offset expenses incurred or believed likely to be incurred through the children's participation. Meaningful age-appropriate compensation for children, such as toys or books, should also be provided.
- It is important to inform parents of situations in which the researchers will have to violate confidentiality: for example, the existence of mandatory reporting of child abuse/neglect.

Informed consent (see Chapter 4)

- Ensuring that participants understand the nature of the research, their rights, and what they are consenting to is essential.
- Informed consent must make clear both the individual risks and benefits of participating in the research, as well as providing a realistic account of the possible scientific and social risks and benefits of the research. It is critical for researchers to conceptualize consent as an ongoing process. The basic tenets of informed consent should be ensured throughout the course of a research study. This may involve ongoing assessments of research comprehension or reminders to the participants about the nature of the research.
- There are special reasons for caution when dealing with substance-dependent candidates, given their generally lower levels of educational attainment and lower

socioeconomic status, the health issues and psychological effects associated with addiction, and the comorbidities that many of them suffer.

- It is important to make clear the kinds of research results that will be shared with participants and the types of results that will not be shared.
- It is also necessary to make clear the kinds of protections to ensure privacy and confidentiality that will be in place, and what the limitations of those protections are. Also potential participants should be made aware of the situations in which information will have to be disclosed to third parties.
- Researchers must make clear during consent that there will not be diagnostic or clinical treatment as part of the study, but that other things might be found that are incidental to the research.
- Conducting the informed consent procedure may be of little use without adequate validation to determine whether potential research participants heard, understood, and can recall what they were told.
- There is a need to explore options for increasing understanding and retention of the components of informed consent. Some of the options include simplifying the structure and content of consent materials to improve readability, using audiovisual techniques, and appointing an independent third party or "research intermediary" to advocate on behalf of the research subject. An ongoing consent process, such as corrected feedback, is another option. Corrected feedback involves assessing an individual's knowledge and comprehension of the informed consent information and providing participants with corrected feedback about incorrect items. More research is necessary to evaluate the effectiveness of each of these options.

Informed consent for research with children (see Chapter 5 and Box 15.2)

- It is necessary to obtain consent from a legally authorized representative, such as a guardian or close family member, before enrolling children in an addiction study.
- Children should participate in the informed consent process as fully as is possible, given their age and cognitive development. Although children may not be able legally to provide informed consent, it is important to secure their assent (i.e., agreement) to participate in the research. All dissent by child participants should be respected.
- Where there is a risk of re-identification, research should be limited to children who are able to understand and meaningfully consent to the research.
- Where there is no risk of re-identification, the child's assent and parent/guardian consent might be sufficient.
- Consent for blanket reuse of stored data and biological samples from children should never be solicited. If children's genetic information or samples are stored in a biobank for potential reuse, their consent should be reobtained at adulthood before use. If consent is not provided, the samples or information should be destroyed (see also Chapter 8).

The problem of reuse in future research (see Chapters 6 and 8)

- There is no single rule as to whether informed consent is legally required for research using stored samples in biobanks under the Common Rule (US Federal Policy for the Protection of Human Subjects; Subpart A of 45 CFR 46 [56FR28003]) or the US Health

---

Box 15.2 Special issues involving children in addiction genetics research

- Selection of children should be representative of the sample population.
- Children in state care should neither be excluded nor deliberately targeted.
- In most circumstances a parent or legal guardian must provide informed consent (see the informed consent checklist in Box 15.3) for the child to participate, and the child must assent to being willing to participate in the research; children should participate in the informed consent process as fully as is possible, given their age and cognitive development.
- Payments to parents designed to encourage the participation of children should be avoided, owing to the risk of them coercing the children to participate.
- Procedures need to be in place to deal with mandatory reporting of neglect and/or abuse.
- Consent for blanket reuse of stored data and biological samples from children should never be solicited.
- Reuse of stored data or biological samples from children requires "re-consent" from the individual at the age of majority, with samples and data destroyed if re-consent is not achieved.
- Parents should be informed that some incidental findings will not be shared, including misattributed paternity.

Insurance Portability and Accountability Act (HIPAA) standards for the protection of individually identified information. There is a need to update these standards to make them more appropriate and relevant to research using genetic samples in biobanks.

- Soliciting blanket or general consent for the storage and reuse of data and materials facilitates future research but raises serious ethical issues. Research participants may not fully understand the implications of the agreement to reuse their genetic data. In addition, it is not possible for individuals to anticipate future research applications, some types of which may be objectionable to them.
- Tiered or layered consent is more ethically appropriate. Tiered consent entails giving subjects several options for providing consent for reuse of their samples and data, such as no reuse, use for research limited to specific diseases or topics, and/or use acceptable/not acceptable for use in commercial research. Tiered consent can also allow participants to decide whether to allow that their samples or data be shared with other researchers. Researchers using a tiered consent protocol will need to keep track of what subjects have consented to, but this requirement can be handled electronically.

Sharing information about research findings

- Participants should be informed about whether they will receive individualized genetic or medical information or just the aggregate research results.
- Findings of uncertain or no clinical importance should not be communicated to the research participants. In most cases the individual research results will not be clinically meaningful or useful, and therefore inappropriate to share with participants. This should be communicated during consent.
- Participants should be offered publications or reports summarizing the main research findings.

Box 15.3 Informed consent checklist

- Assess the capacity of each research candidate to provide meaningful consent.
- Consent should be conceptualized as an ongoing process, including:
  (1) appropriate modalities for improvement in understanding and retention, such as corrected feedback, video, etc.
  (2) the ongoing right to refuse to participate and to withdraw from participation
  (3) use of a research intermediary/third-party research participant advocate.
- Informed consent must make clear both the individual risks and benefits of participating in the research, as well as give a realistic account of the possible scientific/social risks and benefits of the research.
- The informed consent process needs to make clear that participating in a study is not a substitute for treatment or clinical diagnosis.
- Mechanisms should be in place to direct participants to clinicians if the participants so desire.
- Make clear what kinds of research results will be shared with participants and what kinds of results will not be shared (e.g., individuals will not be told their status regarding alleles).
- Make clear what kinds of protections regarding privacy will be in place, and what the limitations of those protections are.
- Make clear when information will have to be disclosed to third parties (e.g., mandatory reporting of suspected child abuse).
- Make clear the potential for incidental findings, what they are and how they will be dealt with (e.g., advise and assist the individual to seek clinical treatment).

- Researchers should have a procedure in place that includes contact details of appropriate health-care professionals should something of clear clinical importance be discovered (e.g., medical conditions or other psychological conditions).

Protecting privacy and confidentiality (see Chapters 6, 7, and 8)

- Researchers who gather sensitive data through genetic studies of addiction should use all available means to protect the confidentiality and security of their data. Strategies for protecting data should be relative to the risks.
- The US does not have a comprehensive law for the protection of health privacy. The Common Rule and the HIPAA are inconsistent in both the degree of detail required and the substance of the protections.
- US guidelines rely heavily on de-identification as a major strategy for protecting privacy and confidentiality, but de-identification alone is inadequate to fully protect genetic privacy. Individuals can be identified from a "de-identified" genomic database with access to 30 to 80 statistically independent single nucleotide polymorphisms. It is also possible to re-identify de-identified health records by matching phenotypes associated with the DNA to identified phenotypes from other databases with genomic information.
- Coded de-identification alone is never adequate to protect privacy. Full anonymization (at the point of collection) is better, but given how few data are necessary to uniquely identify individuals, it will not guarantee protection of privacy.
- In the absence of a well-considered legal framework for regulating privacy in genetic research on alcohol dependence and other addictions, research subjects need to be

informed about the specific measures that will be used to protect their privacy and the likely effectiveness of each as part of the informed consent process to enable them to calculate the risks and benefits of participating in the research.

- Certificates of Confidentiality issued by the US National Institutes of Health provide one means to attempt to protect the privacy of research subjects. Certificates of Confidentiality are issued to institutions or universities where the research is conducted to allow the investigator to refuse to disclose identifying information in any civil, criminal, administrative, legislative, or other proceeding at the federal, state, or local level. Alone, however, they are inadequate to protect privacy: Certificates of Confidentiality are untested legally, and they do not prevent voluntary or quasi-voluntary disclosures. Because Certificates' protections are based on US federal laws, they do not cover research in other countries. There may also be differences between the institution and researcher over whether to resist disclosure (e.g., from courts), and institutions may not be willing to resist a court order.

Biobanks and the storage of data

- It is impossible to guarantee absolute confidentiality/privacy when biological samples are banked or large amounts of genomic or other data are stored. This is importantly different from research in which information/samples are used once and the data can be fully anonymized.
- Strategies to attempt to protect the privacy and confidentiality of genomic information stored in biobanks include software protections on particularly sensitive data (such as storing aggregate information only) and sequestering of sensitive information: only releasing the data relevant to the particular research project and that has been approved by the research subject through tiered consent.
- We recommend against blanket consent for future use of stored materials or data.
- Tiered consent is more ethically appropriate; uses outside those envisioned by the tiered consent process should require re-consenting.

Funding sources (see Chapter 10)

- Researchers engaged in genetics research on addiction should not accept funding from producers of products associated with addictive consumption. Corporations that trade in legalized addictive consumption products seek to position themselves as legitimate businesses, but they differ from other corporations in their capacity to generate harm.
- Moral jeopardy/ethical risk is generated when researchers or research organizations committed to the public good opt to receive funding from addictive consumptions in ways that generate real or perceived conflicts of interest, which in turn can jeopardize their research, autonomy, and academic integrity. Five of the main risks researchers confront in accepting funding from the makers of products associated with addictive consumption are: (1) the possibility of contributing to sales of these products; (2) the possibility of improving the producer's public profile; (3) reputational risks or damage to an individual or institutional reputation; (4) the loss of academic independence; and (5) the disillusionment of staff.
- Key indicators in assessing the extent of ethical risk associated with accepting industry funding from corporations involved in the production of addictive substances are:

(1) the extent to which the primary purpose of the research activity clashes with the primary purpose of the activities of the donor corporation; and (2) the level of harmfulness associated with the particular product. Note that most research into individual risk factors for addiction will be incompatible with the goal of reducing the population-level costs (in health and money) of addiction.

- Corporations that produce addictive products support research on genetic explanations for addiction and disease because such an interpretation is consistent with policies that remove responsibility from industry products and their marketing strategies. There is also the hope that genetic explanations may result in weaker regulations and controls on the availability and marketing of harmful substances. Also, by spending significant amounts of money on scientific research, industries can portray themselves as "good corporate citizens."

- Approaches to minimize the effects of conflict of interest in addiction research that have been applied include: (1) the drafting of voluntary guidelines and consensus statements to serve as a guide for research scientists and professional organizations, one usual feature of which is the disclosure of all potential conflicts of interest; (2) ethical analysis and awareness training using ethical analysis techniques; and (3) total bans on acceptance of industry funding for research.

- There are a number of ways in which money from the alcohol, tobacco, gambling, and pharmaceutical industries becomes available. The link to funding by these industries is not always clear or apparent because the source of the funding may be camouflaged or channeled through third-party organizations. Money from producers of addictive substances that comes via other sources is unlikely to be sufficiently "cleaned" and to be sufficiently free from the implications of accepting funding from makers of addictive products.

- There are reasons to be cautious about accepting corporate funding more generally, including from the pharmaceutical industry, for research on the genetics of addiction. Researchers should consider: what type of research gets funded; whether there is freedom to choose direction; who controls the publication of the results (funding with strings attached regarding publication is funding that should be rejected); how the results will be used and interpreted; and who will profit from the results.

Translation and interpretation of genetic research on addiction

Communication of scientific results

Public understanding (see Chapter 11)

- Expect problems communicating research findings: the lack of scientific literacy in the general public and the weak basic understanding of genetics in particular, coupled with the complexity of behavioral genetics conceptually and empirically, complicate the communication of research findings. Many members of the public have a simplistic and deterministic view of genetic contributions to disorders. The media's tendency to portray genetic susceptibility in a deterministic manner and to overhype and/or to erroneously describe discoveries also contributes to misunderstandings – including overly optimistic expectations and overinterpretations.

- One common misunderstanding of genetic research is the belief that having a genetic predisposition to a disorder means one either has, or is likely to develop, the disorder.
- The challenge for public education on genetic research will be to better explain the personal and public health implications of polygenic disorders in which individual alleles weakly predict risk and interact with each other and with environmental factors.
- Researchers have an ethical responsibility not to promote popular misunderstandings and a professional responsibility not to oversell their research results. This calls for humility in professional publications, grant proposals, and in publicly reporting research results. It also requires working with institutional publicity departments to minimize misunderstandings and overinterpretation of research results. In addition, there is a need to anticipate the role the media will play and to seek to minimize the likely misreporting by resisting media pressure to simplify and overstate findings. Note: few studies in this field have conclusive findings.
- Survey results suggest that the US public is generally optimistic about genetic research and its benefits.
- Evidence from studies indicates that genetic explanations for alcohol dependence have been growing in popularity and are distributed across a wide segment of the population (see Chapter 13).

Impact of genetic explanations on self-understanding of addicted individuals (see Chapters 11 and 12)

- As noted above, we argue that at this time there is no good reason to test anyone in a clinical setting, nor should people get tested commercially for a potential predisposition to alcohol dependence or other forms of addiction. Hence no one ought to have individual information about his or her alleles potentially associated with addiction. However, as they might, it is important to anticipate how receiving genetic testing results could affect the self-understanding of addicted individuals.
- It is often assumed that conveying genetic risk information will prompt individuals to change their behavior in desired directions, but addicted individuals may interpret genetic risk information in a deterministic way and believe they are powerless to change their behavior or risk of addiction. There is also the possibility that if persons are told or believe they are at lower genetic risk of addiction disorders, they may be less motivated to change their behavior.
- Genetic explanations may be particularly useful as a coping mechanism among individuals who perceive a risk of substance dependence and who hold fatalistic views about health. Genetic explanations may also be attractive to individuals when they sense that the behavioral changes required to reduce the actual risk are difficult to enact and/or when they experience threats to their self-image due to stigmas associated with a condition.
- There is no research available indicating whether genetic explanations change the willingness of addicted individuals to enter treatment. There is a speculative possibility that persons who know they have a higher genetic risk may be less inclined to seek treatment because they believe their disorder is incurable. More research is needed on this topic.

Impact of genetic explanations on public understanding

- One risk of understanding addiction as primarily genetic rather than having an important environmental component is that it will encourage public policymakers and members of the public not to accord sufficient importance to environmental factors.
- There is the possibility that people assuming themselves to have low genetic risk will believe themselves to be immune to becoming addicted. This could encourage them to be comfortable about using more dependence-forming harmful substances. There needs to be additional research on this potential risk (see Chapter 11).
- The existing level of stigma directed at addicted persons is high – even more extreme than when compared with highly stigmatized psychiatric disorders.
- Proponents of a biomedical view of addiction believe that highlighting biological and genetic basis will reduce the degree to which addicted persons are held responsible for their addictions, thereby reducing stigmatization and discrimination of persons with addiction. However, the limited evidence available suggests that geneticization may increase rather than decrease stigmatization. Increasing genetic explanations for addictions may be layered on top of personal blame, thus subjecting addicted persons and their families to the negative consequences associated with both personal guilt and genetic explanations. There is a need for further research on the effect of genetic causal attribution on stigma (see Chapter 12).

Public health and policy implications (see Chapter 14)

- At present the potential for genetic research on alcohol, nicotine, and drug dependence to be useful in preventing these disorders seems doubtful. In addition, research identifying genes predictive of addiction liability and treatment responses may be misused or misinterpreted in ways that harm individual and population health.
- Successful public health interventions have tended to be social interventions and not individual biomedical interventions (which have had limited meaningful impact on public health).
- Addiction genetics research usually directs attention away from social factors (that are associated with differences in addiction rates) and toward factors internal to individuals (individual heavy users or addicts). This tends to focus interventions away from social factors and toward individual biomedical interventions.
- Industry's support of research on genetic factors related to addiction to tobacco, alcohol, and gambling is intended to focus attention away from the availability of the addictive substance and toward the individuals who are addicted. This change in focus makes continued use and availability of the product to be socially acceptable, and implies that a focus on "problem users" is sufficient to improve public health. Evidence suggests that such an approach in isolation is ineffective.
- Population-level research into environmental correlates to harmful use and addiction (especially social factors) should be actively pursued and health policy should focus on the social and environmental changes known to be successful in reducing harm.
- Public investment in genetic research into addiction needs to be based on a realistic assessment of the likely benefits it will provide; these benefits do not currently and are very unlikely in the future to include meaningful improvements in population-level

Box 15.4 Priorities for addiction research

- Social policy correlates to harmful use and social policy changes likely to decrease harmful use, including broad social determinants of health, income inequality, and social opportunity.
- The influences on the probability of problem users seeking treatment; how we can make it more likely that problem users will seek treatment.
- Broad assessments of successful treatments that examine all approaches to reducing harmful drug use, including population-level approaches as well as biomedical interventions. Note: this is one area in which genetic research on correlates to successful treatments may be of some use, but caution is needed, as it shifts the focus toward biomedical modalities and away from other treatment options.
- Research on the ways that addiction genetic research influences:
  (1) addicted individuals' self-understanding
  (2) stigma and understanding of addicts and addiction
  (3) funding for addiction research more generally (e.g., does genetic research on addiction make research into the social determinants of addiction rates harder to fund?)
  (4) influence on public policy – Does it make certain policies harder (or easier) to implement? Does it make some policies seem (perhaps inappropriately) more or less likely to be successful?
  (5) clinicians' understanding of addiction and willingness to use the results of addiction genetics research in clinical practice, including willingness to try new interventions.
- Research on the effective communication of genetic research in general, and addiction genetics research in particular, to the lay public and to clinicians and social workers involved with addicted populations. How to ensure that the results of research are interpreted accurately and not over- or misinterpreted?
- Ways to improve process of informed consent, including increasing subject understanding and retention, and improving the recruitment process – for example, more research into the compensation of subjects, more research into particular techniques for making consent into an effective process, etc.

health (however they may be of great intellectual interest, with possible economic spin-offs, and may someday have implications for individual clinical decision making, e.g., applications to pharmacogenetics).

Priorities for addiction research

The physical and psychological harms and financial costs associated with addiction and addictive behavior are real and serious. The priorities listed in Box 15.4 seem to us to be the key areas in which more research is necessary and is likely to have a substantial impact.

Index

Printed in the United States
by Baker & Taylor Publisher Services